Directory of
THERAPEUTIC ENZYMES

Edited by

Barry M. McGrath

National University of Ireland
Galway, Ireland

Gary Walsh

University of Limerick
Limerick, Ireland

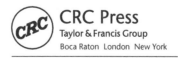

CRC Press
Taylor & Francis Group
Boca Raton London New York

CRC Press is an imprint of the
Taylor & Francis Group, an **informa** business

Published 2006 by CRC Press
Taylor & Francis Group
6000 Broken Sound Parkway NW, Suite 300
Boca Raton, FL 33487-2742

©2006 by Taylor & Francis Group, LLC
CRC Press is an imprint of Taylor & Francis Group, an Informa business

First issued in paperback 2019

No claim to original U.S. Government works

ISBN-13: 978-0-367-45408-1 (pbk)
ISBN-13: 978-0-8493-2714-8 (hbk)

**Visit the Taylor & Francis Web site at
http://www.taylorandfrancis.com**

**and the CRC Press Web site at
http://www.crcpress.com**

Library of Congress Cataloging-in-Publication Data

Directory of therapeutic enzymes / [edited by] Barry M. McGrath and Gary Walsh.
    p. ; cm.
  Includes bibliographical references and index.
  ISBN-13: 978-0-8493-2714-8 (alk. paper)
  ISBN-10: 0-8493-2714-8 (alk. paper)
    1. Enzymes-Therapeutic use Catalogs. [DNLM: 1. Enzymes-therapeutic use. QU 135 D5985 2006]
I. McGrath, Barry M. II. Walsh, Gary, Dr.

RM666.E55D57 2006
615'.35--dc22   2005012902

Preface

Today myriad enzymes are used for various industrial, analytical, and therapeutic purposes. In the context of this publication, they form a significant subcategory of modern biopharmaceuticals. Thus, we aim to overview these therapeutic enzymes, focusing in particular on more recently approved products produced by recombinant means.

This book is primarily aimed at those in the biopharmaceutical/biotechnology industries who wish to gain a comprehensive understanding of enzyme-based therapeutic products. The publication also will be of direct relevance to students undertaking advanced under-graduate/postgraduate programs in relevant aspects of the biological sciences, as well as to researchers in these areas.

Chapter 1 provides a summary overview of applied enzymology, while Chapter 2 focuses upon the theory and applications of enzyme engineering. Between them, these chapters set an appropriate backdrop for the remaining 11 chapters, which focus upon actual enzyme products that have now gained regulatory approval for general medical use. Chapters 3 through 13 highlight the manifold applications of approved therapeutic enzymes, including use in the treatment of blood-clotting disorders, certain cancers, and a variety of genetic disorders.

As editors, we wish to extend our sincere gratitude to all contributing authors and to our publisher, Taylor & Francis. Finally, we wish to dedicate this book to our parents, Hugh and Deirdre McGrath and Bina and the late John Walsh.

Contributors

Barngrover, Debra   Therapeutics Operation Management, Genzyme Corporation, Cambridge, Massachusetts

Bayol, Alain   Analytical Department, Sanofi-Synthelabo Recherche, Labège, France

Bras, Jean-Marc   Analytical Department, Sanofi-Synthelabo Recherche, Labège, France

Brun, Nikolai   Novo Nordisk A/S, Bagsvaerd, Denmark

Couderc, René   Functional Genomic Department, Sanofi-Synthelabo Recherche, Labège, France

Demeester, Joseph   Laboratory of General Biochemistry and Physical Pharmacy, Faculty of Pharmacy, Ghent University, Ghent, Belgium

De Smedt, Stefaan C.   Laboratory of General Biochemistry and Physical Pharmacy, Faculty of Pharmacy, Ghent University, Ghent, Belgium

Edmunds, Tim   Therapeutic Protein Research, Genzyme Corporation, Framingham, Massachusetts

Erhardtsen, Elisabeth   Novo Nordisk A/S, Bagsvaerd, Denmark

Ferrara, Pascual   Functional Genomic Department, Sanofi-Synthelabo Recherche, Labège, France

Grinnell, Brian W.   Biotechnology Discovery Research, Lilly Research Laboratories, Eli Lilly and Co., Indianapolis, Indiana

Kakkis, Emil   BioMarin Pharmaceutical Inc., Novato, California

Klausen, Niels Kristian   Novo Nordisk A/S, Bagsvaerd, Denmark

Körholz, Dieter   Department of Pediatrics, University of Leipzig Clinic and Policlinic for Children and Adolescents, Leipzig, Germany

Lascombes, Françoise   Clinical and Exploratory Pharmacology, Sanofi-Synthelabo Recherche, Nancy, France

Loison, Gérard   Functional Genomic Department, Sanofi-Synthelabo Recherche, Labège, France

Loyaux, Denis   Functional Genomic Department, Sanofi-Synthelabo Recherche, Labège, France

Macias, William L.   Lilly Laboratory for Clinical Reseach, Lilly Research Laboratories, Eli Lilly and Co., Indianapolis, Indiana

Mauz-Körholz, Christine   Division of Pediatric Hematology and Oncology, Clinic and Policlinic for Children and Adolescents, University of Leipzig Medical Center, Leipzig, Germany

McGrath, Barry M.   Gene Therapy Group, Regenerative Medicine Institute, National University of Ireland, Galway, Ireland

O'Connell, Shane   Chemical and Environmental Sciences Department, University of Limerick, Limerick, Ireland

Persson, Egon   Novo Nordisk A/S, Bagsvaerd, Denmark

Rexen, Per   Novo Nordisk A/S, Bagsvaerd, Denmark

Sanders, Niek N.   Laboratory of General Biochemistry and Physical Pharmacy, Faculty of Pharmacy, Ghent University, Ghent, Belgium

Shanley, Nancy   Department of Applied Science, Limerick Institute of Technology, Moylish, Limerick City, Ireland

Wahn, Volker   Clinic for Children and Adolescents, Uckermark Medical Center, Schwedt/Oder, Germany

Walsh, Gary   Industrial Biochemistry Program, University of Limerick, Limerick, Ireland

Yan, S. Betty   Lilly Laboratory for Clinical Research, Lilly Research Laboratories, Eli Lilly and Co., Indianapolis, Indiana

Contents

1

Applied Enzymology: An Overview

Nancy Shanley and Gary Walsh

CONTENTS

1.1 Introduction

Several thousand enzymes have been identified to date. This group of biomolecules first found industrial application in the early 1900s. Today, a myriad enzymes are employed for industrial, analytical, and therapeutic purposes [1–3]. While the following sections of this book focus specifically upon therapeutic uses of enzymes, this chapter provides a summary overview of their additional applied uses, offering a framework for the interested reader to better understand the entire application range of these versatile biomolecules.

Enzymes are biological catalysts. They speed up the rate of biochemical reactions by several orders of magnitude (see Table 1.1) and function under relatively mild conditions of pH and temperature [4]. With the exception of a small group of catalytic RNA molecules [5], all enzymes are protein-based. They are globular proteins, typically soluble

TABLE 1.1

Rate Enhancement Produced by Selected Enzymes

Enzyme	Rate Enhancement
Carbonic anhydrase	10^6
Chorismate mutase	10^6
Triose phosphate isomerase	10^9
Carboxypeptidase A	10^{11}
AMP nucleosidase	10^{12}
Phosphoglucomutase	10^{12}
Succinyl CoA transferase	10^{13}
Staphylococcal nuclease	10^{14}
Orotidine monophosphate decarboxylase	10^{17}

in aqueous-based solutions, and sensitive to environmental conditions such as changes in temperature and pH. Enzymes are high-molecular mass molecules, ranging from 13 to 500 kDa, although many fall within the 30 to 100 kDa range. They generally display a high degree of specificity with respect to the substrate(s) with which they interact. The region of the enzyme where the substrate is transformed to form the product is known as the active site. Some enzymes also require the presence of a nonprotein cofactor at the active site in order to maintain catalytic activity.

1.1.1   History of Enzymology

The study of enzymes began in earnest toward the end of the 18th century. Much of the initial work upon these molecules stemmed from digestive physiological research that focusing upon the ability of stomach secretions to digest meat and saliva to convert starch into sugars. The scientist Frederick Kuhne [28] proposed the term "enzyme" in 1878. In 1884, Jokichi Takamine [28] was awarded a patent for a product termed "Taka-diastase," the active component of which was an amylolytic enzyme derived from *Aspergillus oryzae* grown on rice. Purification of enzymes began in the 1920s. Urease, for example, was first purified and crystallized in 1926, while pepsin, trypsin, and several other digestive enzymes were crystallized in the 1930s (Figure 1.1). By then, scientists were also attempting to use crude enzyme preparations for a variety of industrial and medical purposes. But in many instances, such early attempts met with limited success, largely due to an incomplete understanding of the nature of enzymes themselves in terms of substrate specificity and the influence of environmental parameters upon enzyme activity.

1.1.2   Classification of Enzymes

Enzymes may be grouped into families on the basis of a number of different criteria. They may be classified according to the type of substrate they transform. They are often named simply by adding "ase" to the end of the substrate name, hence the general classifications of "protease," "carbohydrase," "lipase," "pectinase," etc. Polymer-degrading enzymes are also often classified as "endo-" or "exo-" acting, depending upon the position of the bonds within the substrate attacked by the enzyme.

The most comprehensive and internationally recognized method of enzyme classification is based upon the type of reaction catalyzed [6]. Using this system, enzymes are assigned to one of six basic categories: oxidoreductases, transferases, hydrolases, lyases, isomerases, and ligases (see Table 1.2).

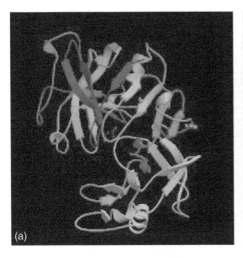
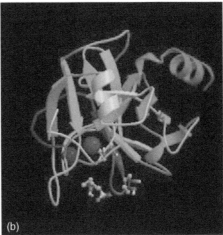

FIGURE 1.1
The three-dimensional structure of (a) porcine pepsin and (b) porcine trypsin. (Courtesy of the protein databank, http://www.pdb.org. Entry ID numbers 3PEP and 1S81, respectively. With permission.)

TABLE 1.2
Classification of Enzymes According to the Reaction Catalyzed

Grouping	Reaction Catalyzed
Oxidoreductases	Catalyze oxidation–reduction reactions such as CH→C–OH, or overall removal or addition of hydrogen atom equivalents, for example: CH (OH)→C=O
Transferases	Mediate the transfer of various chemical groups, such as aldehyde, ketone, acyl, sugar, phosphoryl, etc. from one molecule to another
Hydrolases	Catalyze hydrolysis reactions, i.e., the transfer of various functional groups to water
Lyases	Catalyze additions to, or formation of, double bonds such as C=C, C=O, and C=N
Isomerases	Catalyze various types of isomerations, including racemization reactions
Ligases	Mediate the formation of C–C, C–O, C–S, and C–N bonds, usually via condensation reactions coupled to ATP cleavage. Often termed synthetases

1.1.3 Applied Enzymology

Today, enzymes find a broad range of applications within industry, medicine, and as analytical reagents [1–3]. The major enzyme preparations used for therapeutic purposes are summarized in Table 1.3 and are discussed further in the forthcoming chapters. The enzymes used for analytical or industrial purposes are summarized below. But, before specific enzymes and their applications are considered, the more general issues of enzyme sources, methods of manufacture, and enzyme immobilization should be discussed first.

1.2 Enzymes: Sources and Production

Enzymes that have found applied use have traditionally been sourced from a range of microbial, plant, and animal species [3,7]. Traditionally, most therapeutic enzymes are extracted directly from the natural source, i.e., from animal or human tissue. In most instances, enzymes used for diagnostic and in particular for industrial purposes have been sourced from microorganisms. This producer microorganism is classified as generally

TABLE 1.3

Major Enzymes Used for Therapeutic Purposes

Enzyme	Therapeutic Application
Tissue plasminogen activator (tPA)	Thrombolytic agent
Urokinase	Thrombolytic agent
(Activated) protein C	Severe sepsis
DNase	Cystic fibrosis
Glucocerebrosidase	Gaucher's disease
α-galactosidase	Fabry's disease
Urate oxidase	Hyperuricemia
Asparaginase	Cancer treatment, most notable childhood leukemia
Factor VIIa	Hemophilia
Factor IX (protease zymogen)	Hemophilia
α-iduronidase	Mucopolysaccharidosis I (MPS I)
Pancreatin/lactase/α-amylase/proteases	Used as digestive aids
Hyaluronidase	Various potential uses for myocardial infarction, cancer therapy, and in anesthesia for eye surgery
Superoxide dismutase	Oxygen toxicity, anti-inflammatory agent
Various proteases, including papain, collagenase, and trypsin	Debriding agents (cleansing of wounds)

recognized as safe (GRAS)). GRAS microorganisms are nonpathogenic, nontoxic, and generally do not produce antibiotics. Microorganisms represent an attractive source of enzymes (and indeed, many other proteins) because they can be cultured on a large scale over a short time-span by well-established methods of fermentation. Accordingly, they can produce an abundant, regular supply of the desired enzyme product.

The advent of genetic engineering has facilitated the production of virtually any protein in recombinant production systems, with associated potential benefits in terms of production levels and, potentially, product safety [7]. A range of enzyme products are now produced by recombinant means. Recombinant enzymes used for industrial and diagnostic purposes are generally produced in engineered microbial systems, whereas many therapeutic enzymes are produced in animal cell lines, a consequence of the need for post-translational modifications.

Most enzymes (both recombinant and nonrecombinant) produced by fermentation and cell culture are secreted directly by the producing cells into the culture medium. Extracellular production displays process advantages, by obviating the necessity of lysing (disrupting) the cells in order to bring about the release of the protein (enzyme) of interest, thereby simplifying downstream processing. Whole cells can be removed by simple filtration or centrifugation of the extracellular medium.

In a few instances, the enzyme of interest is produced intracellularly. Accordingly, it is necessary to disrupt the cells upon completion of fermentation and cell harvesting. This releases not only the enzyme of interest, but also the entire intracellular content of the cell. Subsequent purification procedures to obtain the final enzyme product are thereby rendered more complicated. Examples of intracellular enzymes that have found industrial application include asparaginase, penicillin acylase, and glucose isomerase.

The complexity of downstream processing undertaken after initial enzyme recovery or extraction depends upon the required specification of the final product. Bulk industrial enzymes generally require minimal or no further purification, and the final product is generated by concentration of crude extract, excipient addition, and drying (if required). Therapeutic enzymes, on the other hand, are invariably purified to homogeneity before final formulation, a process requiring multiple high-resolution chromatographic steps. Processing of enzymes used for analytical purposes generally falls somewhere between

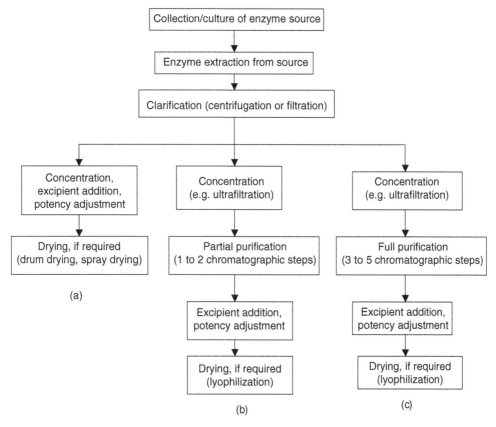

FIGURE 1.2
An overview of a generalized manufacturing scheme for (a) industrial grade, (b) analytical, and (c) therapeutic enzymes.

these two extremes, with most such enzymes being partially purified. An overview of downstream processing of these enzyme products is provided in Figure 1.2.

1.2.1   Immobilized Enzymes

Enzymes are expensive to produce. It therefore makes economic sense, where practicable, to recover the enzyme after it carries out its intended function, so that it can be reused or recycled. Enzyme immobilization technology makes this possible. Immobilized enzymes often display increased stability due to the fact that their support material can provide protection from pH and temperature changes in the surrounding environment.

Enzymes can be immobilized by a variety of techniques, for example, adsorption, encapsulation, covalent attachment, and entrapment of the enzyme [8,9] (Figure 1.3). Entrapment is achieved by incubating the enzyme along with gel monomers (e.g., acrylamide or methacrylic acid) and then promoting gel polymerization. The gel pore size must be large enough to allow free passage of enzyme reactants and products but small enough to retain the entrapped enzyme molecules. Industrially, polymeric gel beads containing the immobilized enzyme are usually packed into columns. As they pass down the column, the substrate molecules diffuse into the beads and are converted into the product by the trapped enzyme. Penicillin acylase and glucose isomerase are examples of two enzymes that are used industrially in an immobilized state. Glucose isomerase catalyzes the interconversion

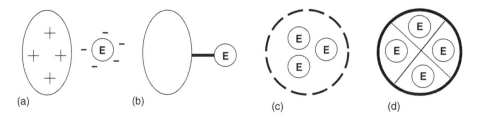

FIGURE 1.3
Enzymes may be immobilized by methods of (a) adsorption, (b) covalent attachment, (c) encapsulation, and (d) entrapment.

of glucose to fructose, both of which are widely used in the production of sweets, jams, soft drinks, etc. Fructose is twice as sweet as glucose, so smaller quantities of fructose can be used to achieve the same degree of sweetness in food products.

1.3 Enzymes Used for Analytical Purposes

Almost 100 enzymes now find routine analytical application in the detection and quantification of analytes of medical, environmental, or industrial significance [10,11]. These enzymes are obtained from a variety of animal, plant, and microbial sources. Most of these enzymes are produced by direct extraction from native producer sources, although some (e.g., alkaline phosphatase) are produced mainly by genetic engineering. The annual world market for analytical enzymes has well surpassed the €100 million mark. In the context of therapeutic enzymes, this may seem modest. Enzymes used for analytical (and industrial) purposes, however, have a much lower cost of production and sales value per unit of activity than therapeutic proteins.

It is not usually necessary to purify enzyme-based diagnostic reagents to homogeneity. However, it is essential that the purification procedure involved removes any proteins or other molecules present in the initial preparation that might interfere with the assay.

1.3.1 Enzymes in Clinical Chemistry

The substrate specificity of enzymes and their catalytic efficiency render these biomolecules attractive as analytical reagents. In most instances, the enzyme employed is one that uses the target analyte directly as a substrate. Changes in the concentration of substrate (or appearance of easily quantifiable product) are then monitored, usually spectrophotometrically. The magnitude of the signal generated is directly proportional to the concentration of the target analyte.

Biochemical research continues to increase our understanding of normal and abnormal metabolic activity. A variety of enzyme preparations have been used as diagnostic reagents in the *in vitro* clinical diagnostics sector for many years (see Table 1.4). Clinical chemistry is the detection, monitoring, and quantitation of a broad variety of marker substances present in clinical biological samples. Substances of diagnostic value include metabolic products such as urea, glucose, cholesterol, or steroid hormones. Other diagnostic markers of higher molecular mass include specific proteins that may be released from damaged tissue or whose normal concentration is altered due to abnormal metabolism. Diagnostic tests that detect viruses and microorganisms have also been developed.

TABLE 1.4

Some Enzymes Used Directly or Indirectly as Diagnostic Reagents — Their Sources and Likely Applications

Enzyme	Source	Application
Acetyl cholinesterase	Bovine erythrocytes	Analysis of organophosphorous compounds such as pesticides
Alcohol dehydrogenase	Yeast	Determination of alcohol levels in biological fluids
Alkaline phosphatase	Calf intestine and kidney, Recombinant (*Picca* sp.)	Conjugation to antibodies allows its use as an indicator in ELISA systems
Arginase	Beef liver	Determination of L-arginine levels in plasma and urine
Ascorbate oxidase	*Cucurbita* sp.	Determination of ascorbic acid levels; eliminates interference by ascorbic acid
Cholesterol esterase	Pig/beef pancreas, *Pseudomonas* sp., Recombinant (*Streptomyces* sp.)	Determination of serum cholesterol levels
Creatine kinase	Rabbit muscle, beef heart, pig heart	Diagnosis of cardiac and skeletal malfunction
Glucose-6-phosphate dehydrogenase	Yeast, *Leuconostoc mesenteroides*	Determination of glucose and ATP in conjunction with hexokinase
Glucose oxidase	*Aspergillus niger*	Determination of glucose in biological samples in conjunction with peroxidase; a marker for ELISA systems
Glutamate dehydrogenase	Beef liver	Determination of blood urea nitrogen in conjunction with urease
Glycerol kinase	*Candida mycoderma, Arthrobacter* sp.	Determination of triglyceride levels in blood in conjunction with lipase
Glycerol-3-phosphate dehydrogenase	Rabbit muscle	Determination of serum triglycerides
Hexokinase	Yeast	Determination of glucose in body fluids
Peroxidase	Horseradish	Indicator enzyme for reactions in which peroxide is produced
Phosphoenolpyruvate carboxylase	Maize leaves	Determination of CO_2 in body fluids
Urease	Jack bean	Determination of blood urea nitrogen; marker enzyme for ELISA systems
Uricase	Porcine liver	Determination of uric acid
Xanthine oxidase	Buttermilk	Determination of xanthine and hypoxanthine in biological fluids

Reproduced from Walsh, G., *Proteins: Biochemistry and Biotechnology*, John Wiley & Sons, Chichester, UK, 2001. With permission from John Wiley & Sons.

Dehydrogenase and oxidase enzymes are the most common substances used for analytical purposes. Dehydrogenases catalyze the following general reaction type:

$$S + NAD^+ \rightarrow P + NADH + H^+$$

NADH absorbs at 340 nm whereas NAD^+ does not, thereby allowing spectrophotometric monitoring of the generation of NADH. The amount of NADH produced bears a direct stoichiometric relationship with the concentration of the substrate (the analyte whose concentration is to be determined) that is present.

Oxidases represent a second class of enzyme often utilized for analytical purposes. However, unlike dehydrogenases, none of the oxidase reaction products is easily measurable. This difficulty may be overcome by the inclusion of a second "linker" enzyme in the assay system. The linker enzyme is chosen on the basis of its ability to utilize one of the products of the primary reaction as a substrate and, in turn, to generate an easily detectable product. A specific example of such a diagnostic system is that of the glucose oxidase/peroxidase system, widely used to determine blood glucose concentrations. In this reaction sequence, the first reaction is catalyzed by glucose oxidase, while the second is catalyzed by peroxidase:

$$Glucose + O_2 + H_2O \rightarrow gluconic\ acid + H_2O_2$$

$$2H_2O_2 + 4\text{-aminophenazone} + phenol \rightarrow quinoneimine + 4H_2O$$

The dye quinoneimine, a reaction product, absorbs at 520 nm, allowing spectrophotometric determination of its concentration produced. This same reaction strategy can be used to detect and quantify additional analytes. For example, a combination of cholesterol oxidase and peroxidase may be used to determine cholesterol concentrations.

1.3.2 Enzymes Used in Immunoassay Systems

A selection of enzymes also find analytical application as reporter groups for immunoassays. Owing to the specificity of antibody–antigen interaction, antibodies are often used to detect and quantify target analytes against which they have been produced [12]. Such immunoassay-based systems now find routine use for a variety of clinical, industrial, and environmental purposes (e.g., the detection and quantification of specific drugs or other analytes in blood, or the detection and quantification of pesticides in food or environmental samples).

The binding of an antibody to an antigen is an event that is itself not readily detectable. One common strategy to overcome this difficulty is to conjugate an easily detectable reporter group to the antibody. Initially, radioactive tags were commonly used for this purpose (radioimmunoassay). More recently, the use of enzyme-based reporter groups (enzyme immunoassay) has become more common. Enzymes may be covalently coupled to antibodies by a variety of relatively straightforward chemical procedures, for example, by incubation with bifunctional cross-linking reagents such as glutaraldehyde. Enzymes capable of converting a chromogenic substrate into a readily detectable colored product (which is therefore easily detected and quantified by spectrophotometry) are most commonly used, for example, alkaline phosphatase isolated from calf stomach. This enzyme can catalytically dephosphorylate *p*-nitrophenylphosphate (PNPP), yielding inorganic phosphate and *p*-nitrophenol. The latter product is yellow, absorbing maximally at 405 nm. Additional enzymes for which chromogenic substrates are available and which, therefore, have been used as reporter groups in immunoassays include β-galactosidase (lactase), urease, and glucose oxidase. Enzyme immunoassays of various different formats have been designed and commercialized. The principle of one such assay type is illustrated in Figure 1.4.

1.3.3 Enzyme-Based Biosensors

In an immobilized format, enzymes can be used as the biological-sensing element of biosensors (Figure 1.5). Biosensors are analytical devices capable of detecting and quantifying specific target analytes often present in complex samples [13,14]. They consist of a biological component, most often an enzyme, immobilized onto a transducer. A transducer is

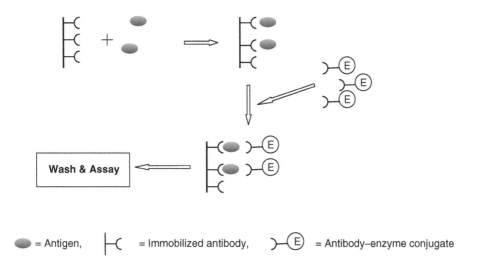

FIGURE 1.4
An overview of the principles and operation of a noncompetitive enzyme-linked immunosorbant assay (ELISA).

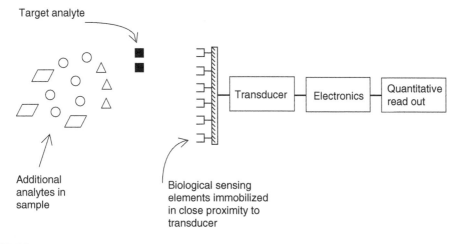

FIGURE 1.5
Basic biosensor design. (Reproduced from Walsh, G., *Proteins: Biochemistry and Biotechnology*, John Wiley & Sons, Chichester, UK, 2001., With permission from J. Wiley & Sons.)

a device that senses one form of energy and converts it to another. The transducer can, for example, be an electrode that converts the biochemical signal generated by the enzyme reaction (e.g., changes in concentration of substrate or product, absorbance, etc.) into a quantifiable electrical signal. The electrical signal generated by the transducer is related to the concentration of the analyte. A standard curve can be constructed from readings obtained when the electrode is immersed in standard solutions containing known concentrations of the analyte.

Most enzyme biosensors use either membrane-based enzyme entrapment, or the enzyme is covalently bound to the inside of a nylon tube. The stability of the electrode is dependent on the stability of the enzyme, which is partially dependent on the method of immobilization. Many enzyme electrodes are available to detect, for example, glucose, urea, creatine, and pyruvate in clinical samples. However, only the glucose biosensor has been widely commercialized.

There are many advantages associated with the use of biosensors as analyte detection and quantitation systems: (1) they are highly specific; (2) they are cost-effective (mainly because they are reusable); (3) no additional reagents are required to make measurements; (4) the assay sample need not be pretreated (e.g., removal of particulate matter etc. is not necessary); (5) they are flexibe (portable biosensors can be used in the field for multiple samples); and (6) they are not complicated to operate, (i.e. technical training is not essential).

1.4   Enzymes Used for Industrial Purposes

By the turn of the 20th century, the annual worldwide sales value of industrial enzymes stood at US$1.5 billion. Protein-degrading (proteolytic) enzymes (proteases) represent the most significant single group of industrial enzymes currently in use and were one of the first enzyme groups to find applied use [7]. Currently, the annual sales value of proteases represents over half of the total sales revenue generated by all industrial enzyme sales combined. Carbohydrate-degrading enzymes (carbohydrases) account for much of the remainder. A comprehensive review of all industrial enzymes and their uses is well beyond the scope of this chapter. Instead, we focus upon industrial proteases as a representative group, followed by a summary of carbohydrases and other enzymes of applied use.

1.4.1   Detergent Proteases

Proteases first found applied use in the food and detergent industries. These continue to be important areas. Currently, proteases also find numerous applications in leather processing and as therapeutic agents. Table 1.5 provides an overview of their industrial uses.

Economically, the most significant single use of proteases is their incorporation into detergents [7]. They facilitate the removal of "biological" dirt, which is mainly protein-based. Obviously, the characteristics of the proteases must be compatible with standard washing conditions. Accordingly, the most successful detergent proteases are stable at alkaline pH values; at relatively high temperatures; and in the presence of bleach, surfactants, and sequestering agents. Screening of proteases from a wide range of sources has identified members of the bacterial subtilisin subfamily as the most appropriate for detergent application [15,16]. Typically, they are optimally active at temperatures between 45 to 65°C and in the pH range of 9 to 12. Many such subtilisins have been modified by genetic engineering with the general aims of increasing their thermal stability as well as improving their resistance to oxidation.

TABLE 1.5

Industrial Sectors in Which Protease Enzymes are Applied

Industry/Process	Application
Laundry detergent additive	Promotes catalytic degradation of protein-based clothing stains
Leather manufacture	To dehair animal hides and to soften (bate) leather
Cheese manufacture	To coagulate casein
Meat processing	To tenderize meat
Beverage industry	Stabilization of some beers
Baking	To alter dough characteristics

1.4.2 The Application of Proteases in the Food and Drink Industry

Rennin (also known as chymosin) is an important commercial protease that is used in the manufacture of cheese. This enzyme catalyzes limited cleavage of kappa casein, the main protein in milk. The destabilized casein micelles then precipitate to form curds. These coagulate, and the remaining liquid (termed whey) is removed. The curd is further processed, ultimately yielding cheese.

The enzyme rennin has a molecular mass of 35 kDa and contains 323 amino acids. It exists in two isoenzyme forms, both with optimal activity at approximately pH 4.0. In its natural state, it is produced by the fourth stomach of suckling calves. Calf rennin catalyzes the proteolytic cleavage of a single peptide bond in casein, which lies between the amino acids phenylalanine and methionine at positions 105 and 106, respectively. In an effort to overcome source availability and cost issues, a variety of alternative proteases have been screened. These proteases, mainly of microbial origin, have met with limited success. Very few induce satisfactory curd formation. An alternative approach involves genetic engineering. Rennin cDNA has been expressed in a variety of microbial species, including *Escherichia coli* and *Trichoderma reesei*. In 1990, recombinant rennin became the first recombinant enzyme to be approved for human use as a food ingredient by the Food and Drug Administration (FDA). The recombinant protein product displays biological properties that are essentially identical to those of the native calf rennin.

In the meat industry, tenderness of the meat product is an extremely desired attribute. Toughness of meat is mainly caused by the connective tissue collagen. Older animals have significantly more collagen, and crucially, more cross-linked collagen than their younger counterparts. Cooking meat from older animals brings about only partial collagen solubilization. Accordingly, the cooked meat remains tough. Storage of fresh carcasses in a cold room for up to 10 d, postslaughter, can maximize tenderness. This conditioning or aging process results in the release of proteolytic and other hydrolytic enzymes, as the integrity of some muscle cells (i.e., the meat) breaks down. Papain, a plant-derived cysteine protease, is used in the meat industry to artificially tenderize meat from older animals. A papain solution may be injected into the animal about 30 min prior to slaughter. This facilitates an even body distribution of the proteolytic enzyme. The papain is injected in its oxidized form, which is inactive. After slaughter, physiological changes in the animal bring about a reducing environment in the tissues. The papain is then converted into its reduced form, which is catalytically active.

Proteases also find application in the brewing industry. The cooling of beer after brewing can often promote the formation of haze. This haze is made up of mainly protein, carbohydrate and polyphenolic compounds. The addition of proteases to the beer removes the haze, as the insoluble, mainly protein-based particles are converted to their fully soluble products.

Fungal proteases are employed in the baking industry. They are used to modify the protein components of flour, thereby altering the texture of the dough. Gluten, the main protein fraction of flour, is in fact a complex of two proteins, gliadin and glutenin. When flour is wetted during the preparation of dough, gluten binds with water and expands to form a lattice-type structure. This can make the dough resistant to stretching. However, the inclusion of low amounts of neutral fungal proteases from *Aspergillus oryzae* results in a limited degradation of the gluten lattice, greatly improving the ability of the dough to stretch. This in turn facilitates better retention of carbon dioxide, which is produced by yeast fermentation. Overall, this influences the pore structure of leavened bread and allows the dough to rise uniformly when it is being baked.

The low-calorie sweetener aspartame is actually a dipeptide, consisting of the amino acids L-aspartic acid and phenylalanine, linked by a peptide bond. It is about 200 times sweeter than sucrose (table sugar) and is used extensively in the diet drink and confectionary industry. It may be synthesized chemically or enzymatically. However, chemical synthesis is expensive, owing to the need to preserve amino acid stereospecificity. Accordingly, enzymatic synthesis, which automatically preserves stereospecificity, is the method of choice. A neutral metalloprotease named thermolysin (from *Bacillus thermoproteolyticus*) is used in its production. Under controlled conditions, the protease carries out peptide bond synthesis rather than hydrolysis.

1.4.3   Additional Applications of Proteases

The production of leather from animal hides involves several steps, many of them using enzymes. Overall, the process involves the removal of lipid, water, and some surface protein (e.g., hair) from the animal skin, followed by partial disruption of the collagen (which comprises about 30% of the animal skin) and its subsequent cross-linking during tanning. Several proteases are used during leather manufacture, including animal pancreatic proteases and microbial proteases. The enzymes help to degrade and remove unwanted skin components. There are environmental benefits associated with the use of enzymes because of the obvious reduction in chemical treatments required and a consequent drop in the amount of chemical pollutant waste that would otherwise be generated.

Additional uses of proteolytic enzymes include the cleaning of contact lenses and the removal of unwanted body hair. Contact lenses adsorb various solutes present in tear fluid. This necessitates regular cleaning of their surfaces, otherwise they might become less transparent and more uncomfortable to wear. The major solutes in tear fluid include proteins (antibodies and lysozyme), mucins (high-molecular mass glycoproteins, which have a lubricant function) and lipids. Proteases, or a combination of proteases and lipases, are very effective in the removal of such deposits. The cleaning process entails the immersion of the contact lenses in the enzyme-containing fluid for a few hours, followed by rinsing of the lens with saline solution. This rinsing step is vital, both to remove the enzyme breakdown products as well as any active enzyme remaining on the lens surface, before it is placed back in the eye.

The plant protease papain also has limited application in delaying or preventing hair regrowth on the body and legs. The enzyme degrades the growing hair (α-keratin) and loosens the hair follicle. Since it is of nonhuman origin, papain can provoke an allergic response in some people.

1.4.4   Carbohydrases and Additional Industrial Enzymes

Carbohydrases represent the second most economically significant grouping of industrial enzymes. These include amylolytic enzymes, pectinases, and to a lesser extent, cellulases (Table 1.6). A combination of microbial-derived α-amylases, glucoamylase, and debranching enzymes (pullulanases and isoamylases) are capable of degrading all the glycosidic bonds linking individual glucose monomers present in starch [17,18]. These enzymes are employed industrially to convert starch into glucose syrup, a much more valuable commodity. The glucose syrup produced by this enzymatic process is usually passed through a reactor containing immobilized glucose isomerase, which isomerizes almost 50% of the glucose molecules to fructose [19]. This further increases the product's (i.e., high-fructose corn syrup) value as a food sweetener, as fructose is twice as sweet as glucose.

Pectin-degrading enzymes constitute yet another family of commercially useful carbohydrases. A combination of microbial-derived pectinases (mainly pectin methyl esterases, and polygalacturonidases, and pectin lyases) are capable of almost completely degrading pectin, a plant structural carbohydrate that binds adjacent cells together. Treatment of fruit with

TABLE 1.6

Representative Carbohydrases Used Industrially and Their Actual Applications

Enzyme	Reaction Catalyzed	Industrial Use
α-amylases	Random hydrolysis of internal α 1-4 glycosidic linkages of starch	Production of glucose syrup from starch Brewing aid Laundry detergent additive Textile desizing Fruit juice processing
Glucoamylase	Sequential hydrolysis of starch glycosidic bonds, releasing glucose	Production of glucose syrup from starch
Starch debranching enzymes	Hydrolysis of α 1-6 glycosidic linkages at starch molecule branch points	Production of glucose syrup from starch
Glucose isomerase	Isomerization of glucose to fructose	Conversion of a glucose syrup into a glucose–fructose mix
Lactase	Hydrolysis of lactose, yielding glucose and galactose	Production of lactose hydrosylate which may be used as a food ingredient
Pectic enzymes	Hydrolysis of various bonds of the carbohydrate polymer pectin	Enhanced extraction of fruit juices Clarification of cloudy juices to produce sparkling juices
Cellulolytic enzymes	Hydrolysis of various bonds within cellulose	Adjunct to pectinases in fruit juice extraction/clarification Stonewashing of denim Detergent additive Paper deinking

pectinases significantly improves the yield of fruit juice recovered upon mechanical pressing. Furthermore, pectin forms an important component of suspended molecular aggregates that constitute "haze" in juice extracts. Addition of pectinases, through degradation of the pectin, helps clarify the juice, thereby producing sparkling or clear fruit juices [20].

Cellulases are a family of enzymes capable of degrading cellulose to glucose and short chains of glucose (oligosaccharides) [21,22]. Various technical and economic complications have thus far conspired to prevent the production of glucose syrup directly from cellulolytic material on an industrial level. However, microbial cellulase preparations are employed for a number of industrial purposes, of which denim stonewashing and paper deinking are two of the more interesting. Formerly, stonewashing of denim was undertaken (as the name suggests) by washing the denim in the presence of pumice stones. By promoting a very partial hydrolysis of the cellulolytic fibres on the denim surface, the cellulases release some of the surface dye, thereby giving the garment a faded look. Cellulolytic-based paper deinking works on the same principle. Enzymatic degradation of the surface cellulose fibers of paper releases trapped ink molecules. This is a significantly more environment-friendly means of paper deinking than the alternative chemical-based process.

In addition to carbohydrases, a number of other enzymes have found significant industrial application. These include lipases, which are used as laundry detergent additives as well as for the purpose of altering the flavor of certain (lipid-containing) foodstuffs, including some cheeses, and removing "pitch" (waxes and triglycerides) from wood pulp [23].

Microbial amino acylase is used in the production of L-amino acids, while penicillin acylase continues to play a central role in the production of semisynthetic penicillins [24]. Microbial cyclodextrin glycosyltransferase is utilized to produce cyclodextrins, cyclic oligosaccharides derived from starch, which have found various pharmaceutical and allied applications. A growing number of enzymes are also produced for use as reagents in molecular biology. These include restriction endonucleases as well as DNA ligase and DNA polymerase [25].

1.5   The Future of Industrial Enzymes

Both the range and market value of industrial enzymes will undoubtedly continue to increase over the coming years. Ongoing research and, in particular, the advent of genomics and proteomics continues to reveal new enzymes from various sources that may prove industrially useful. Extremophiles (microorganisms that live under extreme environmental conditions) constitute a rich source of novel, potentially useful enzymes [26,27]. Many enzymes derived from hyperthermophiles, for example, function optimally at temperatures well in excess of 80°C. In some instances, undertaking an enzyme-mediated industrial process at elevated temperatures might have distinct advantages (e.g., if the reactants were significantly less soluble at lower temperatures, or to reduce the viscosity of processing fluids).

It is now well established that many enzymes retain catalytic activity and display altered catalytic characteristics when placed in organic solvents. Again, such an approach may prove industrially useful in circumstances where, for example, a reactant is sparingly soluble or insoluble in aqueous media but soluble in organic media [7].

Enzyme engineering will also significantly impact upon the field of applied enzymology. As increasing understanding of the molecular relationship between enzyme function and structure develops, researchers will be increasingly able to modify structure in order to tailor function. Several detergent enzymes now in general use have been engineered in order to render them oxidation resistant, as mentioned earlier. Without doubt, an increasing proportion of future industrial, analytical, and therapeutic enzymes will be tailored through protein engineering. The principles and applications of enzyme engineering are discussed in Chapter 2.

Enzymes have proven themselves to be among the most prominent of all biological molecules, both scientifically and commercially, and their application in medicine and industry will continue to expand over the years to come.

References

1. Gerhartz, W., *Enzymes in Industry: Production and Applications*, VCH, Weinheim, Germany, 1998.
2. Godfrey, T. and West S., *Industrial Enzymology*, 2nd ed., Macmillan, Basingstoke, UK, 1996.
3. Uhlig, H., *Industrial Enzymes and their Applications*, Wiley Interscience, New York, 1998
4. Fersht, A., *Enzyme Structure and Mechanism*, 2nd ed., W.H. Freeman, New York, 1985.
5. Joyce, G.F., Nucleic acid enzymes: Playing with a fuller deck, *Proc. Natl. Acad. Sci. USA*, 95, 5845–5847, 1998.
6. Dixon, M. and Webb, E.C., *Enzymes*, 2nd. ed., Academic Press Inc., New York, 1964.
7. Walsh, G., *Proteins: Biochemistry and Biotechnology*, John Wiley & Sons, Chichester, UK, 2001.
8. Bickerstaff, G., *Immobilization of Enzymes and Cells*, Humana Press, New York, 1996.
9. Tischer, W. and Wedekind, F., Immobilized enzymes; Methods and applications. *Biocatalysis— from discovery to application*, 200, 95–126, 1999.
10. Burkhard-Kresse, G., Analytical uses of enzymes, in *Biotechnology, a Multi-Volume Treatise*, 2nd ed., Vol. 9, VCH, Weinheim, 1995. pp. 138–163.
11. Kopetzki, E., et al., Enzymes in diagnostics: Achievements and possibilities of recombinant DNA technology, *Clin. Chem.*, 40, 688–704, 1994.
12. Edwards, R., *Immunodiagnostics*, Oxford University Press, Oxford, 1999.
13. Ngo, T., *Biosensors and their Applications*, Plenum Press, New York, 2000.
14. Scheller, F., et al., Research and development in biosensors, *Curr. Opin. Biotechnol.*, 12, 35–40, 2001.

15. Bott, R., *Subtilisin Enzymes*, Plenum, New York, 1995.

16. Bryan, P., Protein engineering of subtilisin, *Biochem. Biophys. Acta – Prot. Struct. Mol. Enzymol.*, 1543, 203–222, 2000.

17. Guzman-Maldonado, H. and Paredes-Lopez, O., Amylolytic enzymes and products derived from starch: A review, *Crit. Rev. Food Sci. Nutr.*, 35, 373–403, 1995.

18. James, J. and Lee, B., Glucoamylases: Microbial sources, industrial applications and molecular biology, a review, *J. Food Biochem.*, 21, 1–52, 1997.

19. Bhosale, S., et al., Molecular and industrial aspects of glucose isomerase, *Microbiol. Rev.*, 60, 280–300, 1996.

20. Kashyap, D., et al., Applications of pectinases in the commercial sector: A review, *Bioresource Technol.*, 77, 215–227, 2001.

21. Tsao, G., *Recent Progress in Bioconversion of Ligocellulolytics*, Springer-Verlag, Godalming, 1999.

22. Himmel. M., et al., Cellulases for commodity products from cellulosic biomass. *Curr. Opin. Biotechnol.*, 10, 358–364.

23. Pandey, A., et al., The realm of microbial lipases in biotechnology, *Biotechnol. Appl. Biochem.*, 29, 119–131, 1999.

24. Shewale, J., et al., Penicillin acylases — Applications and potential, *Proc. Biochem.*, 25, 97–103, 1990.

25. Steitz, T., DNA polymerases; Structural diversity and common mechanisms. *J. Biol. Chem.*, 274, 17395–17398, 1999.

26. Horikoshi, K., *Extremophiles*, John Wiley and Sons, Chichester, UK., 1998.

27. Hough, D. and Danson, M., Thermozymes, biotechnology and structure: Function relationships, *Extremophiles*, 2, 179–183, 1998.

28. Sears, A. and Walsh, G., Industrial enzyme applications, in Biotechnology in the Feed Industry, Lyons, T.P., Ed. Alltech Technical Publications, KY, USA, 1993, pp. 373–394.

2

Enzyme Engineering

Barry M. McGrath

CONTENTS

2.1   Introduction

Enzymes catalyze a myriad of chemical transformations, often with great specificity, exquisite control, and remarkable rate enhancements, forming the basis for metabolism in all living organisms [1,2]. Enzymes have been used by humankind for millennia for a wide variety of biotechnological purposes, including the production of foodstuffs such as cheese, bread, wine, and beer. Currently, enzymes are used for a multitude of applications in a number of diverse areas ranging from detergent manufacturing to the production of fuels and pharmaceuticals, from food and feedstuff manufacturing to cosmetics production, as medicinal products, and as tools for research and development [3–8].

Increasingly, enzymes are being used as biocatalysts in manufacturing bulk chemicals, pharmaceutical and agrochemical intermediates, active pharmaceuticals, and food ingredients [9–13]. Enzymes offer a number of advantages over chemical catalysts in that they are derived from natural and renewable resources, are biodegradable, typically operate under mild conditions of temperature and pH, and generally offer exquisite selectivity in both reactant and product stereochemistry [14,15]. Despite the tremendous potential offered by enzymes as biocatalysts, applications are frequently hampered by evolution-led catalytic traits [16]. Enzymes have evolved to catalyze specific reactions under certain environmental conditions. From an industrial point of view, many enzymes are not readily amenable to industrial-scale use due to the extremes of temperature, pressure, pH, and other conditions used in such processes.

Industry is interested in finding and creating applications for new enzymes that have desirable properties and are not easily accessible or found in nature. Traditionally, this approach has involved sourcing new enzymes with improved properties from microbial sources [14]. The inability to cultivate the vast majority of microorganisms present in microbial niches [17–19] has often hampered this approach, and has focused research efforts on developing new technologies to exploit the genomes of microbes without prior cultivation [14,20–23], while simultaneously, efforts to engineer the properties of existing enzymes continue to grow. It is the latter area which is the subject of this brief review.

The past two decades have witnessed intensive industrial and academic research attempts to develop techniques to engineer enzymes to meet industrial demands, to replace traditional chemical catalysts used widely throughout industry, and to broaden the scope of enzyme applications [9,14,15]. Perhaps subtilisin, a bacterial serine protease, best illustrates the multiple goals of enzyme engineering. Subtilisin has been used for many years as a key component of many detergents, in addition to being used in many other applications in industry. Thus far, mutations in over 50% of the 275 amino acid (aa) residues of subtilisin have been reported in the literature, resulting in improvements in subtilisin's overall catalytic activity, mechanism of action, stability (thermal and pH), substrate specificity, surface activity, folding mechanisms, and in the evolution of new activities for subtilisin (see [24] and references therein for a comprehensive review).

2.2 Improving Enzymes by Engineering

Initial attempts to improve enzyme properties involved introducing random mutagenesis into source organisms by physical and chemical mutagens, natural recombination, and protoplast fusions. One major disadvantage associated with these techniques is that they randomly affect the entire genome of microbes producing the relevant enzyme. Consequently, a small number of genotype variants created using these techniques will result in mutations in the gene of interest. Thus, high-throughput screening (HTS) methods are required to select variants with interesting or improved desired properties. Furthermore, these traditional techniques do not enable the specific alteration of certain protein properties. Modern attempts to engineer enzymes take advantage of the increasing knowledge of enzyme structure, function, and mechanism of action that has been acquired in recent times, enabling the specific alteration of certain enzyme characteristics. Bioinformatics (for predicting structure and function), advances in protein chemistry, and developments in molecular biology and recombinant DNA technologies have all impacted enormously upon the rapidly expanding field of enzyme engineering (see [25] for a historical review of protein engineering).

Modern enzyme engineering efforts exploit the fact that the functional properties of enzymes reside in the structure of the protein. The three-dimensional structure of a protein is largely determined by the sequence of aas that comprise the protein, which can readily be altered employing modern molecular biology procedures. Enzyme engineering consists of approaches that alter protein structure, usually by modifying existing aas, by deleting or introducing aas into a given protein sequence. These changes can be made by altering the corresponding nucleotide sequence of the gene encoding the enzyme. The approaches for generating enzymes with altered properties primarily consist of (1) modulating enzyme properties by the exchange of a single or a few aas or (2) exchanging functional domains between related enzymes, creating hybrid enzymes.

Generally speaking, two distinctive strategies can be used to introduce changes into the aa sequence of an enzyme [26–28]. Rational design relies on extensive and in-depth knowledge of the particular enzyme's structure, in addition to knowledge about the relationships between sequence, structure, and function [29,30]. In sharp contrast, directed evolution approaches enable enzyme optimization in the absence of structural or mechanical information, by testing many different variants using various evolutionary algorithms [14,15,31–38]. Both of these genetic techniques have their advantages and disadvantages relative to specific enzyme engineering applications, and are discussed further in Sections 2.3–2.4. For comprehensive reviews and comparisons of these strategies, see [26–28]. The advances that have occurred in molecular biology techniques since the 1970s have facilitated the development of many innovative, new tools for the enzyme engineer. Both rational design and directed evolution strategies are discussed in more detail in the next sections.

2.2.1 Rational Design

Rational design (or rational redesign) attempts to understand enzyme structure and function at a complete mechanistic level so that desired changes can be effected by calculation from first principles (see Figure 2.1 and [25,27,29,30,39–41] for reviews). Precise aa changes are preconceived based on a detailed knowledge of the enzyme structure, function, and mechanism, and are typically introduced using site-directed mutagenesis (SDM) (see Figure 2.2). Since the first descriptions of this technique in the literature [42–45], SDM has emerged as a very powerful tool enabling the modification of the primary aa sequence of any protein, and remains the cornerstone of many rational design attempts. The first examples of using SDM to modify enzyme structure were reported in 1982 for a β-lactamase and tyrosyl-transfer RNA synthetase [46–48]. Since that time, SDM has had a major impact on engineering some of the key properties of enzymes, such as altering substrate specificity (reviewed in [29,40,49] and Section 2.3.3), enhancing enzyme stability ([29,30,41,50], and Section 2.3.2), and improving overall catalytic activity ([25,29,39] and Section 2.3.1). For comprehensive reviews of the dramatic effects of rational design on key enzymatic properties, see [25,29,30,39–41] and references therein.

The increasing number of databases of high-resolution protein structures and sequences (for instance, see [51]),[1] coupled with the growth in protein molecular modeling programs

---

[1] For further information on the expanding growth of protein structure and analysis, visit www.expasy.org. The ExPASy (Expert Protein Analysis System) proteomics server of the Swiss Institute of Bioinformatics (SIB) is dedicated to the analysis of protein sequences and structures as well as 2-D PAGE.

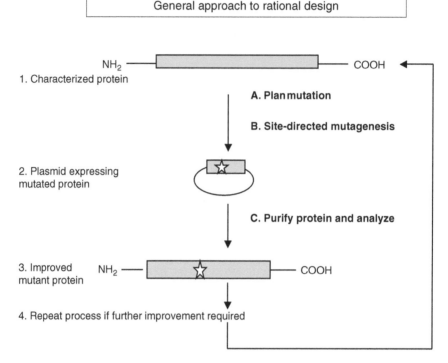

FIGURE 2.1

Overview of rational design process. Step 1: The protein of interest is characterized, and a strategy for rationally introducing specific amino acid (aa) changes is planned on the basis of the known protein structure (A). The desired aa changes are typically introduced using site-directed mutagenesis (SDM) (B). Step 2: A plasmid expressing the mutated protein is created and transformed into an appropriate host (e.g., *E. coli*), and the mutated protein is purified and analyzed for desired properties (C). Step 3: If the mutant protein displays the desired properties, it is isolated. Step 4: The wild-type or variant protein may be subjected to further rounds of SDM and analysis to improve further desired characteristics.

([52–55] and reviewed in [39]), is making rational design an increasingly efficient tool for engineering enzymatic properties. Rational design remains an important component of the protein engineer's toolbox, and its usefulness will no doubt become more apparent as more in-depth knowledge of various industrial and medicinal enzymes accrues. Concomitantly, rational design is complementing our basic understanding and appreciation of fundamental enzymology. Rational design has tremendous potential for the much sought-after area of *de novo* protein enzyme design [39]. Furthermore, as discussed in Section 2.4, rational design has expanded and is predicted to continue to expand the usefulness of enzymes as medicinal products, an area of tremendous potential economic and health benefits. Despite the fact that rational design has had a tremendous impact on protein and enzyme engineering, the strategy usually requires detailed understanding of the structures and mechanisms. However, this information is not available for the vast majority of enzymes, and even if it was, the actual molecular basis of the desired function may not be [56]. These limitations on rational design have prompted the development of some innovative new technologies, such as directed evolution.

2.2.2   Directed Evolution

Despite the ever-growing body of knowledge surrounding enzyme structure and function, it is quite clear that various aspects of enzyme function cannot be predicted [57]. Rational

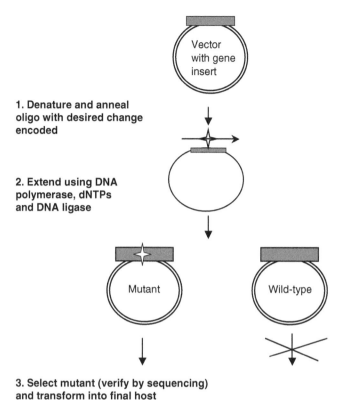

1. Denature and anneal oligo with desired change encoded

2. Extend using DNA polymerase, dNTPs and DNA ligase

3. Select mutant (verify by sequencing) and transform into final host

FIGURE 2.2
Schematic diagram outlining the general approach adopted to alter the amino acid (aa) sequence by site-directed mutagenesis. The DNA fragment encoding the wild-type (unaltered) protein of interest is cloned into a plasmid vector. An appropriate oligonucleotide (oligo) is designed, the ends of which are complementary to the nucleotide (nt) sequence of the gene, while the central portion of the oligo contains an altered nt sequence corresponding to the desired change in the protein (marked with a star). The dsDNA is denatured to make the template strand available for hybridization with the mutagenic oligo (Step 1). The addition of dNTPs, DNA polymerase, and DNA ligase enables DNA synthesis, forming closed circular molecules (Step 2). The mutated plasmid is selected, and the desired change is verified (by sequencing). The mutant plasmid is selected and transformed into a final host strain (Step 3), where large amounts of the mutant protein can be produced using standard recombinant methods.

design approaches to enzyme engineering are not particularly suited to generating enzymes in a random, selection-driven manner [32]. In direct contrast to rational design, the technique of directed evolution requires minimal knowledge of the enzyme mechanism and of how the enzyme structure relates to its function [26–28,52,56]. Directed evolution approaches involve either random mutagenesis of the gene encoding the enzyme or recombination of gene fragments encoding homologs of the enzyme in question, followed by stringent selection and screening processes for identifying enzymes with desired properties. In this respect, the directed evolution approach mimics Darwinian evolution. In contrast to the natural evolution of species, which can take millions of years, directed evolution approaches can be performed in any modern molecular biology laboratory in a matter of weeks or months, and with an unlimited number of parents [33,37,38].

Directed evolution is essentially a two-step procedure (Figure 2.3):

1. Generation of initial diversity, followed by cloning this library into an appropriate expression vector and host organism
2. Screening and selection of the library of mutants created in step 1 to obtain an enzyme with the desired altered trait(s)

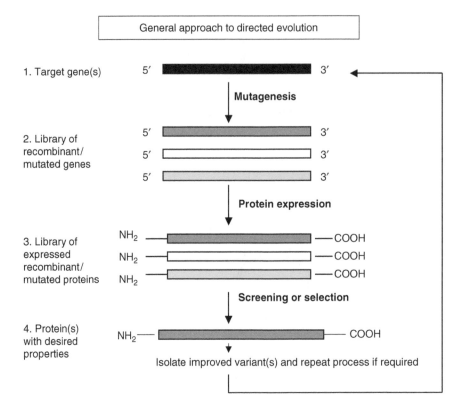

FIGURE 2.3

Overview of directed evolution process. Step 1: The wild-type (wt) gene encoding the protein of interest is isolated. Step 2: The wt gene is subjected to random mutagenesis creating a library of mutated wt variants. Step 3: The library of variants are expressed in an appropriate host. Step 4: Variants of the wt protein are screened for improved desired characteristics and the best variant(s) are selected. These improved variants may undergo several rounds of mutagenesis and screening before a variant displaying the desired traits is selected.

In many ways, step 2 is most challenging, as without an effective screening strategy, the ability to isolate useful clones generated in step 1 is severely diminished (techniques to create diversity are briefly outlined in Section 2.2.2.1). The maxim that "you get what you screen for" [38] is applicable to all directed evolution experiments, and is discussed further in Section 2.2.2.2. The subsequent brief reviews focuses primarily on recent reports in the literature concerning the successes witnessed over the past decade with directed evolution experiments to enhance some of the key features of enzymes, namely, catalytic activity (Section 2.3.1), stability (Section 2.3.2), and specificity (Section 2.3.3).

2.2.2.1   Techniques to Generate Diversity

What follows is a very brief overview of some of the recent developments concerning techniques for creating molecular diversity. This rapidly developing field is gaining tremendous attention from both academic and industrial researchers. For recent and more comprehensive reviews of this fascinating subject area, some excellent review articles [31,57] and recent books on the topic have been published (see [37,38,58], and references therein for detailed protocols of directed evolution library creation methods).

Broadly speaking, the methods for generating enzyme-encoding libraries can be divided into three categories:

1. *In vivo* random mutagenesis techniques
2. *In vitro* random and directed oligonucleotide-based methods introducing changes at positions throughout the gene sequence
3. *In vitro* recombination methods

The first techniques used to create molecular diversity principally involved chemical and physical mutagenic agents. However, these methods randomly affect the entire genome of microbes producing the relevant enzyme(s). Random mutagenesis can be achieved through *in vivo* recombination via replication in mutator strains. Numerous mutator *Escherichia coli* and yeast strains, defective in repair systems, have been utilized to generate variants of a wild-type enzyme encoding gene. New techniques that enable targeting of the mutagenesis to a specific gene have been described (see [59,60,61] for examples of *E. coli* and yeast strains). Recently, several mutator plasmids have also been created for this purpose [62,63].

The early 1990s marked the beginning of a new era in terms of creating molecular diversity *in vitro*. Error-prone polymerase chain reaction (ep-PCR) is a technique that has gained widespread use as a method for generating random mutagenesis *in vitro* [64,65]. Ep-PCR protocols are modifications of standard PCRs, designed to enhance the natural error rate of the polymerase by using a low-fidelity DNA polymerase in combination with reaction conditions that further decrease the fidelity of the polymerase. Conditions reducing fidelity include varying the ratios of nucleotides used, altering initial template concentration, increasing or decreasing the number of PCR cycles, and using higher concentrations of $MgCl_2$ than standard PCRs. $MnCl_2$ can also be used to enhance the error rate [66]. The products generated using ep-PCR are variants of the original template that contain random point mutations along the full-length genes. One drawback associated with ep-PCR is the biased occurrence of aas as a result of single-base replacements in the triplet codons. An elegant methodology for circumventing this bias has been reported by Murakami et al. [67,68], termed random insertion/deletion (RID) mutagenesis. RID enables the deletion of an arbitrary number of consecutive bases at random positions, and, at the same time, insertion of a specific or random sequence of an arbitrary number into the same position.

Some sophisticated random mutagenic strategies have been developed recently, such as GeneReassembly™ and Gene Site Saturation Mutagenesis™ (GSSM), which enable the creation of comprehensive directed mutagenesis libraries. For instance, the GSSM technique [69] creates a library of all possible codon variants in a gene to each of its 63 alternatives, thereby enabling access to all 19 aa side-chain variants at each aa residue in a protein sequence. This technique has proven very effective at enhancing both pH and thermal tolerance [70,71], and in enhancing enantioselectivity [72]. For comprehensive reviews of these and other emerging technologies, see [14,31,57,58].

Tremendous random diversity can be achieved through *in vitro* recombination methods, based upon the random rearrangement of genetic information among parental genes. Perhaps the biggest influence on directed evolutionary techniques was the pioneering work of Frances H. Arnold (Caltech, Pasadena, California, USA) and Willem P. Stemmer (Maxygen Inc., Redwood city, California, USA), among others, who developed recombination-based methods that heralded a new era of rapid development and growth in enzyme engineering. DNA shuffling, an *in vitro* recombination technique devised by Stemmer, has had a major impact on enzyme engineering strategies since its introduction more than 10 years ago. The initial description [73] and application [74] of the technique utilized single genes, with introduced point mutations as the source of diversity. The libraries of variants are created by firstly cleaving the initial population of molecules into random fragments, which are then reassembled after cycles of denaturation, annealing, and extension by polymerase. Diversity arises through random point mutations resulting from the polymerase reaction (Figure 2.4A; see [73–75] for detailed protocols). An alternative source of diversity is to use naturally occurring homologous genes (Figure 2.4B), providing functional diversity [76]. This approach accelerates evolution as naturally occurring homologs are preenriched for functional diversity, because deleterious variants have been selected against over millions of years of evolution [75]. Numerous modifications of the family DNA shuffling technique have been described (see, for example, [75,77–80]) since the initial description by Crameri et al. [76]. Other techniques, based on similar methodologies to DNA shuffling, have also been reported. For instance, Zhao et al. [81] have developed a simple and efficient technique for *in vitro* mutagenesis and recombination of nucleotide sequences, known as the staggered extension process (StEP). This process, like DNA shuffling, can be used to promote recombination between mutant genes. Another technique, known as random chimaeragenesis on transient templates (RACHITT) [82], is conceptually very similar to DNA shuffling and StEP, and claims to overcome some of the limitations encounted with other DNA shuffling techniques (Table 2.1 and [82,83]).

One disadvantage of the family DNA shuffling-based techniques is the requirement for the parent genes being recombined to share considerable (~60%) homology. Several modifications and refinements of the original recombination-based techniques have appeared in recent years that do not require such high levels of homology (Table 2.1). For instance, the techniques of sequence homology-independent protein recombination (SHIPREC) [84] and incremental truncation for the creation of hybrid enzymes (ITCHY) [85] lead to the formation of hybrids, which are single-point fusions of unrelated sequences. The initial

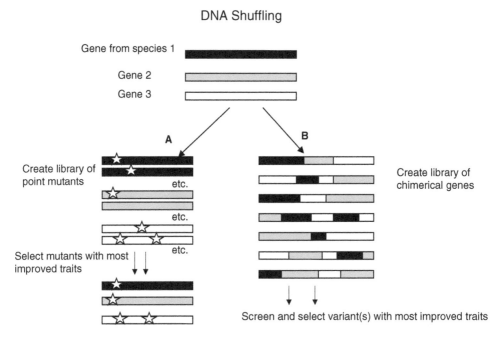

FIGURE 2.4

Overview of DNA shuffling process [73,74]. Genes encoding the enzymes of interest are isolated and cloned. In single gene shuffling [73,74] (pathway A), mutant libraries of each of the genes are created using DNA shuffling. The variant enzymes are expressed in an appropriate host, screened for improved properties, and those variants displaying the desired improved properties are selected. In family DNA shuffling [76] (pathway B), homologs of the desired gene-encoding enzyme are recombined together, creating a library of hybrid genes. These chimeras are expressed in an appropriate host, screened for improved properties, and those variants displaying the desired improved properties are selected.

TABLE 2.1
Directed Evolution Techniques (DNA Recombination-Based Methods)

Method	Pros	Cons	Ref.
1. Exon shuffling	No sequence homology required; High percentage of folded proteins; Maintains structural domains; Can use varied parent genes	Restricted to intron-containing genes (not applicable to prokaryotic genes)	[80]
2. Family DNA shuffling	Combines useful mutations and loses harmful mutations; Can use multiple parent genes to increase the diversity and fitness of a library	Relies on sequence homology	[76]
3. RACHITT	Crossovers occur in regions of short (0–5 bases) sequence homology; Single hybridization event reduces the mismatching sometimes seen in PCR-based methods	Incomplete degradation by λ exonuclease affects quality of ssDNA substrate, which is critical; Additional steps require upfront phagemid cloning and preparation of ss gene fragments and template DNA	[82], [83]
4. Family shuffling with ssDNA	May reduce parental sequence reproduction and favor the formation of chimeras	Additional steps in phage compared with family shuffling; May be unnecessary with most proteins or in experiments with effective screens	[78], [79]
5. StEP	Comparable diversity to other DNA-shuffling formats; Simple, single-tube method with no fragment purification	Relies on sequence homology; Project-specific optimization of PCR conditions can be time-consuming and limit robustness of the method	[81]
6. CLERY	Useful for screening proteins expressed in yeast	Additional steps; No advantage to *in vitro* family shuffling unless proteins are to be screened in yeast	[60]
7. SHIPREC	Creates hybrid library of two unrelated genes; No sequence homology required so junctions are randomly distributed; Researchers preselect full-length hybrids	Only one crossover per hybrid per round (low diversity library, but may iterate or combine with homologous recombination methods to improve crossovers); Limited to two parents of equal length; Low-fitness hybrids (two thirds may contain frame-shift); May induce aa deletions or duplications at junctions	[84]
8. ITCHY	Same pros as for SHIPREC; Researchers preselect functional hybrids with auxotrophic *E. coli*	Same cons as for SHIPREC; Parent gene length is not conserved in hybrids	[85]
9. THIOITCHY	Same pros as for ITCHY; More efficient and easier than ITCHY	Same as for ITCHY; dNTP analogs remain in hybrid and may interfere with other DNA-binding proteins	[86], [87]

Note: Methods 1–6 exploit homologous recombination; Methods 7–9 are based on ligation. ssDNA = single-stranded DNA.
Adapted from Kurtzman, A.L. et al., *Curr. Opin. Biotechnol.*, 12, 361–370, 2001.

version of ITCHY was performed via timed exonuclease digestions, and proved difficult to optimize; it subsequently led to the development of THIO-ITCHY, in which initial templates are created with phosphothioate linkages, incorporated at random points along the length of the gene [86,87]. More recently, a nonhomologous recombination technique, termed SCRATCHY, which combines features of ITCHY and DNA shuffling, has been described [88,89]. Although these techniques do not require much detailed knowledge of the protein structure, such information can be utilized in the design of crossover points, as illustrated by the recently described technique known as structural-based combinatorial protein engineering (SCOPE) [90].

Compared with oligonucleotide-based or *in vivo* random mutagenesis, the key advantage of *in vitro* recombination methods is the ability to accumulate beneficial mutations while simultaneously removing deleterious mutations [27,33,81]. Since the description of the first DNA recombination-based techniques, a multitude of techniques based on the recombination model have been developed, with many industrial and academic researchers striving to improve or modify the basic techniques. Some excellent reviews of new patented and widely available techniques that have emerged in recent years have been reported [37,57,58], including techniques based on oligonucleotide-driven randomization, whole-gene randomization, and homology-dependent and homology-independent recombination techniques. Also, numerous reports of computational methods seek to complement laboratory-based techniques by identifying useful sequence space to be probed during directed evolution experiments. This concept of *in silico* design and screening has proven very useful in reducing the redundancy of enzyme libraries and enabling more useful sequence space to be explored. Some examples include computer programs that identify specific aa residues in a protein more tolerant to mutagenesis [91], and others such as Xencor's patented protein design automation (PDA®) technology [92,93]. It is difficult to be comprehensive, because new techniques are constantly emerging; for more in-depth reviews of the growing area of computational methods to aid protein engineering experiments, see [31,36,52,53,57,58,94] and references therein.

It is also worth noting that the various recombination-based DNA shuffling techniques are not just limited to creating diversity in single protein structures. DNA shuffling has been used to adapt whole organisms to excel under foreign conditions associated with commercial process conditions [95], to evolve murine leukemia viruses with broader cell tropisms [96], to create retroviruses with improved stability and yields under processing conditions [97], in the evolution of new metabolic pathways [98], and in the *de novo* molecular evolution of an Archael DNA fragment with unknown function (lacking ampicillin resistance) to confer ampicillin resistance on an *E. coli* strain [99].

2.2.2.2   Screening and Selection

The previous section briefly outlined some of the numerous methods that are available for the first step of any directed evolution experiment — creating the initial genetic diversity. Perhaps the most challenging step in any directed evolution experiment is finding those proteins that perform the desired function according to specified criteria among the created library of mutant sequences [38]. In parallel with the development of methods to create diversity, numerous technological advances have been made in HTS to enable rapid screening of libraries of mutant proteins.

Some of the key features associated with any effective screening method are that they (1) should be high throughput (to enable detection of useful variants), (2) are highly sensitive to the desired function, (3) are reproducible, (4) are robust, and (5) enable easy detection [38]. Typically, screening an enzyme library involves analysis of variants that are arranged on microtiter plates (usually 96- or 384-well plates), on Petri dishes, or by other means and are then analyzed by functional assays [38,100]. HTS can be performed with whole cells, cell lysates, or partially purified proteins. Some recent innovative developments in enzyme screening and assay methods are reviewed elsewhere [38,101–109].

Alternatively, selection of an improved enzyme involves coupling the desired trait to those variants possessing the specific trait. Selections offer the advantage of isolating functional proteins from very large libraries (frequently $\geq 10^7$ clones) simply by growing a population of cells under selective conditions. However, the expressed enzyme must confer a significant biological advantage, which limits the range of enzymes and properties that can be assessed [100,110]. *In vivo* selection protocols are the most convenient but require that the expressed enzyme directly confers a significant biological advantage [38,100,111]. Consequently, numerous *in vitro* selection protocols have been developed which directly link the phenotype and genotype. Phage display [112–114] remains the most common technique for *in vitro* selection, while other tools, such as water-in-oil *in vitro* compartmentalization, have emerged as very powerful alternative selection tools linking phenotype with genotype for the directed evolution of enzyme properties [115–118]. Comprehensive reviews of recent developments in *in vitro* selection techniques have been reported [31,38,101,111].

2.2.3 Combining Rational Design and Directed Evolution

The two principal strategies employed for genetic manipulation of an enzyme's primary aa sequence, rational design and directed evolution, which approaches the goal of engineering from different perspectives, are by no means mutually exclusive. In recent years, a number of papers have appeared in the literature which employ rational design and directed evolution strategies in combination, particularly in cases where a certain amount of knowledge of the enzyme's structure is known, or where a region of the protein structure is known to affect a particular property such as substrate binding for instance.

One of the first examples illustrating the power of using this combined approach used directed evolution to augment a rational design attempt to engineer a novel function into an α/β-barrel enzyme by completely converting the activity of indole-3-glycerol-phosphate synthase (IGPS) into that of an efficient phosphoribosyl-anthranilate isomerase (PRAI). Structure-based design was employed to modify the IGPS α/β-barrel by incorporating the basic design of the PRAI loop system, yielding a hybrid variant with very low PRAI activity. This variant served as a scaffold for subsequent directed evolution engineering using DNA shuffling and StEP. Genetic selection (agar plate-based) was then employed to select a variant with increased PRAI activity. The final engineered variant obtained displayed six-fold higher activity than wild-type PRAI and had no IGPS activity, while retaining 28% identity to PRAI and 90% identity to IGPS [118].

Since then, an ever-increasing number of reports combining rational design and directed evolution approaches to alter enzyme performance have appeared in the literature. These have included combined approaches to improve overall catalytic activity [119–121], altering the substrate [122,123] and product specificity [124] of various enzymes, enhanced thermostability [125–129], and enhanced resistance to natural enzyme inhibitors [130] (see Section 2.3). It has been predicted that future enzyme engineering strategies will employ a combination of both directed evolution and rational design strategies [25–29,35,39,41,125–127,131,132].

2.2.4 Other Techniques

Manipulations of protein properties at the genetic level, by directed evolution and rational design techniques, have led to dramatic advances in engineering enzymes. Although overshadowed to some extent by these advances, both physical and chemical means of modifying enzymes still remain very useful strategies for the optimization of enzyme properties, as does the addition of stabilizers. Physical modification, for instance through immobilization onto solid supports, has proven very effective at enhancing enzyme stability (some examples are listed in Section 2.3.2). One major goal of chemical modification is to increase enzyme stability and activity (Sections 2.3.1 and 2.3.2), and has proven very effective in achieving these goals, particularly in nonaqueous environments (Section 2.3.2.2). As this review focuses primarily on recent advances in enzyme engineering by manipulation at the genetic level, the interested reader is referred to some recent reviews on chemical modification of proteins [50,133–138]. For a review of physical and chemical approaches to engineering lipases, which are widely used in the detergent industry and increasingly so in the production of optically pure compounds, see [139,140].

2.3   Engineered Enzyme Properties

Properties of enzymes that have been improved include increased catalytic performance (increase activity), thermostability and stability in unusual environments (e.g., organic solvents or extremes of pH), altered selectivity/specificity, evolution of new activities, susceptibility to proteases, and solubility. The following section highlights recent examples in some of these areas.

2.3.1   Catalytic Activity

Improving the catalytic efficiency of an enzyme is a common goal in protein engineering. Rational design, directed evolution, and other techniques have been used successfully to improve biocatalyst activity and turnover properties, and some examples are given below.

Notable rational design successes in improving catalytic turnover have been reported (reviewed in [25,29,100]). For instance, the turnover of superoxide dismutase (one of the fastest known enzymes) was improved using rational design approaches [141], while the turnover of papain for nitrile hydratase was increased 10^4-fold relative to the wild-type by replacement of an active site residue (Q19E) [142]. Knowledge of aa residues involved in catalysis can aid the design of new, improved active sites by means of rational design. For example, deacetoxycephalosporin C synthase (DAOCS) from *Streptomyces clavuligerus* catalyzes the ring expansion of penicillin to form cephalosporin, and has potential industrial uses in synthesizing new cephalosporin antibiotics. The C-terminus was known to be critical to DAOCS activity. Chin et al. [143] explored the role of asparagine residue 304 (N304) by substituting N304 with other aas. One mutant, N304L, displayed increased activity for penicillin and penicillin analogs ranging from 130 to 420%, relative to the wild-type. Other mutants such as N304K and N304R exhibited even more improved activity (up to 730% that of the wild-type). Replacement of N304 with aas bearing aliphatic or basic side-chains is thought to incorporate favorable hydrophobic or charged interactions between the variant enzymes and their substrates, thus enhancing enzyme activity [143].

Directed evolution techniques have also proven adept at enhancing enzyme activity (reviewed in [14,32,36]). Directed evolution studies have frequently concluded that beneficial mutations do not necessarily occur in the enzyme's active site, and that residues outside the active site can play important roles in determining catalytic activity [56]. For example, amylosucrase from *Neisseria polysaccharea* is a glucosyltransferase that catalyzes the formation of glucose polymers from sucrose [144]. Unique among enzymes belonging to its class, amylosucrase can produce an amylase-like glucan consisting solely of α-1,4-

linked glucose residues. Unlike other similar enzymes, amylosucrase does not require the addition of expensive activated sugars. It has numerous potential industrial applications as a polysaccharide-synthesizing or -modifying agent. Its potential has been limited by its low catalytic efficiency on sucrose, low stability, and side reactions producing sucrose isomers. Using ep-PCR, DNA shuffling, and appropriate selection, Van der Veen et al. [144] generated two amylosucrase variants with vastly improved properties more suited to industrial synthesis conditions compared to the wild-type enzyme. The specific activities were over five-fold greater than the wild-type, and both displayed greatly improved catalytic efficiency. Both variants had two aa substitutions outside the active site of the enzyme, which would have been difficult to predict using a rational design approach.

Some impressive examples of using directed evolution and high-throughput screening strategies to improve catalytic turnover have been reported. Using ep-PCR and DNA shuffling, a variant of the *Pseudomonas diminuta* MG organophosphohydrolase, a nerve agent degrader, was selected using cell surface display and a colorimetric assay. The variant showed a 25-fold increase in turnover [145]. Selection of a large mutant library by *in vitro* compartmentalization yielded a phosphotriesterase variant exhibiting a 63-fold higher k_{cat} than the parent enzyme [117].

Rational design and directed evolution have been combined to improve catalytic activity. A five-fold increase in the activity of a carbon–carbon bond-forming side reaction of benzoylformate decarboxylase was reported using both strategies [121]. Ep-PCR generated a mutant (L476G), with a five-fold greater carboligase activity than the parent. Saturation mutagenesis was then applied to Leu476 that yielded an additional eight variants with both improved catalytic activity and enantioselectivity than the parent.

2.3.2 Enzyme Stability

Enzymes are increasingly used for a wide range of industrial applications (reviewed in [4,5,9,14,15,32]). The increasing use of biocatalysts in industry is dependent on developments that improve enzyme performance under process conditions. Enzymes have evolved to catalyze specific reactions under certain environmental conditions. From an industrial point of view, many enzymes are not readily amenable to industrial-scale use, due to the extremes of temperature, pressure, pH, and other conditions used in such processes. Thus, the ability to engineer increased stability into enzymes such that they can be readily applied to industrial processes is desirable.

2.3.2.1 Thermostability

Many industrial processes occur at elevated temperatures. Enzyme thermostability is of major industrial importance, as the use of biocatalysts in industry is dependent, in many instances, on the enzyme's ability to tolerate or function at elevated temperatures. Intensive efforts have been made in academic and industrial laboratories in recent years to improve enzyme thermostability (reviewed in [41,50,110,127,128,146]). Strategies used to improve protein thermostability include directed evolution approaches, rational design methods, consensus sequence approaches, and chemical modification and addition of stabilizers. The following section highlights some of the more recent successes reported using these techniques.

Studies of hyperstable enzymes detected in extreme environmental conditions have revealed that enzymes have utilized numerous strategies to evolve thermostability. A multitude of long-range and local interactions determine enzyme stability at elevated temperatures [127,146]. Two important general stabilizing strategies have been observed in hyperstable enzymes: (1) the presence of large surface networks of electrostatic interactions and (2) a tendency of hyperstable enzymes to be multimeric. In practice, however, such properties are difficult to engineer into a protein.

Attempts to design enzyme thermostability rationally have utilized several approaches with some successes, including mutations aimed at reducing the entropy of unfolded proteins (by introducing disulfide bridges or by increasing Pro residues), increasing the number of α-helices through Gly$\rightarrow$Ala substitutions, and engineering of salt bridges [30,41,127]. Table 2.2 highlights some of the successes achieved using rational design principles to improve enzyme stability at elevated temperatures. Despite these successes, no simple set of rules for predicting thermostability have been devised as yet, thereby limiting the ability of rational design to engineer thermostability.

Directed evolution techniques have proven very adept at modifying the thermostability of commercially important enzymes. The advances in techniques for generating diversity (Section 2.2.2.1), coupled with advances in high-throughput screening for thermostability [14,147,148], has led to the development of many biocatalysts with improved thermostability (reviewed in [12,32,41,50]). For instance, a variant of subtilisin, widely used as a detergent protease, was developed displaying a 1200-fold increase in half-life at 60°C [149,150]. A peroxidase developed for use in the detergent industry was improved by directed evolution to display a 174-fold increase in thermostability at 50°C [151]. Adaptation of enzymes to colder temperatures using directed evolution have been reported [152–154].

Many of the earlier attempts at improving enzyme thermostability using directed evolution or rational design strategies came with a concomitant reduction in catalytic activity. One explanation for this trade-off is that during evolution, enzymes have adjusted the strength and number of stabilizing interactions to optimize the balance between rigidity (for stability) and flexibility (for activity) [110]. Some recent examples illustrate that it is now possible to alter thermostability without any detrimental effect on catalytic activity (Table 2.3).

Lehmann et al. [127] and Lehmann and Wyss [128] have introduced a semirational strategy, the consensus approach, for engineering thermostability into proteins. This approach hypothesizes that at a given position in a protein sequence, conserved aa residues contribute more than average to stability than nonconsensus aa residues. Thus, substitution of the nonconserved aas may be a feasible course of action for increasing thermostability. Using this approach, an improved phytase, a commercially important animal feed additive, was designed [129]. By aligning homologous sequences of 13 wild-type phytases from fungal sources, key residues were identified that were thought to contribute to thermostability. A synthetic consensus phytase was constructed from this data that was 15 to 26°C more stable than all the parent phytases. In addition, gains in thermostability did not compromise the catalytic activity of the phytase. Other examples of utilizing the consensus approach have been reported, highlighting the potential of using this approach as an additional tool for engineering and understanding thermostability in enzymes [155,156].

Manipulation of protein properties at the genetic level by directed evolution, rational design, and other techniques, has led to dramatic advances in engineering enzyme thermostability, as outlined previously. Although overshadowed by these advances, chemical modification remains a very useful technique, as does the technique of addition of stabilizers (reviewed in [50]). Protein structures can be stabilized by forming intramolecular crosslinks, such that the internal crosslink can prevent protein unfolding under stressful conditions. One form of this involves crosslinking small protein crystals with gluteraldehyde. These crosslinked enzyme crystals (CLECs) display increased operational and storage stabilities relative to untreated enzymes. Glucoamylase hydrolyzes starch and is used extensively in the starch, glucose, and fermentation industries. Typically, immobilized glucoamylase preparations are used to reduce operation costs and downtime, but have the disadvantage of reduced thermostability over nonimmobilized forms. To overcome these

TABLE 2.2

Some of the Successes Achieved Using Rational Design to Improve Enzyme Thermostability

Enzyme	Amino Acid (aa) Changes and Rationale	Modified Characteristics	Ref.
Aspergillus niger phytase (EC 3.1.3.8)	A 31-aa sequence from *Aspergillus terreus* phytase was substituted by corresponding region from *A. niger* phytase	$t_{1/2}$ at 49°C 308 min, wild type $t_{1/2}$ at 49°C of 53 min	[243]
Thermolysin-like protease (Boilysin) (EC 3.4.24.28)	Eight aa substitutions in regions known to contribute to protein stability including G8C and N60C which led to formation of an extra disulfide bridge	$t_{1/2}$ at 100°C 170 min (parent completely inactive at 100°C)	[244]
Pyroglutamyl peptidase I (EC 3.4.19.3)	S185C substitution led to formation of an additional disulfide bond	30°C increase in thermal stability relative to wild-type	[245]
Alkaline protease (AprP) (EC 3.4.21.63)	S331D substitution eliminated autolytic cleavage site at Ser331	$t_{1/2}$ at 60°C doubled in variant relative to wild-type	[246]
Pyrroloquinoline quinone glucose dehydrogenase (EC 1.1.99.17)	Replacement of Ser331 with Cys, Met, Leu, Asp, Asn, His or Lys increased thermostability, S331K showed greatest increase	Eight-fold increase in $t_{1/2}$ at 55°C relative to wild-type	[247]
Penicillin G acylase (EC 3.5.1.11)	Replacement of basic surface residues with alanine	Two- to three-fold increase in $t_{1/2}$ at 55°C relative to wild-type	[164]
Penicillin G acylase (EC 3.5.1.11)	Increasing lysine content on enzyme surface to increase multipoint covalent attachment of enzyme to support	Immobilized variants show 4 to 11 times more stability at temperatures from 4 to 60°C	[248]

TABLE 2.3

Some Recent Examples of Altering Enzyme Thermostability Using Directed Evolution Technologies

Enzyme	Application	Methods[a]	Amino Acid (AA) Changes	Modified Characteristics[b]	Enhancement Factor[c]	Ref.
Lipase B from *Candida antarctica* (EC 3.1.1.3)	Resolution of commercially important compounds	ep-PCR	Variant 1 = 2, variant 2 = 3	Both variants show a 20-fold increase in $t_{1/2}$ at 70°C compared to wild-type	Variants show a 3- to 10-fold increase in k_{cat}/K_m	[248]
Xylanase (EC 3.2.1.8)	Food or fuel production, brewing, feed supplements	GSSM, gene reassembly	6	Increase in maximum thermal tolerance 60–90°C	Variant displays a higher (~1.1-fold) activity	[71]
Esterase from *Pseudomonas fluorescens* KCTC 1767	Production of commercially valuable (*S*)-ketoprofen	ep-PCR, StEP	3	Variant retains 30 and 10% of activity at 50 and 55°C, respectively (parent inactive at 50°C)	1.5-fold higher activity, 1.2-fold increase in k_{cat}/K_m	[250]
Maltogenic amylase from *Thermus* spp. (EC 3.2.1.133)	Widespread use in starch industry	DNA shuffling	7	T_{opt} increase by 15 to 75°C, increase in $t_{1/2}$ at 80°C from 5.3–172 min	Reduced K_m, k_{cat}/K_m slightly reduced	[251]
Fructosyl-amino acid oxidase (EC 1.5.3)	Diabetes diagnosis	*In vitro* mutagenesis in *E. coli* XL1-Red	6	T_{opt} increase by 10°C, activity at 50°C increased 20%, stable at 45°C (parent unstable > 37°C)	1.5-fold increase in k_{cat}/K_m	[252]
E. coli phytase (EC 3.1.3.26)	Animal feed supplement	GSSM	8	100% activity at 62°C, 27% activity after 10 min at 85°C, T_m increase. of 12°C	k_{cat}/K_m activity unchanged in variant	[70]
Pseudomonas putida formaldehyde dehydrogenase (EC 1.2.1.46)	Formaldehyde detoxification	ep-PCR	1	T_{opt} decrease by 10°C (to 37°C),	1.5-fold increase in k_{cat}/K_m at 37°C	[153]

[a] Methods of generating diversity include error-prone PCR (ep-PCR), gene site saturation mutagenesis (GSSM), staggered extension process (StEP).

[b] $t_{1/2}$ = half-life; T_m = melting temperature; T_{opt} = optimal temperature.

[c] Enhancement in activity relative to the wild-type enzyme.

disadvantages, glucoamylase CLECs were developed which displayed enhanced thermo-stability and significantly increased activity at higher temperatures [157]. This technique has been applied to various enzymes including lipases, subtilisin, and thermolysin (reviewed in [158]).

Attachment of the protein to multiple sites of a suitable polymer is another chemical modification approach to enhance enzyme thermostability. Gómez et al. [159] used such an approach to improve the thermostability of a yeast invertase. By covalently attaching the invertase to the carbohydrates chitosan and pectin, the half-life of invertase at 65°C increased from 5 min to 5 h, and from 5 min to 2 d, respectively [159, 160]. Pig kidney D-aa oxidase is unstable above 55°C, and is used as a liquid assay reagent for analytical deter-mination of D-aas. Attachment of the enzyme to dextran ensured stability up to 75°C, with an overall improvement in catalytic activity [161]. Immobilization of enzymes onto solid supports is another viable method for enhancing thermostability. Glucose oxidase is used in glucose biosensors with various applications including monitoring glucose concentra-tions in food and fermentation processes. Enhancing the thermostability of glucose oxi-dase is relevant to its practical applications for online process monitoring. Using glass beads treated with 4% silane, the thermostability of glucose oxidase was enhanced to tol-erate temperatures up to 75°C while displaying a 180% increase in activity, relative to the untreated enzyme [162].

2.3.2.2   Stability in the Presence of Organic Solvents

The ability of enzymes to function in the presence of organic solvents would greatly broaden the scope of enzyme use to many industrial processes [16,163]. Biocatalyst-enhancement technologies have been developed in recent years to improve the functional-ity of enzymes in the presence of organic solvents. Directed evolution approaches have been used successfully to enhance enzyme stability in numerous nonnatural solvents (reviewed in [9,16,163]). In contrast, rational engineering has not been as effective in achiev-ing this goal, due to the difficulty in predicting which aa residues contribute to stability, but some successes have been reported [164,165]. Chen and Arnold [166] used sequential ran-dom mutagenesis to generate subtilisin E variants, which showed enhanced turnover in dimethylformamide (DMF) when compared to aqueous medium. Directed evolution was used to generate several variants of phospholipase A_1 with enhanced stability and activity in organic solvents [167]. The activity of para-nitrobenzyl esterase in the presence of 30% DMF was improved 50-fold using random mutagenesis [168]. Directed evolution has been successfully employed to generate a horseradish peroxidase variant that displayed enhanced stability in the presence of hydrogen peroxide, sodium dodecyl sulfate (SDS), and salts [169].

Biocatalysts with improved functionality in organic solvents have also been devel-oped using chemical modification techniques [50,163]. Modification of glycoside hydro-lases, including mannosidase, glucosidase, and glucosaminidase, was achieved by lipid coating the enzymes such that the activity of these enzymes was greatly enhanced in isopropyl ether [170]. Chemical modification of a catalase by addition of Brij-35, a sur-factant, increased the activity 200-fold in tricholoroethylene and 15-fold in aqueous media, when compared to the nonmodified catalase [171]. Penicillin G acylase is used widely in the production of synthetic penicillin-based antibiotics [165]. Encapsulation of crosslinked enzyme aggregates into a polymeric matrix significantly increased the enzyme's stability in the presence of organic solvents, with an observed increase in reac-tion rates and yields [172]. Altering the reaction media by addition of various excipients (e.g., nonbuffer salts) is an alternative strategy to enhance enzyme performance in non-aqueous media [173].

2.3.3   Enzyme Specificity

The use of enzymes in industry, academia, and medicine could be broadened considerably by altering specificity. Enzyme engineering attempts to alter the enzyme's substrate and product range, alter the stereoselectivity, and evolve new activities.

2.3.3.1   Altering Substrate Specificity

The rational design approach has been used successfully to alter the substrate specificity of various enzymes (reviewed in [29,174]). Some recent examples include introducing a single-point mutation into the *Candida antarctica* lipase B (CALB), which is sufficient to enable CALB to make carbon–carbon bonds [175]. The substrate preference of D-2-deoxy-ribose-5-phosphate aldolase (DERA) was engineered using rational design principles to accept nonphosphorylated substrates, while the natural substrates of DERA are phosphorylated [176]. Using a combination of chemical modification and rational design, a protease subtilisin from *Bacillus lenteus* was redesigned for use in peptide synthesis [177]. Introduction of a cysteine residue, followed by chemical modification, expanded the substrate range of the subtilisin enabling the synthesis of combinatorial libraries of D- and L-peptides.

The directed evolution approach has proven very successful in altering enzyme substrate and product specificity [14,32–35]. Some impressive examples of altering enzyme substrate specificity with nonnatural substrates have been reported. For instance, β-glucuronidase was evolved in the laboratory into a β-galactosidase, using ep-PCR and DNA shuffling [178]. The evolved enzyme hydrolyzes a β-galactoside substrate 500 times more efficiently than the wild-type, and displayed a 52 million-fold inversion in specificity. Directed evolution applied to an *E. coli* tyrosyl-tRNA synthetase generated an enzyme capable of incorporating novel aa into proteins [179].

Enzymes involved in DNA recognition, manipulation, and synthesis provide a multitude of tools for genomic analysis, genetic engineering, molecular biology, and gene therapy [180]. Ghadessy et al. [181] report the directed evolution of *Taq* DNA polymerases using the technique of compartmentalized self-replication (CSR) to enhance the stability of *Taq* polymerase. *Taq* polymerases with expanded substrate spectrums were subsequently generated using CSR [182]. The *Taq* polymerases extended mismatched sequences, in addition to acquiring the ability to process a diverse range of noncanonical substrates while maintaining high catalytic turnover, processivity, and fidelity. The extended substrate spectrum of the evolved *Taq* polymerases has a wide range of biotechnological applications [182]. Xia et al. [183] report applying directed evolution to evolve a DNA polymerase into an efficient RNA polymerase. Restriction enzymes are an indispensable tool for molecular biologists. The ability to engineer restriction endonucleases with altered recognition sequences is needed for biotechnology and medical applications [180]. The substrate range of the promiscuous restriction endonuclease *Bst*YI was narrowed using directed evolution. The variant endonuclease displayed a 12-fold increase in DNA sequence specificity [184]. Recombinase enzymes integrate, excise, and move DNA by catalyzing cleavage and rejoining of DNA strands at specific sites. Site-specific recombinases have recently been applied to experimental biology, biotechnology, and gene therapy. Several recent reports describe the directed evolution of prokaryotic recombinases to insert into mammalian cells [185–187], with applications as tools for modifying the genomes of eukaryotic cells [188]. For example, Sclimenti et al. [186] report the evolution of phage ΦC31 integrase to target a specific DNA sequence in the human genome. The wild-type phage integrase recombines sequences in a semirandom fashion in the human genome. Using DNA shuffling and screening strategies, an integrase with improved integration frequency and narrower target-site specificity was generated.

2.3.3.2 Altered Product Specificity

The application of enzymes as biocatalysts to assist the industrial manufacturing of fine chemicals and pharmaceuticals can be broadened significantly by developing tailor-made biocatalysts for specific processes [16]. The flavor compound, strawberry furanone, is a high-value fine chemical that is widely used in the food industry. Currently, furanone is produced synthetically from expensive 2,5-hex-3-ynediol. Newman et al. [189] report the use of directed evolution to enable the enzymatic synthesis of furanone from the relatively inexpensive *p*-xylene. A bacterial toluene dioxygenase operon was subjected to DNA shuffling to improve the biotransformation of a range of aromatic compounds. An increase in the substrate specificity and selectivity of the toluene dioxygenase system was achieved, such that an alternative, commercially viable, enzyme-driven preparation of furanone is now available [189]. Other commercially relevant biocatalysts, optimized by directed evolution, providing potential alternatives to expensive chemocatalytic reactions have also been recently reported. Saturation mutagenesis is used to optimize a dioxygenase for producing quinone derivatives used as precursors for food, pharmaceutical and industrial compounds [190]. Saturation mutagenesis was also used to develop a toluene-*o*-monooxygenase for enhanced naphthol production and chloroform degradation [191]. DNA shuffling and saturation mutagenesis were used in combination to develop a toluene-*o*-xylene monooxygenase for the synthesis of catechols and other industrially important products [192].

2.3.3.3 New Substrate Activity

Engineering novel substrate specificity is a major challenge. Several recent reports have emerged illustrating the significant advances made in this area using directed evolution and screening strategies. Using a combination of rational design and directed evolution, Altamirano et al. [118] report the evolution of novel substrate activity of an α/β-barrel protein by switching the activity of indole-3-glycerol-phosphate synthase to a phosphoribosylanthranilate isomerase. Another impressive example is the directed evolution of ampicillin resistance from a functionally unrelated DNA fragment [99]. These reports, suggest that evolving novel substrate specificities can be achieved using directed evolution in particular.

2.3.3.4 Stereoselectivity

The use of biocatalysts is increasing rapidly in many key industrial processes [14,32,174,193,194]. The ability to obtain high stereoselectivities, and hence enantiomerically pure compounds with biocatalysts is of key importance in the production of chemicals and key ingredients and products in the pharmaceutical and agrochemical industries. Large-scale industrial applications of biocatalysts include using lipases for the production of enantiopure alcohols and amides, esterases and amidases for enantiopure aas, nitrilases for the production of enantiopure carboxylic acids, and acylases for the production of new semisynthetic β-lactam antibiotics [8,9,16,164]. Many new developments are expected in this area in the years ahead [4,13,15].

Many strategies have been used to control stereoselectivity during biocatalysis, including modifying the substrate or through solvent engineering, by changing the reaction conditions or by a combination of chemocatalysis and biocatalysis (reviewed in [195,196]). All these strategies do not involve modification of the biocatalyst. In contrast, genetic engineering approaches (rational design and directed evolution) alter the primary structure of the enzyme. Subtle changes in enzyme structure and even changes in reaction conditions can influence enantioselectivity [110]. Such changes are very difficult to predict however, and thus attempts at rationally engineering enantioselectivity are rare (see [174], for a review of rationally designed enantioselective enzymes). In contrast, directed evolution approaches have proven extremely successful in altering enantioselectivity [193], aided by the recent developments in high-throughput enantioselective screening systems [197–199]. Table 2.4 highlights some recent examples of altering enzyme enantioselectivity using a directed evolution approach together with high-throughput screening systems (see [193,200] for recent reviews).

2.3.4   Other Properties

In addition to modifying key enzyme traits such as activity, specificity, and selectivity, directed evolution has been used to modify other traits such as protein expression. Microbial hosts are normally used to express enzymatically active proteins for analysis. In many cases, active enzymes are not expressed efficiently in microbial hosts, owing to difficulties in posttranslational modifications, formation of disulfide bridges and proper protein folding [201]. For instance, horseradish peroxidase contains four disulfide bridges, which are difficult to form in certain microbial hosts, with the result that active, soluble enzyme is not easy to obtain. Lin et al. [202] applied directed evolution to overcome this and tried to improve the folding efficiency of horseradish peroxidase in *E. coli*. Ep-PCR was used to generate a library of variants that identified one mutant (A225A) with improved folding efficiency in *E. coli*. An improved α-amylase displaying an altered pH optimum and high levels of heterologous expression in a *Pseudomonas* host system was developed using directed evolution [203].

Recent enzyme optimization reports using directed evolution illustrate that it is possible to simultaneously alter multiple enzyme properties. Examples include improving both thermostability and catalytic activity (Table 2.3); phytases with enhanced thermostability, pH tolerance and catalytic activity [70]; improved catalytic activity and altered substrate specificity [204]; and improved oxidative stability and thermostability [205]. A particularly impressive example of improving several characteristics in a convergent manner was reported for subtilisin. DNA family shuffling of 26 subtilisin genes yielded variants with improved activity at 23°C, enhanced thermostability, increased resistance to organic solvents, and greater pH tolerance [206].

2.4   Engineering Therapeutic Enzymes

2.4.1   Introduction

Advances in understanding the molecular principles and mechanisms of many disease conditions have led to the realization that many proteins have tremendous potential as therapeutic agents. Many enzymes are emerging as viable therapeutics for a variety of conditions due to the fact that enzymes are catalytic (which enhances potency), and that many of them display exquisite specificity and affinity for their substrates [207].

The idea of using enzymes as therapeutics was proposed 40 years ago [208], but the first enzyme to receive approval for use as a human medicine did not appear until relatively recently. Adenosine deaminase (ADA; marketed as Adagen®; generic name: pegademase bovine) was the first enzyme to receive FDA approval for the treatment of a particular type of severe combined immunodeficiency disorder (SCID) in 1990. As

TABLE 2.4

Examples of Directed Evolution Approaches to Altering Enantioselectivity

Enzyme	Substrate(s)	Mutagenesis Method	Screen	Amino Acid (AA)	Changes in Evolved Enzyme[a]		Ref.
					Enantioselectivity Effect		
Nitrilase (EC 3.5.5.1)	3-Hydroxyglutaryl nitrile	GSSM	MS	1	ee = 87.8 to 98.1%		[72]
Lipase (EC 3.1.1.3)	(RS)-ethyl 3 phenylbutyrate	SIMPLEX	Spectrophotometric	4	Inversion of enantioselectivity from (S)-form ($E_S = 33$) to (R)-form ($E_R = 38$)		[253]
Lipase (EC 3.1.1.3)	p-Nitrophenyl 2-methyldecanoate	ep-PCR, cassette mutagenesis, DNA family shuffling	Spectrophotometric	11	Inversion of enantioselectivity from (S)-form ($E_S = 1.1$) to (R)-form ($E_R = 30$)		[254–256]
Esterase (EC 3.1.1.3)	Bromo-2-methylpropanoate (S1), ethyl-3-phenyl-butyrate(S2)	Saturation mutagenesis	Spectrophotometric	1	$E = 12$ to 19 (S1), and $E = 3.5$ to 12 (S2)		[257]
Aldolase (EC 4.1.2.4)	D-fructose-1,6 bisphosphate (FBP)	DNA shuffling and ep-PCR	Spectrophotometric	4	Reversed stereochemistry producing FBP instead of tagatose-1, 6-bisphosphate		[258]
Hydantoinase (EC 3.5.2.2)	D-MTEH	Saturation mutagenesis and ep-PCR	Spectrophotometric	1	Inversion of enantioselectivity from $ee_D = 40$ to 20%		[259]
Monoamine oxidase (EC 1.4.3.4)	α-methylbenzyl amine	E. coli XL1-Red mutator strain	Colorimetric	1	Deracemization of α-methylbenzyl amine yielding the (R)-form in 93% ee		[260] [261]
Epoxide hydrolase (EC 3.3.2.3)	Glycidyl phenyl ether	ep-PCR	ESI-MS	1	$E = 4.6$ to 10.8 for (S)-form		[262]

[a] Changes in evolved variant relative to wild-type enzyme.

Abbreviations: D-MTEH = D-5-(2-methylthioethyl) hydantoin; ee = enantiomeric excess; E = enantiomeric selectivity factor; GSSM = gene site saturation mutagenesis; MS = mass spectrometry; SIMPLEX = single-molecule-PCR-linked *in vitro* expression; ESI-MS = electrospray ionization mass spectrometry.

reviewed throughout this book and elsewhere [207,209–211], an increasing number of enzymes have been developed, tested in clinical trials, and marketed for use, with many more currently in development as therapeutic agents. In the past decade, the therapeutic applications of enzymes have expanded considerably to treat a variety of diseases and conditions, including certain cancers, blood-clotting disorders, infectious diseases, and a variety of genetic conditions [207].

2.4.2   Engineering Therapeutic Enzymes

Despite the undeniable clinical and commercial success of therapeutic enzymes, virtually any therapeutic protein, including enzymes, can benefit from engineering to improve its clinical and safety profiles [212–217]. In addition to engineering the traditional features of enzymes, such as stability, specificity, and catalytic activity, engineering therapeutic enzymes aims to improve other biological and clinical parameters, such as the serum half-life, the efficacy of different therapeutic mechanisms of action, potential for deleterious side effects and increased immunogenicity, and endogenous protease susceptibility [212]. Consequently, engineering efforts to improve the properties of therapeutic enzymes are becoming increasingly prevalent. Table 2.5 summarizes most of the engineered therapeutic enzymes currently approved for use in U.S. and European markets. Most engineering attempts thus far have set out to enhance the half-life, alter the immunogenicity, and generate a faster- or slower-acting product. Several strategies exist for improving therapeutic enzyme performance. Therapeutic enzyme engineering can involve alteration of the enzyme's primary aa sequence, modification of the glycocomponent of a glycosylated protein, or the covalent attachment of chemical entities such as polyethylene glycol [209]. The next sections present a brief overview of some of the technologies and strategies employed to improve the key biological parameters of therapeutic enzymes, and to discover novel therapeutic enzymes.

2.4.2.1   Alteration of Primary AA Sequence

Rational design of therapeutic enzymes has emerged as a key technique in enhancing therapeutic enzymatic performance in the clinical setting. Generally, enzymes used as drugs would typically have been studied in-depth and their mechanism of action will be well established. Thus, rational design, the hypothesis-driven strategy to solve problems that beset many therapeutic enzymes, is widely used to enhance enzyme performance [217]. Identification of key aa residues involved, for example, in substrate binding or catalytic activity, could be altered by SDM and variants assayed for enhanced performance in a clinical setting.

An elegant example of applying rational design to improve a therapeutic enzymes clinical performance has recently been described by Berg et al. [218], who have redesigned activated protein C (APC). APC is an antithrombotic, antiinflammatory serine protease that plays a central role in vascular homeostasis and provides a vital feedback mechanism to attenuate blood coagulation. An approved drug form of this enzyme (drotrecogin alfa; tradename: Xigris®; developed by Lilly) has been used widely to reduce mortality in patients with severe sepsis (reviewed extensively in Chapter 4). However, APC is downregulated *in vivo* by the serine proteases (serpins), protein C inhibitor (PCI), and α1-antitrypsin (α1-AT). These serpins initially act as substrates for APC, then as irreversible inhibitors of APC by binding to and inactivating APC. Consequently, APC has a very short half-life *in vivo*, a feature that workers at Lilly thought amenable to engineering using rational design. Despite the fact that no high-resolution structural model of APC was available, computer modeling of APC–substrate complexes was used to identify key aa

TABLE 2.5

Some of the Currently Approved (United States and Europe) Engineered Therapeutic Enzymes

Enzyme	Product Name (Company)	Indication	Modification(s)	Property	Ref.
Adenosine deaminase (EC 3.5.4.4)	Adagen (Enzon)	SCID	Attached polyethylene glycol (PEGylated)	Increased circulatory half-life	[235], [240]
D-asparaginase (EC 3.5.1.11)	Oncaspar (Enzon)	Certain cancers	PEGylated L-asparaginase	Increased circulatory half-life; reduced immunogenicity	[240], [263]
Glucocerebrosidase (EC 3.2.1.45)	Cerezyme (Genzyme)	Gaucher's disease (types I, II, and III)	A495→H and modified carbohydrate content	Improved intake by target cells	[229]
Tissue plasminogen activator (tPA) (EC 3.4.21.68)	Retavase (Centocor/Boehringer)	Thrombolytic agent	Removal of 3 of the 5 domains of native tPA	Increased circulatory half-life	[219]
TPA (3.4.21.68)	TNKase (Genentech/Roche)	Thrombolytic agent	T103→A, G299→A	Increased half-life and enhanced specificty	[220]

residues involved in binding to the serpin inhibitors. Application of SDM to introduce a L194S substitution produced an APC variant with six-fold increase in plasma half-life and a five-fold decrease in inactivation by the serpins *in vitro* (when compared to wild-type APC). Introduction of a T245S substitution preserved the anticoagulant functions of APC without introducing any negative effects on plasma half-life *in vitro*. By combining the L194S and T245S substitutions, the APC variant has been shown to exhibit a significantly longer half-life *in vivo* in rabbits and monkeys, and is currently in development by Lilly [218]. This example illustrates that application of rational design can significantly improve the pharmacological properties of a therapeutic, while simultaneously preserving the desired biological functions through the rational, hypothesis-driven introduction of a minimal number of changes to the primary sequence of the protein.

As discussed in detail in Chapter 3, tissue plasminogen activator (tPA) is a serine protease that triggers activation of the fibrinolytic system by activating plasminogen. tPA has proven effective in the emergency treatment of myocardial infarction. Native human tPA is a 527-aa serine protease with five structural domains, each of which displays specific functions. Extensive knowledge of the structure and mechanism of action of tPA has enabled the development of engineered forms of tPA, which display significant improvements over the wild-type form (Table 2.5). Retavase® (rapilysin) is an engineered form of tPA (marketed by Boehringer-Mannheim/Centocor), which consists of only two of the five structural domains of native tPA, and displays a much longer circulatory half-life than native tPA, while removal of the other three domains does not impact negatively upon tPA's use as a thrombolytic agent [219]. Another engineered form of tPA, TNKase® (tenecteplase; marketed by Genentech/Roche) was developed by introducing aa substitutions into different regions of the native tPA (Table 2.5). The net effect of these substitutions is that the tPA variant displays enhanced specificity for fibrin binding, resulting in reduced plasma clearance (longer half-life) and increased resistance to a natural tPA inhibitor, plasminogen activator inhibitor 1 [220].

Mammalian DNase (EC 3.1.21.1) is a phosphodiesterase that catalyzes the hydrolysis of DNA and is currently used in the treatment of cystic fibrosis (CF), and is also being developed for treatment of a variety of other conditions including systemic lupus erythematosus, as a debriding agent, and also for the treatment of certain cancers (see Chapter 5). Pulmozyme® (Genentech), a form of DNase, has been approved since the early 1990s for the treatment of CF. Owing to the extensive efforts made in recent years to understand the enzyme and its mechanism of action, an extensive body of knowledge has been accrued, enabling the rational design of more active variants. Knowledge of the DNA-binding domain of DNase enabled workers at Genentech to create hyperactive DNase variants showing >10,000-fold higher activity than wild-type DNase, by introducing basic aa's at selected positions in the DNA-binding region, which enhances the interaction of DNase with the negatively charged phosphates on the DNA backbone [221,222].

The aforementioned examples of tPA and DNase illustrate how knowledge of a protein's structure, function, and mechanism can lead to the rational redesign of the primary sequence enabling the development of variants with improved clinical properties. It has been anticipated that similar rational engineering attempts will dramatically improve many therapeutic enzymes and enable the development of novel therapeutic enzymes [206,212,217]. Directed evolution technologies have made a huge impact on the development of many biocatalysts of industrial and commercial significance, especially in terms of improving key enzyme traits such as stability, specificity, and catalytic activity (as outlined in Section 2.3). Directed evolution has yet to make a similarly spectacular impact upon enhancing the performance of therapeutic enzymes. When developing therapeutic enzymes, traditionally it was attempted by introducing minimal changes to the primary aa sequence, due to altered pharmacokinetic (PK) and immunogenic properties associated with gross primary sequence changes [217]. However, some examples have been reported, which illustrate the potential that directed evolution technologies hold for tailoring key properties of therapeutic enzymes.

One enzyme undergoing development with potential human therapeutic applications is butyrylcholinesterase (BChE), a naturally occurring human serum detoxification enzyme, which breaks down acetylcholine. It has potential uses in the treatment of acute cocaine toxicity and addiction, as BChE has been shown to hydrolyze cocaine. However, the naturally occurring form of BChE in human serum has poor affinity for cocaine as a substrate. Workers at Applied Molecular Evolution used directed evolution technologies to generate two mutations within wild-type BChE [223]. The double-mutant variant (AME-359) has a greater affinity for cocaine and hydrolyzes cocaine with 40-fold improved k_{cat} relative to wild-type BChE. Other variants displaying even greater efficiency in hydrolyzing cocaine have also been generated and are currently in preclinical development [224,225].

Another example of the potential of directed evolution technologies to enhance therapeutic enzyme performance is provided in the case of thymidine kinase (TK) (EC 2.7.1.21), from herpes simplex virus (HSV) types I and II. HSV-TK has been used in several clinical trials as a "suicide" gene for killing cancer cells, and also as an agent to enhance the effects of the anti-HIV drug AZT [226]. Using repeated rounds of DNA shuffling of two viral TKs (from HSVI and HSVII), in combination with high-throughput screens to select TKs that conferred on *E. coli* higher sensitivity to the drug AZT, evolved TKs were isolated that exhibited 7- to 44-fold higher selectivity (k_{cat}/K_M) towards AZT (vs. the natural substrate thymidine) relative to the wild-type viral TKs [227]. The best mutant was a complex chimera formed by ten crossovers between the two parental genes and contained five nonparental aa mutations. This chimera differs from HSVI-TK at 22 aas and from HSVII-TK at 86 aa residues [228]. Such variants may prove useful for anti-HIV gene therapy, and similar approaches could enhance the performance of other enzyme–pro-drug combinations [227].

2.4.2.2 Modification of Glycocompent

Many proteins undergo glycosylation after translation, which is often critical to the protein's biological activity. Simple strategies to engineer glycosylated enzymes involve either modifying the carbohydrate content of the attached sugars or modification of the glycosylation site, often leading to dramatic effects in the enzyme performance as a therapeutic agent. For instance, glucocerebrosidase is a lysosomal enzyme involved in the degradation of glycolipids. Ceredase® (imiglucerase), a form of placental glucocerebrosidase, has been approved for use in the treatment of Gaucher disease, a lysosomal storage disease, characterized by a lack of glucocerebrosidase (see Chapter 6 for an extensive review of glucocerebrosidase). Recombinant DNA technology enabled the development of Cerezyme® (Table 2.5), a modified form of glucocerebrosidase, which is specifically targeted to the cell type most affected by the disease, while unmodified glucocerebrosidase is quickly removed from the bloodstream [229]. A further example of modifying the carbohydrate component of a therapeutic enzyme is that of the previously mentioned Retevase, a modified form of tPA (Section 2.4.2.1). In addition to removing three of the five native tPA domains, Retevase is produced in *E. coli*, and hence is unglycosylated. This lack of glysoylation, in addition to removal of certain protein domains, is thought to confer a significantly longer half-life upon the variant tPA [219]. Modifying the carbohydrate component of many protein-based therapeutic agents has proven an effective strategy for improving performance in the clinical setting, and its usefulness is expected to grow considerably in the years ahead [209,210].

2.4.2.3 Chemical Modification

Polyethylene glycol (PEG) is a highly flexible and soluble polymer that has gained widespread scientific and regulatory acceptance as a chemical modifier of therapeutic proteins [230]. The process of attaching PEG to a protein (PEGylation) has often benefited the pharmacokinetic profiles of many therapeutic proteins and enzymes primarily by increasing the effective size of a protein. PEGylation has also been shown to reduce immunogenicity and aggregation of many protein therapeutics [230–232]. Typically, the PEG moiety is attached to the N-terminus region of the protein or to cysteine residues. It is thought that attachment of PEG increases the half-life of the therapeutic protein by reducing its systemic clearance [232].

The first approved therapeutic enzyme, adenosine deaminase (ADA), received approval for the treatment of a particular type of severe combined immunodeficiency disorder (SCID). ADA cleaves excess adenosine present in SCID patients and reduces the toxicity to the immune system of elevated adenosine levels. Adagen contains a PEG moiety attached to the ADA. The net effect of PEGylation is that the modified ADA shows an increased half-life and reduced immunogenicity relative to the unmodified form [233]. PEG-modified forms of various other therapeutic enzymes are also on the market (see Table 2.5). For instance, Oncaspar® (pegaspargase; developed by Enzon Inc.) is a PEG-modified form of L-asparaginase (L-Asp), which is used to treat acute lymphoblastic leukemia in children (see Chapter 9 for a review of asparaginase). The PEG-modified form of L-Asp displays a significant increase in serum half-life, and reduced immunogenicity compared with unmodified forms of L-Asp [234].

Various other PEGylated therapeutic enzymes for a variety of conditions are currently being developed for human therapy (Table 2.6). Recently, a PEGylated form of arginine deiminase (ADI), an arginine-degrading enzyme, has been shown to be effective in inhibiting human melanomas and hepatocellular carcinomas, which are auxotrophic for arginine due to lack of arginosuccinate synthethase activity. The PEGylated ADI (PEG-ADI), despite showing a reduced activity, had an increased serum half-life and displayed reduced immunogenicity, relative to wild-type, unmodified ADI [235,236]. In recently completed phase I and II studies, PEG-ADI showed impressive results in reducing detectable plasma arginine levels [237]. PEG-ADI is currently undergoing phase I testing for malignant melanomas and phase III testing of PEG-ADI for hepatocellular carcinomas is in progress [238].[2] Urate oxidase is used to treat hyperuricemia, gout, and tumor lysis syndrome (reviewed in Chapter 8). Two other PEG-modified forms of urate oxidase are currently in the development process, both of which display reduced immunogenicity and increased half-life relative to the unmodified form [238–240].

2.4.3 Future Prospects

Since the introduction of the first therapeutic enzyme over a decade ago, many more enzymes have been approved for therapeutic applications to treat a variety of conditions including blood-clotting disorders, infectious diseases, certain cancers, and a variety of genetic conditions. As the molecular mechanisms underlying many disease conditions continue to be elucidated, it is expected that the application of the enzyme as a drug will also increase (see Table 2.6 for some enzymes currently in development for therapeutic purposes).

Enzyme engineering applied to therapeutic enzymes attempts to improve the clinical performance of existing enzymes. Chemical modification techniques, particularly

---

[2] Phoenix Pharmacologics Inc. (Lexington, Kentucky, USA) are developing PEG-modified forms of arginine deiminase (ADI-PEG-20) and urate oxidase (Uricase-PEG-20).

TABLE 2.6

Some Engineered Therapeutic Enzymes Currently in Development

Enzyme	Company	Indication	Modification(s)[a]	Modified Enzyme Traits[b]	Ref.
Arginine deiminase (EC 3.5.3.6)	Phoenix Pharmacologics	Malignant melanomas, hepatocellular carcinomas	PEGylation	Increased half-life, reduced immunogenicity	[235–238]
Activated protein C (EC 3.4.21.69)	Lilly	Anticoagulant and inflammatory used for severe sepsis	L194S and T254S substitutions	Increased resistance to endogenous proteases	[218]
Butyrylcholinesterase (EC 3.1.1.8)	Applied Molecular Evolution/Lilly	Cocaine addiction and toxicity	A328T and T332A substitutions	40-fold increase in k_{cat}; 250-fold improvement in potency	[224], [225], [242]
DNase (EC 3.1.21.1)	Genentech	Cystic fibrosis, certain cancers, systemic lupus erythematosus, debriding agent,	Modification of DNA-binding domain by substitution with six basic amino acid residues	> 10,000-fold increase in activity	[221], [222]
Urate oxidase (EC 1.7.3.3)	Savient Pharmaceuticals/ Mountain View Pharmaceuticals	Gout, tumor lysis syndrome, hyperuricemia	PEGylation	Increased half-life, reduced immunogenicity	[239]
Urate oxidase (EC 1.7.3.3)	Phoenix Pharmacologics	Gout, tumor lysis syndrome, hyperuricemia	PEGylation	Increased half-life, reduced immunogenicity	[238]

a   Abbreviations used include PEGylation (addition of polyethylene glycol).

b   Modifications of engineered enzymes relative to unmodified forms.

PEGylation, have proven very effective in enhancing therapeutic enzyme performance, and the emergence of several companies specializing in applying PEG technology to protein biopharmaceuticals is a testament to this fact [239,240].[3,4] As our knowledge of protein structure and mechanism of enzymatic action continues to grow, so will the application of rational engineering attempts to improve existing therapeutic enzymes, and in the design of new therapeutic uses for enzymes [93,217]. Directed evolution technologies, although proven to be very effective at engineering industrially relevant biocatalysts (for which simple, rapid screening methods and assays are available), are yet to make such an impact in engineering therapeutic enzymes (which typically involve more complicated and time-consuming assays). The advances in technologies in high-throughput assays, coupled with the advances in directed evolution technologies, suggest that directed evolution will emerge as a very powerful strategy to engineer enzymes for therapeutic applications, and also in the design of novel enzyme therapeutics [212,213,216]. Several companies specializing in applying directed evolution techniques to therapeutic proteins, including enzymes, have emerged recently [241,242].[5,6]

2.5 Conclusions

The use of enzymes in industry continues to grow at a rapid rate. The application of protein engineering strategies will continue to expand the use of enzymes for industrial, technical, and medicinal uses. The past decade, in particular, has witnessed some remarkable progress in developing new technologies to enhance enzyme activity, specificity, and stability (among other enzymatic features), and in applying these improved enzymes for a myriad of applications. This chapter merely touches the tip of the iceberg in terms of applying engineering principles to enzymes, as reflected by the huge growth of reports in the literature in recent years describing enzyme engineering efforts. As our knowledge of protein structure, function, and mechanism of action continues to expand, coupled with the rapid development in engineering technologies, the ability to improve existing enzymes and to tailor enzymes to our specific needs appears to be very promising. Use of the enzyme as a therapeutic agent also continues to grow rapidly. Chemical modification continues to be a powerful tool in improving the clinical performance of many enzymes. The genetic approaches to engineering enzymes, namely directed evolution and rational design techniques, hold tremendous potential to expand the usefulness and efficacy of may preexisting therapeutic enzymes to specific clinical applications, and also in the design and development of novel therapeutic enzymes.

---

[3] Savient Pharmaceuticals Inc. (East Brunswick, New Jersey, USA) and Mountain View Pharmaceuticals Inc. (Menlo Park, California, USA) are developing a PEG-modified urate oxidase (Puricase).

[4] Enzon Pharmaceuticals Inc. (Bridge water, New Jersey, USA), which holds a number of patents on PEG technology, have developed and are developing a number of PEG-modified therapeutic enzymes including Adagen® (PEG-modified adenosine deaminase — the first approved therapeutic enzyme in the United States) and Oncospar® (PEG-modified L-asparaginase).

[5] Direvo Biotech AG (Cologne, Germany) applies a patented directed evolution technology (the DIREVO Process) to the optimization of industrial and therapeutic proteins, industrial, technical and therapeutic enzymes.

[6] Applied Molecular Evolution (San Diego, CA, U.S.A.) specializes in applying a patented directed molecular evolution technology (AMEsystem™) to the discovery, optimization, and development of human biotherapeutics, including some therapeutic enzymes.

References

1. Georgiou, G. and DeWitt, N., Enzyme beauty, *Nat. Biotechnol.*, 17, 1161–1162, 1999.
2. Radzicka, A. and Wolfenden, R., A proficient enzyme, *Science*, 267, 90–93, 1995.
3. Godfrey, T. and West, S. (Eds.), *Industrial Enzymology*, 2nd ed., Macmillan Press, London, 1996.
4. Kirk, O., Borchert, T.V., and Fuglsang, C.C., Industrial enzyme applications, *Curr. Opin. Biotechnol.*, 13, 345–351, 2002.
5. Van Beilen, J.B. and Li, Z., Enzyme technology: An overview, *Curr. Opin. Biotechnol.*, 13, 338–344, 2002.
6. Kirst, H.A., Yeh, W.-K., and Zmijewski, M.J., Jr. (Eds.), *Enzyme Technologies for Pharmaceutical and Biotechnological Applications*, Marcel Dekker Inc., New York, 2001.
7. Walsh, C.W., Enabling the chemistry of life, *Nature*, 409, 226–231, 2001.
8. Schmid, A., et al., The use of enzymes in the chemical industry in Europe, *Curr. Opin. Biotechnol.*, 13, 359–366, 2002.
9. Schoemaker, H.E., Mink, D., and Wubbolts, M.G., Dispelling the myths — biocatalysts in industrial synthesis, *Science*, 299, 1694–1697, 2003.
10. Aehle, W., (Ed.), *Enzymes in Industry — Production and Applications*, 2nd ed., Wiley-VCH, Weinheim, 2004.
11. Jaeger, K.-E., Protein technologies and commercial enzymes. White is the hype-biocatalysts on the move, *Curr. Opin. Biotechnol.*, 15, 269–271, 2004.
12. Koeller, K.M. and Wong, C.-H., Enzymes for chemical synthesis, *Nature*, 409, 232–240, 2001.
13. Roberts, S.M., Biocatalysts in synthetic organic chemistry, *Tetrahedron*, 60, 499–500, 2004.
14. Robertson, D.E. and Steer, B.A., Recent progress in biocatalyst discovery and optimization, *Curr. Opin. Chem. Biol.*, 8, 141–149, 2004.
15. Cherry, J.R. and Fidanstef, A.L., Directed evolution of industrial enzymes: An update, *Curr. Opin. Biotechnol.*, 14, 438–443, 2003.
16. Burton, S.G., Cowan, D.A., and Woodley, J.M., The search for the ideal biocatalyst, *Nat. Biotechnol.*, 20, 37–45, 2002.
17. Amann, R.I., Ludwig, W., and Schleifer, K.H., Phylogenetic identification and *in situ* detection of individual microbial cells without cultivation, *Microbiol. Rev.*, 59, 143–169, 1995.
18. Pace, N.R., A molecular view of microbial diversity and the biosphere, *Science*, 276, 734–740, 1997.
19. Handelsman, J. and Smalla, K., Techniques. Conversations with the silent majority, *Curr. Opin. Biotechnol.*, 6, 271–273, 2003.
20. Jacobsen, J., Lyndolph, M., and Lange, L., Culture independent PCR: An alternative enzyme discovery strategy, *J. Microbiol. Methods*, 60, 63–71, 2005.
21. Streit, W., Daniel, R., and Jaeger, K.-E., Prospecting for biocatalysts and drugs in the genomes of non-cultured organisms, *Curr. Opin. Biotechnol.*, 15, 285–290, 2004.
22. Zengler, K., et al., Cultivating the uncultured, *Proc. Natl. Acad. Sci. USA*, 99, 15681–15686, 2002.
23. Lorenz, P., et al., Screening for novel enzymes for biocatalytic processes: Accessing the metagenome as a resource of novel functional sequence space, *Curr. Opin. Biotechnol.*, 13, 572–577, 2002.
24. Bryan, P.N., Protein engineering of subtilisin, *Biochim. Biophys. Acta*, 1543, 203–222, 2000.
25. Brannigan, J.A. and Wilkinson, A.J., Protein engineering 20 years on, *Nat. Rev. Mol. Cell Biol.*, 3, 964–970, 2002.
26. Van Regenmortel, M.H.V., Are there two distinct research strategies for developing biologically active molecules: Rational design and empirical selection? *J. Mol. Recog.*, 13, 1–4, 2000.
27. Chen, R., Enzyme engineering: Rational redesign versus directed evolution, *Trends Biotechnol.*, 19, 13–14, 2001.
28. Bornscheuer, U.T. and Pohl, M., Improved biocatalysts by directed evolution and rational protein design, *Curr. Opin. Chem. Biol.*, 5, 137–143, 2001.
29. Cedrone, F., Ménez, A., and Quéméneur, E., Tailoring new enzyme functions by rational design, *Curr. Opin. Struct. Biol.*, 10, 405–410, 2000.
30. Eijsink, V.G.H., et al., Rational engineering of enzyme stability, *J. Biotechnol.*, 113, 105–120, 2004.
31. Lutz, S. and Patrick, W.M., Novel methods for directed evolution of enzymes: Quality, not quantity, *Curr. Opin. Biotechnol.*, 15, 291–297, 2004.

32. Turner, N.J., Directed evolution of enzymes for applied biocatalysis, *Trends Biotechnol.*, 21, 474–478, 2003.
33. Woodyer, R., Chen, W., and Zhao, H., Outrunning nature: Directed evolution of superior biocatalysts, *J. Chem. Education*, 81, 126–133, 2004.
34. Tao, H. and Cornish, W.W., Milestones in directed enzyme evolution, *Curr. Opin. Struct. Biol.*, 13, 500–505, 2003.
35. Zhao, H., Chockalingam, K., and Chen, Z., Directed evolution of enzymes and pathways for industrial biocatalysis, *Curr. Opin. Biotechnol.*, 13, 104–110, 2002.
36. Dalby, P.A., Optimising enzyme function by directed evolution, *Curr. Opin. Struct. Biol.*, 13, 500–505, 2003.
37. Arnold, F.H. and Georgiou, G., (Eds.), *Directed Enzyme Evolution Library Creation: Methods and Protocols*, Vol. 231, Humana Press, Totowa, NJ, 2003.
38. Arnold, F.H. and Georgiou, G., (Eds.), *Directed Enzyme Evolution: Screening and Selection Methods*, Vol. 230, Humana Press, Totowa, NJ, 2003.
39. Bolon, D.N. et al., *De novo* design of biocatalysts, *Curr. Opin. Chem. Biol.*, 6, 125–129, 2002.
40. DeSantis, G. and Jones, J.B., Towards understanding and tailoring the specificity of synthetically useful enzymes, *Acc. Chem. Res.*, 32, 99–107, 1999.
41. Van den Burg, B. and Eijsink, V.G.H., Selection of mutations for increased protein stability, *Curr. Opin. Biotechnol.*, 13, 333–337, 2002.
42. Shortle, D. and Nathans, D., Local mutagenesis: A method for generating viral mutants with base substitutions in preselected regions of the viral genome, *Proc. Natl. Acad. Sci. USA*, 75, 2170–2174, 1978.
43. Razin, A., et al., Efficient correction of a mutation by use of chemically synthesized DNA, *Proc. Natl. Acad. Sci. USA*, 75, 4268–4270, 1978.
44. Mueller, W., et al., Site-directed mutagenesis in DNA: Generation of point mutations in cloned β-globin complementary DNA at the positions corresponding to amino acids 121 to 123, *J. Mol. Biol.*, 124, 343–358, 1978.
45. Hutchison, C.A., III et al., Mutagenesis at a specific position in a DNA sequence, *J. Biol. Chem.*, 253, 6551–6560, 1978.
46. Dalbadie-McFarland, G., et al., Oligonucleotide-directed mutagenesis as a general and powerful method for studies of protein function, *Proc. Natl. Acad. Sci. USA*, 79, 6409–6413, 1982.
47. Sigal, I.S., Harwood, B.G., and Arentzen, R., Thiol β-lactamase: Replacement of the active site serine of RTEM β-lactamase by a cysteine residue, *Proc. Natl. Acad. Sci. USA*, 79, 7157–7160, 1982.
48. Winter, G., et al., Redesigning enzyme structure by site-directed mutagenesis: Tyrosyl tRNA synthetase and ATP binding, *Nature*, 299, 756–758, 1982.
49. Harris, J. L. and Craik, C.S., Engineering enzyme specificity, *Curr. Opin. Chem. Biol.*, 2, 127–132, 1998.
50. Ó'Fágáin, C., Enzyme stabilization-recent experimental progress, *Enz. Microb. Technol.*, 33, 137–149, 2003.
51. Gasteiger, E., et al., ExPASy: The proteomics server for in-depth protein knowledge and analysis, *Nucleic Acids Res.*, 31, 3784–3788, 2003.
52. Gustaffson, C., Govindarajan, S., and Minshull, J., Putting engineering back into protein engineering: Bioinformatic approaches to catalyst design, *Curr. Opin. Biotechnol.*, 14, 366–370, 2003.
53. Bolon, D.N. and Mayo, S.L., Enzyme-like proteins by computational design, *Proc. Natl. Acad. Sci. USA*, 98, 14274–14279, 2001.
54. Gordon, S.B., Marshall, S.A., and Mayo, S.L., Energy functions for protein design, *Curr. Opin. Struct. Biol.*, 9, 509–513, 1999.
55. Kazlauskas, R.J., Molecular modeling and biocatalysis: Explanations, predictions, limitations, and opportunities, *Curr. Opin. Chem. Biol.*, 4, 81–88, 2000.
56. Arnold, F.H., Combinatorial and computational challenges for biocatalyst design, *Nature*, 409, 253–257, 2001.
57. Neylon, C., Chemical and biochemical strategies for the randomization of protein encoding DNA sequences: Library construction methods for directed evolution, *Nucleic Acids Res.*, 32, 1448–1459, 2004.
58. Robertson, D.E. and Noel, D.R. (Eds.), *Methods in Enzymology: Protein Engineering*, Vol. 388, Academic Press Inc., New York, 2004.

59. Fabret, C., et al., Efficient gene targeted random mutagenesis in genetically stable *Escherichia coli* strains, *Nucleic Acids Res.*, 28, e95, 2000.

60. Abécassis, V., Pompon, D., and Truan, G., High efficiency family shuffling based on multi-step PCR and *in vivo* recombination in yeast: Statistical and functional analysis of a combinatorial library between human cytochrome P450 1A1 and 1A2, *Nucleic Acids Res.*, 28, e88, 2000.

61. Nguyen, A.W. and Daugherty, P.S., Production of randomly mutated plasmid libraries using mutator strains, in *Directed Enzyme Evolution Library Creation: Methods and Protocols*, Vol. 231, Arnold, F.H. and Georgiou, G., Eds., Humana Press, Totowa, NJ, 2003, pp. 39–44.

62. Miyakazi, K., Creating random mutagenesis libraries by megaprimer PCR of whole plasmids (MEGAWHOP), in *Directed Enzyme Evolution Library Creation: Methods and Protocols*, Vol. 231, Arnold, F.H. and Georgiou, G., Eds., Humana Press, Totowa, NJ, 2003, pp. 23–28.

63. Selifinova, O. and Schellenberger, V., Evolution of microorganisms using mutator plasmids, in *Directed Enzyme Evolution Library Creation: Methods and Protocols*, Vol. 231, Arnold, F.H. and Georgiou, G., Eds., Humana Press, Totowa, NJ, 2003, pp. 45–52.

64. Cadwell, R.C. and Joyce, J.F., Randomization of genes by PCR mutagenesis, *PCR Methods Appl.*, 2, 28–33, 1992.

65. Cadwell, R.C. and Joyce, J.F., Mutagenic PCR, *PCR Methods Applic.*, 3, S136–S140, 1994.

66. Cirino, P.C., Mayer, K.M., and Umeno, D., Generating mutant libraries using error-prone PCR, in *Directed Enzyme Evolution Library Creation: Methods and Protocols*, Vol. 231, Arnold, F.H. and Georgiou, G., Eds., Humana Press, Totowa, NJ, 2003, pp. 3–10.

67. Murakami, H., Hohsaka, T., and Sisido, M., Random insertion and deletion of arbitrary number of bases for codon-based random mutation of DNAs, *Nat. Biotechnol.*, 20, 76–81, 2002.

68. Murakami, H., Hohsaka, T., and Sisido, M., Random insertion and deletion mutagenesis, in *Directed Enzyme Evolution Library Creation: Methods and Protocols*, Vol. 231, Arnold, F.H. and Georgiou, G., Eds., Humana Press, Totowa, NJ, 2003, pp. 53–64.

69. Kretz, K.A., et al., Gene site saturation mutagenesis: A comprehensive mutagenesis approach, in *Methods in Enzymology: Protein Engineering*, Robertson, D.E. and Noel, D.R., Eds., Vol. 388, Academic Press Inc., New York, 2004, pp. 3–11.

70. Garrett, J.B., et al., Enhancing the thermal tolerance and gastric performance of a microbial phytase for use as a phosphate-mobilizing monogastric-feed supplement, *Appl. Environ. Microbiol.*, 70, 3041–3046, 2004.

71. Palackal, N., et al., An evolutionary route to xylanase process fitness, *Protein Sci.*, 13, 494–503, 2004.

72. DeSantis, G., et al., Creation of a productive, highly enantioselective nitrilase through gene site saturation mutagenesis, *J. Am. Chem. Soc.*, 125, 11476–11477, 2003.

73. Stemmer, W.P.C., DNA shuffling by random fragmentation and reassembly – *in vitro* recombination for molecular evolution, *Proc. Natl. Acad. Sci. USA*, 91, 10747–10751, 1994.

74. Stemmer, W.P.C., Rapid evolution of a protein *in vitro* by DNA shuffling, *Nature*, 370, 389–391, 1994.

75. Joern, J.M., DNA shuffling, in *Directed Enzyme Evolution Library Creation: Methods and Protocols*, Vol. 231, Arnold, F.H. and Georgiou, G., Eds., Humana Press, Totowa, NJ, 2003, pp. 85–90.

76. Crameri, A. et al., DNA shuffling of a family of genes from diverse species accelerates directed evolution, *Nature*, 391, 288–291, 1998.

77. Zhao, H. and Arnold, F.H., Optimization of DNA shuffling fir high fidelity recombination, *Nucleic Acids Res.*, 25, 1307–1308, 1997.

78. Kikuchi, M., Ohnishi, K., and Harayama, S., Novel family shuffling methods for the *in vitro* evolution of enzymes, *Gene*, 236, 159–167, 1999.

79. Kikuchi, M., Ohnishi, K., and Harayama, S., An effective family shuffling method using single-stranded DNA, *Gene*, 243, 133–137, 2000.

80. Kolkman, J.A. and Stemmer, W.P.C., Directed evolution of proteins by exon shuffling, *Nat. Biotechnol.*, 19, 423–428, 2001.

81. Zhao, H., et al., Molecular evolution by staggered extension process (StEP) *in vitro* recombination, *Nat. Biotechnol.*, 16, 258–261, 1998.

82. Coco, W.M., et al., DNA shuffling method for generating highly recombined genes and evolved enzymes, *Nat. Biotechnol.*, 19, 354–359, 2001.

83. Pelletier, J.N., A RACHITT in our toolbox, *Nat. Biotechnol.*, 19, 314–315, 2001.

84. Sieber, V., Martinez, C.A., and Arnold, F.H., Libraries of hybrid proteins from distantly related sequences, *Nat. Biotechnol.*, 19, 456460, 2001.
85. Ostermeier, M., Shim, J.H., and Benkovic, S.J., A combinatorial approach to hybrid enzymes independent of DNA homology, *Nat. Biotechnol.*, 17, 1205–1209, 1999.
86. Lutz, S., Ostermeier, M., and Benkovic, S.J., Rapid generation of incremental truncation libraries for protein engineering using α-phosphothioate nucleotides, *Nucleic Acids Res.*, 29, E16, 2001.
87. Lutz, S., and Benkovic, S.J., Homology-independent protein engineering, *Curr. Opin. Biotechnol.*, 11, 319–324, 2000.
88. Lutz, S., et al., Creating multiple-crossover DNA libraries independent of sequence identity, *Proc. Natl. Acad. Sci. USA*, 98, 11248–11253, 2001.
89. Lutz, S. and Ostermeier, M., Preparation of SCRATCHY hybrid protein libraries: Size- and in-frame selection of nucleic acid sequences, in *Directed Enzyme Evolution Library Creation: Methods and Protocols*, Vol. 231, Arnold, F. H. and Georgiou, G., Eds., Humana Press, Totowa, NJ, 2003, pp. 143–152.
90. O'Maille, P.E., Bakhtina, M., and Tsai, M.-D., Structure-based combinatorial protein engineering (SCOPE), *J. Mol. Biol.*, 321, 677–691, 2002.
91. Voigt, C.A., et al., Computational method to reduce the search space for directed protein evolution, *Proc. Natl. Acad. Sci. USA*, 98, 3778–3783, 2001.
92. Hayes, R.J., et al., Combining computational and experimental screening for rapid optimization of protein properties, *Proc. Natl. Acad. Sci. USA*, 99, 15926–15931, 2002.
93. See also, Xencor's website: www.xencor.com; for further details on PDA technology, patents, and relevant publications showing the applicability of this technology.
94. Moore, G.L. and Maranas, C.D., Computational challenges in combinatorial library design for protein engineering, *AlChE J.*, 50, 262–272, 2004.
95. Zhang, Y.W., et al., Genome shuffling leads to rapid phenotypic improvement in bacteria, *Nat. Biotechnol.*, 415, 644–646, 2002.
96. Soong, N.W., et al., Molecular breeding of viruses, *Nat. Genet.*, 25, 436–439, 2000.
97. Powell, S.K., et al., Breeding of retroviruses by DNA shuffling for improved stability and processing yields, *Nat. Biotechnol.*, 18, 1279–1282, 2000.
98. Schmidt-Dannert, C., Umeno, D., and Arnold, F.H., Molecular breeding of carotenoid biosynthetic pathways, *Nat. Biotechnol.*, 18, 750–753, 2000.
99. Yano, T. and Kagamiyama, H., Directed evolution of ampicillin-resistant activity from a functionally unrelated DNA fragment: A laboratory model of molecular evolution, *Proc. Natl. Acad. Sci. USA*, 98, 903–907, 2001.
100. Soumillion, P. and Fastrez, J., Novel concepts for selection of catalytic activity, *Curr. Opin. Biotechnol.*, 12, 387–394, 2001.
101. Lin, H. and Cornish, V.W., Screening and selection methods for large-scale analysis of protein function, *Agnew. Chem. Int. Ed. Engl.*, 41, 4402–4425, 2002.
102. Goddard, J.-P. and Reymond, J.-L., Recent advances in enzyme assays, *Trends Biotechnol.*, 22, 363–370, 2004.
103. Goddard, J.-P. and Reymond, J.-L., Enzyme assays for high-throughput screening, *Curr. Opin. Biotechnol.*, 15, 314–322, 2004.
104. Eisenthal, F. and Danson, M., (Eds.), *Enzyme Assays: A Practical Approach*, Oxford University Press, Oxford, 2002.
105. Olsen, M., Iverson, B., and Georgiou, G., High-throughput screening of enzyme libraries, *Curr. Opin. Biotechnol.*, 11, 331–337, 2000.
106. Wahler, D. and Reymond, J.-L., High-throughput screening for biocatalysts, *Curr. Opin. Biotechnol.*, 12, 535–544, 2001.
107. Becker, S., et al., Ultra-high-throughput screening based on cell-surface display and fluorescence-activated cell sorting for the identification of novel biocatalysts, *Curr. Opin. Biotechnol.*, 15, 323–329, 2004.
108. Geddie, M., et al., High throughput microplate screens for directed protein evolution, in *Methods In Enzymology (Protein Engineering)*, Robertson, D.E. and Noel, J.P., Eds., Vol. 388, Academic Press Inc., New York, 2004, pp. 134–145.

109. Lafferty, M. and Dycaico, GigaMatrix: A novel ultrahigh throughput protein optimization and discovery platform, in *Methods In Enzymology (Protein Engineering)*, Robertson, D.E. and Noel, J.P., Eds., Vol. 388, Academic Press Inc., New York, 2004, pp. 119–133.

110. Arnold, F.H., et al., How enzymes adapt: Lessons from directed evolution, *Trends Biochem. Sci.*, 26, 100–106, 2001.

111. Jestin, J.-L. and Kaminski, P.A., Directed evolution and selections for catalysis based on product formation, *J. Biotechnol.*, 113, 85–103, 2004.

112. Fernandez-Gacio, A., Uguen, M., and Fastrez, J., Phage display as a tool for the directed evolution of enzymes, *Trends Biotechnol.*, 21, 408–414, 2003.

113. Soumillion, P. and Fastrez, J., Investigation of phage display for the directed evolution of enzymes, in *Directed Molecular Evolution of Proteins*: Or How to Improve Enzymes for Biocatalysis, Brakmann, S. and Johnsson, K.E. Eds., Wiley–VCH, Weinheim, 2002, pp. 79–110.

114. Hoess, R.H., Protein design and phage display, *Chem. Rev.*, 101, 3205–3218, 2001.

115. Tawfiks, D.S. and Griffiths, A.D., Man-made cell-like compartments for molecular evolution, *Nat. Biotechnol.*, 16, 652–656, 1998.

116. Griffiths, A.D. and Tawfiks, D.S., Man-made enzymes from design to *in vitro* compartmentalisation, *Curr. Opin. Biotechnol.*, 11, 338–353, 2000.

117. Griffiths, A.D. and Tawfiks, D.S., Directed evolution of an extremely fast phosphotriesterase by *in vitro* compartmentalisation, *EMBO J.*, 22, 24–35, 2003.

118. Altamirano, M.M., et al., Directed evolution of new catalytic activity using the α/β-barrel scaffold, *Nature*, 403, 617–622, 2000.

119. Rothman, S.C., Voorhies, M., and Kirsch, J.F., Directed evolution relieves product inhibition and confers *in vivo* function to a rationally designed tyrosine aminotransferase, *Prot. Sci.*, 13, 763–772, 2004.

120. Kim Y.-W., et al., Directed evolution of a glycosynthase from *Agrobacterium* sp. increases its catalytic activity dramatically and expands its substrate repertoire, *J. Biol. Chem.*, 41, 42787–42793, 2004.

121. Lignen, B., et al., Improving the carboligase activity of benzoylformate decarboxylase from *Pseudomonas putida* by a combination of directed evolution and site-directed mutagenesis, *Prot. Eng.*, 15, 585–593, 2002.

122. Peters, M.W., et al., Regio- and enantioselective alkane hydroxylation with engineered cytochromes P450 BM-3, *J. Am. Chem. Soc.*, 125, 13442–13450, 2003.

123. Ni, J., et al., Conversion of a typical catalase from *Bacillus* sp. TE124 to a catalase-peroxidase by directed evolution, *J. Biosci. Bioeng.*, 93, 31–36, 2002.

124. Wang, C.-W. and Liao, J.C., Alteration of product specificity of *Rhodobacter sphaeroides* phytoene desaturase by directed evolution, *J. Biol. Chem.*, 44, 41161–41164, 2001.

125. Priyamvada A., et al., Structural basis of selection and thermostability of laboratory evolved *Bacillus subtilis* lipase, *J. Mol. Biol.*, 341, 1271–1281, 2004.

126. Gupta, R.G., Beg, Q.K., and Lorenz, P., Bacterial alkaline proteases: Molecular approaches and industrial applications, *Appl. Microbiol. Biotechnol.*, 59, 15–32, 2002.

127. Lehmann, M., et al., The consensus concept for thermostability of proteins, *Biochim. Biophys. Acta*, 1543, 408–415, 2000.

128. Lehmann, M. and Wyss, M., Engineering proteins for thermostability: The use of sequence alignments versus rational design and directed evolution, *Curr. Opin. Biotechnol.*, 12, 371–375, 2001.

129. Lehmann, M., et al., From DNA sequence to improved functionality: Using protein sequence comparisons to rapidly design a thermostable consensus phytase, *Prot. Eng.*, 13, 49–57, 2000.

130. He, M., Nie, Y.-F., and Xu, P., A T42M substitution in bacterial 5-enolpyruvylshikimate-3-phosphate synthase (EPSPS) generates enzymes with increased resistance to glyphosate, *Biosci. Biotechnol. Biochem.*, 67, 1405–1409, 2003.

131. Radianingtyas. H. and Wright, P.C., Alcohol dehydrogenases from thermophilic and hyperthermophilic archaea and bacteria, *FEMS Microbiol. Rev.*, 27, 593–616, 2003.

132. Eggert, T., et al., Novel biocatalysts by identification and design, *Biocatal. Biotransf.*, 22, 139–144, 2004.

133. DeSantis, G. and Jones, J.B., Chemical modification of enzymes for enhanced functionality, *Curr. Opin. Biotechnol.*, 10, 324–330, 1999.

134. Davis, B.G., Chemical modification of biocatalysts, *Curr. Opin. Biotechnol.*, 14, 379–386, 2004.
135. Tann, C.M., Qi, D.F., and Distefano, M.D., Enzyme design by chemical modification of protein scaffolds, *Curr. Opin. Chem. Biol.*, 5, 696–704, 2001.
136. Qi, D.F., et al., Generation of new enzymes via covalent modification of existing proteins, *Chem. Rev.*, 101, 3081–3111, 2001.
137. Iwai, H. and Pluckthun, A., Circular β-lactamase: Stability enhancement by cyclizing the backbone, *FEBS Lett.*, 459, 166–172, 1999.
138. Hofmann, R. and Muir, T.W., Recent advances in the application of expressed protein ligation to protein engineering, *Curr. Opin. Biotechnol.*, 13, 297–303, 2002.
139. Bornscheuer, U.T., et al., Optimizing lipases and related enzymes for efficient application, *Trends Biotechnol.*, 20, 433–437, 2002.
140. Villeneuve, P., et al., Customizing lipases for biocatalysis: A survey of chemical, physical and molecular biological approaches, *J. Mol. Catal.*, 9, 113–148, 2002.
141. Getzoff, G.D., et al., Faster superoxide dismutase mutants designed by enhancing electrostatic guidance, *Nature*, 358, 347–351, 1992.
142. Dufour, E., Storer, A.C., and Ménard, R., Engineering nitrile hydratase activity into a cysteine protease by a single mutation, *Biochemistry*, 34, 16382–16388, 1995.
143. Chin, H.S., Goo, K.S., and Sim, T.S., A complete library of amino acid alterations at N304 in *Streptomyces clavuligerus* deacetoxycephalosporin C synthase elucidates the basis for enhanced penicillin analogue conversion, *Appl. Environ. Microbiol.*, 70, 607–609, 2004.
144. Van Der Veen, B.A., et al., Combinatorial engineering to enhance amylosucrase performance: Construction, selection and screening of variant libraries for increased activity, *FEBS Lett.*, 560, 91–97, 2004.
145. Cho, C.M., Mulchandani, A. and Chen, W., Bacterial cell surface display of organophosphorous hydrolase for selective screening of improved hydrolysis of organophosphate nerve agents, *Appl. Environ. Microbiol.*, 68, 2026–2030, 2002.
146. Wintrode, P.L. and Arnold, F.H., Temperature adaptation of enzymes: Lessons from laboratory evolution, *Adv. Prot. Chem.*, 55, 161–225, 2000.
147. Cirino, P. and Georgescu, R., Screening for thermostability, in *Directed Enzyme Evolution: Screening and Selection Methods*, Vol. 230, Arnold, F.H. and Georgiou, G., Eds., Humana Press, Totowa, NJ, 2003, pp. 117–126.
148. Berk, H. and Lebbink, R.J., High-throughput screening of mutant α-amylase libraries for increased activity at 129°C, in *Directed Enzyme Evolution: Screening and Selection Methods*, Vol. 230, Arnold, F.H. and Georgiou, G., Eds., Humana Press, Totowa, NJ, 2003, pp. 127–136.
149. Zhao, H. and Arnold, F.H., Directed evolution converts subtilisin E into a functional equivalent of thermitase, *Prot. Eng.*, 12, 47–53, 1999.
150. Wintrode, P.L., Miyazaki, K., and Arnold, F.H., Patterns of adaptation on a laboratory evolved thermophilic enzyme, *Biochim. Biophys. Acta*, 1549, 1–8, 2001.
151. Cherry, J.R., et al., Directed evolution of a fungal peroxidase, *Nat. Biotechnol.*, 17, 379–384, 1999.
152. Lebbink, J.H.G. et al., Improving low-temperature catalysis in the hyperthermostable *Pyrococcus furiosus* β-glucosidase celB by directed evolution, *Biochemistry*, 39, 3656–3665, 2000.
153. Fujii, Y., et al., The artificial evolution of an enzyme by random mutagenesis: The development of formaldehyde dehydrogenase, *Biosci. Biotechnol. Biochem.*, 69, 1722–1727, 2004.
154. Suzuki, T., et al., Adaptation of a thermophilic enzyme 3-isopropylmalate dehydrogenase to low temperatures, *Prot. Eng.*, 14, 85–91, 2001.
155. Mizayaki, J., et al., Ancestral residues stabilizing 3-isopropylmalate dehydrogenase of an extreme thermophile: Experimental evidence supporting the thermophilic common ancestor hypothesis, *J. Biochem.*, 129, 777–782, 2001.
156. Chen, J. and Stites, W.E., Packing is key selection factor in the evolution of protein hydrophobic cores, *Biochemistry*, 40, 15280–15289, 2001.
157. Abraham, T.E., et al., Crosslinked enzyme crystals of glucoamylase as a potent catalyst for biotransformations, *Carbohyd. Res.*, 339, 1099–1104, 2004.
158. Govardhan, C.P., Crosslinking of enzymes for improved stability and performance, *Curr. Opin. Biotechnol.*, 10, 331–335, 1999.
159. Gómez, L., Ramirez, H.L., and Villalonga, R., Stabilization of invertase by modification of sugar chains with chitosan, *Biotechnol. Lett.*, 22, 347–350, 2000.

160. Gómez, L. and Villalonga, R., Functional stabilization of invertase by covalent modification with pectin, *Biotechnol. Lett.*, 22, 1191–1195, 2000.

161. Bakke, M. and Kajiyama, N., Improvement in the thermal stability and substrate binding of pig kidney D-amino acid oxidase by chemical modification, *Appl. Biochem. Biotechnol.*, 112, 123–131, 2004.

162. Babu, V.R.S., et al., Stabilization of immobilised glucose oxidase against thermal inactivation by silanization for biosensor applications, *Biosens. Bioelectron.*, 19, 1337–1341, 2004.

163. Klibanov, A.M., Improving enzymes by using them in organic solvents, *Nature*, 409, 241–246, 2001.

164. Yang, S., et al., Rational design of a more stable penicillin G acylase against organic cosolvent, *J. Mol. Catal.*, 18, 285–290, 2002.

165. Sio, C.F. and Quax, W.J., Improved β-lactam acylases and their use as industrial biocatalysts, *Curr. Opin. Biotechnol.*, 15, 349–355, 2004.

166. Chen, K. and Arnold, F.H., Tuning the activity of an enzyme for unusual environments: Sequential random mutagenesis of subtilisin E for catalysis in dimethylformamide, *Proc. Natl. Acad. Sci. USA*, 90, 5618–5622, 1993.

167. Song, J.K. and Rhee, J.S., Enhancement of stability and activity of phospholipase A_1 in organic solvents by directed evolution, *Biochim. Biophys. Acta*, 1547, 370–378, 2001.

168. Moore, J. and Arnold, F.H., Directed evolution of a para-nitrobenzyl esterase for aqueous-organic solvents, *Nat. Biotechnol.*, 14, 458–467, 1996.

169. Morawski, B., Quan, S., and Arnold, F.H., Functional expression and stabilization of horseradish peroxidase by directed evolution in *Saccharomyces cerevisiae*, *Biotechnol. Bioeng.*, 76, 99–107, 2001.

170. Mori, T. and Okahata, Y., A variety of lipid-coated glycoside hydrolases as effective glycosyl transfer catalysts in homogenous organic solvents, *Tetrahedron Lett.*, 38, 1971–1974, 1997.

171. Jene, O., Pearson, J.C., and Lowe, C.R., Surfactant modified enzymes: Solubility and activity of surfactant-modified catalase in organic solvents, *Enzyme Microb. Technol.*, 20, 69–74, 2000.

172. Wilson, L., et al., Encapsulation of crosslinked penicillin G acylase aggregates in lentikats: Evaluation of a novel biocatalyst in organic media, *Biotechnol. Bioeng.*, 86, 558–562, 2004.

173. Lee, M.-Y. and Dordick, J.S., Enzyme activation for nonaqueous media, *Curr. Opin. Biotechnol.*, 13, 543–547, 2002.

174. Hult, K. and Berglund, P., Engineered enzymes for improved organic synthesis, *Curr. Opin. Biotechnol.*, 14, 395–400, 2003.

175. Branneby, C., et al., Carbon–carbon bonds by hydrolytic enzymes, *J. Am. Chem. Soc.*, 125, 874–875, 2003.

176. DeSantis, G., et al., Structure-based mutagenesis approaches toward expanding the substrate specificity of D-2-deoxyribose-5-phosphate aldolase, *Bioorg. Med. Chem.*, 11, 43–52, 2003.

177. Matsumoto, K., Davis, B.G., and Jones, J.B., Chemically modified 'polar patch' mutants of subtilisin in peptide synthesis with remarkably broad substrate acceptance: Designing combinatorial biocatalysts, *Chemistry*, 8, 4129–4137, 2002.

178. Matsumura, I. and Ellington, A.D., *In vitro* evolution of beta-glucuronidase into a beta-galactosidase proceeds through non-specific intermediates, *J. Mol. Biol.*, 305, 331–339, 2001.

179. Wang, L., et al., Expanding the genetic code of *Escherichia coli*, *Science*, 292, 498–500, 2001.

180. Collins, C.H., et al., Engineering proteins that bind, move, make and break DNA, *Curr. Opin. Biotechnol.*, 14, 371–378, 2003.

181. Ghadessy, F.J., Ong, J.L., and Hollinger, P., Directed evolution of polymerase function by compartmentalized self-replication, *Proc. Natl. Acad. Sci. USA*, 98, 4552–4557, 2001.

182. Ghadessy, F.J., et al., Generic expansion of the substrate spectrum of a DNA polymerase by directed evolution, *Nat. Biotechnol.*, 22, 755–759, 2004.

183. Xia, G., et al., Directed evolution of novel polymerase activities: Mutation of a DNA polymerase into an efficient RNA polymerase, *Proc. Natl. Acad. Sci. USA*, 99, 6597–6602, 2002.

184. Samuelson, J.C. and Xu, S.Y., Directed evolution of restriction endonuclease *Bst*YI to achieve increased substrate specificity, *J. Mol. Biol.*, 319, 673–683, 2002.

185. Akopian A., et al., Chimeric recombinases with designed DNA sequence recognition, *Proc. Natl. Acad. Sci. USA*, 100, 8688–8691, 2003.

186. Sclimenti, C.R., Thyagarajan, B., and Calos, M.P., Directed evolution of a recombinase for improved genomic integration at a native human sequence, *Nucleic Acids Res.*, 29, 5044–5051, 2001.

187. Santoro, S.W. and Schultz, P.G., Directed evolution of the site specificity of Cre recombinase, *Proc. Natl. Acad. Sci. USA*, 99, 4185–4190, 2002.

188. Thygarajan, B., et al., Mammalian genomes contain active recombinase recognition sites, *Gene*, 244, 47–54, 2000.

189. Newman, L.M., et al., Directed evolution of the dioxygenase complex for the synthesis of furanone flavour compounds, *Tetrahedron*, 60, 729–734, 2004.

190. Keenan, B., et al., Saturation mutagenesis of *Burkholderia cepacia* R34 2,4-dinitrotoluene dioxygenase at DntAc Valine 350 for synthesizing nitrohydroquinone, methylhydroquinone, and methoxyhydroquinone, *Appl. Environ. Microbiol.*, 70, 3222–3231, 2004.

191. Rui, L., et al., Saturation mutagenesis of toluene *ortho*-monooxygenase *Burkholderia cepacia* G4 for enhanced 1-naphthol synthesis and chloroform degradation, *Appl. Environ. Microbiol.*, 70, 3246–3252, 2004.

192. Vardar, G. and Wood, T.K., Protein engineering of toluene-*o*-xylene monooxygenase from *Pseudomonas stutzeri* for synthesizing 4-methylresorcinol, methylhydroquinone, and pyrogallol, *Appl. Environ. Microbiol.*, 70, 3253–3262, 2004.

193. Jaeger, K.-E. and Eggert, T., Enantioselective biocatalysis optimized by directed evolution, *Curr. Opin. Biotechnol.*, 15, 305–313, 2004.

194. Panke, S., Held, M., and Wubbolts, M., Trends and innovations in industrial biocatalysis for the production of fine chemicals, *Curr. Opin. Biotechnol.*, 15, 272–279, 2004.

195. Bornscheuer, U.T., Methods to increase enantioselectivity of lipases and esterases, *Curr. Opin. Biotechnol.*, 13, 543–547, 2002.

196. Turner, N.J., Controlling chirality, *Curr. Opin. Biotechnol.*, 14, 401–406, 2003.

197. Reetz, M.T., New methods for the high-throughput screening of enantioselective catalysts and biocatalysts, *Agnew. Chem. Int. Ed. Engl.*, 41, 1335–1338, 2002.

198. Reetz, M.T., An overview of high-throughput screening systems for enantioselective enzymatic transformations, in *Directed Enzyme Evolution: Screening and Selection Methods*, Vol. 230, Arnold, F.H. and Georgiou, G., Eds., Humana Press, Totowa, NJ, 2003, pp. 259–282.

199. Reetz, M.T., Select protocols of high-throughput *ee*-screening systems for assaying enantioselective enzymes, in *Directed Enzyme Evolution: Screening and Selection Methods*, Vol. 230, Arnold, F.H. and Georgiou, G., Eds., Humana Press, Totowa, NJ, 2003, pp. 283–290.

200. Reetz, M.T., Controlling the enantioselectivity of enzymes by directed evolution: Practical and theoretical ramifications, *Proc. Natl. Acad. Sci. USA*, 101, 5716–5722, 2004.

201. Waldo, G.S., Genetic screens and directed evolution for protein solubility, *Curr. Opin. Chem. Biol.*, 7, 33–38, 2003.

202. Lin, Z., Thorsen, T., and Arnold, F.H., Functional expression of horseradish peroxidase in *E. coli* via directed evolution, *Biotechnol. Progr.*, 15, 467–471, 1999.

203. Richardson, T.H. et al., A novel, high performance enzyme for starch liquefaction. Discovery and optimization of a low pH, thermostable alpha-amylase, *J. Biol. Chem.*, 277, 26501–26507, 2002.

204. Raillard, S., et al., Novel enzyme activities and functional plasticity revealed by recombining highly homologous enzymes, *Chem. Biol.*, 8, 891–898, 2001.

205. Oh, K.H., Nam, S.H., and Kim, H.S., Directed evolution of *N*-carbamyl-D-amino acid amidohydrolase for simultaneous improvement of oxidative and thermal stability, *Biotechnol. Progr.*, 18, 413–417, 2002.

206. Ness, J.E., et al., DNA shuffling of subgenomic sequences of subtilisin, *Nat. Biotechnol.*, 17, 893–896, 1999.

207. Vellard, M., The enzyme as drug: Application of enzymes as pharmaceuticals, *Curr. Opin. Biotechnol.*, 14, 444–450, 2003.

208. De Duve, C., The significance of lysosome in pathology and medicine, *Proc. Inst. Med. Chic.*, 26, 73–76, 1966.

209. Walsh, G., Second-generation biopharmaceuticals, *Eur. J. Pharmaceutics Biopharmaceutics*, 58, 185–196, 2004.

210. Walsh, G., Biopharmaceutical benchmarks — 2003, *Nat. Biotechnol.*, 21, 865–870, 2003.

211. Walsh, G., *Biopharmaceuticals: Biochemistry and Biotechnology*, 2nd ed., Wiley, Chichester, 2003.

212. Lazar, G., et al., Designing proteins for therapeutic applications, *Curr. Opin. Struc. Biol.*, 13, 513–518, 2003.

213. Vasserot, A.P., et al., Optimization of protein therapeutics by directed evolution, *Drug Discovery Today*, 8, 118–126, 2003.
214. Vasserot, A.P. and Watkins, J.D., Expanding the clinical utility of therapeutic proteins: Activated protein C variants with improved pharmacological properties, *Trends Pharmacol. Sci.*, 24, 501–504, 2003.
215. Huisman, G.W. and Gray, D., Towards novel processes for the fine-chemical and pharmaceutical industries, *Curr. Opin. Biotechnol.*, 12, 328–352, 2002.
216. Kurtzman, A.L., et al., Advances in directed protein evolution by recursive genetic recombination: Applications for therapeutic applications, *Curr. Opin. Biotechnol.*, 12, 361–370, 2001.
217. Marshall, S.A., et al., Rational design and engineering of therapeutic proteins, *Drug Discovery Today*, 8, 212–221, 2003.
218. Berg, D.T., et al., Engineering the proteolytic activity of activated protein C improves its pharmacological properties, *Proc. Natl. Acad. Sci. USA*, 100, 4423–4428, 2003.
219. Verstraete, M., Third generation thrombolytic agents, *Am. J. Med.*, 109, 52–58, 2000.
220. Davydov, L. and Cheng, J.W., Tenecteplase, a review, *Clin. Ther.*, 23, 982–997, 2001.
221. Pan, C.Q. and Lazarus, R.A., Hyperactivity of human DNase I variants. Dependence on the number of positively charged residues and concentration, length, and environment of DNA, *J. Biol. Chem.*, 273, 11701–11708, 1998.
222. Pan, C.Q. and Lazarus, R.A., Ca^{2+}-dependent activity of human DNase I and its hyperactive variants, *Protein Sci.*, 8, 1780–1788, 1999.
223. Sun, H., et al., Re-engineering butyrylcholinesterase as a cocaine hydrolase, *Mol. Pharmacol.*, 62, 220–224, 2002.
224. Gao, Y. and Brimijoin, S., An engineered cocaine hydrolase blunts and reverses cardiovascular responses to cocaine in rats, *J. Pharmacol. Exp. Ther.*, 310, 1046–1052, 2004.
225. Pancook, J.D., et al., Application of directed evolution technology to optimize the cocaine hydrolase activity of human butyrylcholinesterase, *FASEB J.*, 17, A565, 2003.
226. Vile, R.G., Thymidine kinases, in *Gene Therapy (Principles and Applications)*, Blankenstein, T., Ed., Birkhäuser Verlag, Basel, 1999, pp. 247–266.
227. Christians, F.C., et al., Directed evolution of thymidine kinase for AZT phosphorylation using DNA family shuffling, *Nat. Biotechnol.*, 17, 259–264, 1999.
228. Stemmer, W.P., Molecular breeding of genes, pathways and genomes by DNA shuffling, *J. Mol. Catal.*, 19–20, 3–12, 2002.
229. Hoppe, H., Cerezyme-recombinant protein treatment for Gaucher's disease, *J. Biotechnol.*, 76, 259–261, 2000.
230. Harris, J.M., et al., Pegylation: A novel process for modifying pharmacokinetics, *Clin. Pharmacokinet.*, 40, 539–551, 2001.
231. Roberts, M.J., Bentley, M.D., and Harris, J.M., Chemistry for peptide and protein PEGylation, *Adv. Drug Del. Rev.*, 54, 459–476, 2002.
232. Greenwald, R.B., et al., Effective drug delivery by PEGylated drug conjugates, *Adv. Drug Del. Rev.*, 55, 217–250, 2003.
233. Hershfield, M., PEG-ADA replacement therapy for adenosine deaminase deficiency; an update after 8.5 years, *Clin. Immunol. Immunopathol.*, 76, 228–232, 1995.
234. Avrami, V.I., et al., A randomized comparison of native *Escherichia coli* asparaginase and polyethylene glycol conjugated asparaginase for treatment of children with newly diagnosed standard-risk acute lymphoblastic leukemia: A children's cancer group study, *Blood*, 99, 1986–1994, 2002.
235. Holtsberg, F.W., et al., Poly(ethylene glycol) (PEG) conjugated arginine deiminase: Effects of PEG formulation on its pharmacological properties, *J. Control. Release*, 80, 259–271, 2002.
236. Curley, S.A., et al., Regression of hepatocellular cancer in a patient treated with arginine deiminase, *Hepatogastroenterology*, 50, 1214–1216, 2003.
237. Izzo, F., et al., Pegylated arginine deiminase treatment of patients with unresectable hepatocellular carcinoma: Results from phase I/II studies, *J. Clin. Oncol.*, 22, 1815–1822, 2004.
238. See www.phoenixpharm.org
239. See www.savientpharma.com and www.mvpharm.com
240. See www.enzon.com
241. See www.direvo.de

242. See www.ame.biz

243. Jermutus, L., et al., Structure-based chimeric enzymes as an alternative to directed evolution: Phytase as a test case, *J. Biotechnol.*, 86, 15–24, 2001.

244. Van Den Burg, B., et al., Engineering an enzyme resistant to boiling, *Proc. Natl. Acad. Sci. USA*, 95, 2056–2060, 1998.

245. Kabashima, T., et al., Enhancement of the thermal stability of pyroglutamyl peptidase I by introduction of an intersubunit disulfide bond, *Biochim. Biophys. Acta*, 1547, 214–220, 2001.

246. Jang, J.W., et al., Enhanced thermal stability of an alkaline protease, AprP, isolated from a *Pseudomonas* sp. by mutation at an autoproteolysis site, Ser-331, *Biotechnol. Appl. Biochem.*, 34, 81–84, 2001.

247. Sode, K., et al., Increasing the thermal stability if the water-soluble pyrroloquinoline quinone glucose dehydrogenase by single amino acid replacement, *Enz. Microb. Technol.*, 26, 491–496, 2000.

248. Abian, O., et al., Stabilization of penicillin G acylase from *Escherichia coli*: Site-directed mutagenesis of the protein surface to increase multipoint covalent attachment, *Appl. Environ. Microbiol.*, 70, 1249–1251, 2004.

249. Zhang, N., et al., Improving tolerance of *Candida antarctica* lipase B towards irreversible thermal inactivation through directed evolution, *Protein Eng.*, 16, 599–605, 2003.

250. Kim, J.-H., et al., Enhanced thermostability and tolerance of high substrate concentration of an esterase by directed evolution, *J. Mol. Catal.*, 27, 169–175, 2004.

251. Kim, Y.-W., et al., Directed evolution of *Thermus* maltogenic amylase toward enhanced thermal resistance, *Appl. Environ. Microbiol.*, 69, 4866–4874, 2003.

252. Sakaue, R. and Kajiyama, N., Thermostabilization of bacterial fructosyl-amino acid oxidase by directed evolution, *Appl. Environ. Microbiol.*, 69, 139–145, 2003.

253. Koga, Y., et al., Inverting enantioselectivity of *Burkholderia cepacia* KWI-56 lipase by combinatorial mutation and high-throughput screening using single-molecule PCR and *in vitro* expression, *J. Mol. Biol.*, 331, 585–592, 2003.

254. Reetz, M.T., et al., Creation of enantioselective biocatalysts for organic chemistry by *in vitro* evolution, *Agnew. Chem. Int. Ed. Engl.*, 36, 2830–2832, 1997.

255. Reetz, M.T., et al., Directed evolution of an enantioselective enzyme through combinatorial multiple-cassette mutagenesis, *Agnew. Chem. Int. Ed. Engl.*, 40, 3589–3591, 2001.

256. Zha, D., et al., Complete reversal of enantioselectivity of an enzyme-catalysed reaction by directed evolution, *Chem. Commun.*, 1, 2664–2665, 2001.

257. Horsman, G.P., et al., Mutations in distant residues moderately increase the enantioselectivity of *Pseudomonas fluorescens* esterase towards methyl 3-bromo-2-methylpropanoate and ethyl 3-phenylbutyrate, *Chemistry*, 9, 1933–1939, 2003.

258. Williams, G., et al., Modifying the stereochemistry of an enzyme-catalyzed reaction by directed evolution, *Proc. Natl. Acad. Sci. USA*, 100, 3143–3148, 2003.

259. May, O., Nguyen, P.T., and Arnold, F. H., Inverting enantioselectivity by directed evolution of hydantoinase for improved production of L-methionine, *Nat. Biotechnol.*, 18, 317–320, 2000.

260. Alexeeva, M., et al., Deracemization of α-methylbenzylamine using an enzyme obtained by *in vitro* evolution, *Agnew. Chem. Int. Ed. Engl.*, 41, 3177–3180, 2002.

261. Carr, R., et al., Directed evolution of an amine oxidase possessing both broad substrate specificity and high enantioselectivity, *Agnew. Chem. Int. Ed. Engl.*, 42, 4807–4810, 2003.

262. Reetz, M.T., et al., Enhancing the enantioselectivity of an epoxide hydrolase by directed evolution, *Org. Lett.*, 6, 177–180, 2004.

263. Kurre, H.A., et al., A pharmacoeconomic analysis of pegasparagase versus native *Escherichia coli* L-asparaginase for the treatment of children with standard-risk, acute lymphoblastic leukaemia: The children's cancer group study (CCG-1962), *J. Pediatr. Hematol. Oncol.*, 24, 175–181, 2002.

3

Tissue Plasminogen Activator-Based Thrombolytic Agents

Gary Walsh

CONTENTS

3.1 Thrombosis and Thrombolytic Therapy

A thrombus, or blood clot, may be described as a solid mass whose constituents are derived from the blood and which forms in the circulatory system [1]. The clot is formed by a complex series of cascading events involving blood coagulation factors, platelets, red blood cells, and interactions with the vessel wall. By obstructing or completely blocking blood flow from the point of formation, the clot deprives downstream tissue of an oxygen supply. In a further complication, fragments (emboli) may break away from the clot, only to obstruct smaller vessels at a point distant from the main clot. Among the most common causes of morbidity and mortality in the Western world are the formation of arterial thrombi (coronary arterial thrombi and cerebral arterial thrombi) and pulmonary emboli.

Therapeutic drugs aimed at minimizing the formation and reformation of such thrombi, or accelerating the removal of thrombi once formed, include antiplatelet agents (which inhibit platelet activation), thrombolytic therapy (which degrades the clot), and the administration of anticoagulants (Table 3.1). Of these, urokinase and tissue plasminogen activator (tPA)-based products display a catalytic mode of action. Urokinase is considered in Chapter 13, while tPA-based products form the focus of the remainder of this chapter.

3.1.1   Fibrinolysis and tPA

The degradation and removal of blood clots from a damaged or diseased blood vessel is termed "fibrinolysis" or the "fibrinolytic process." Fibrinolysis is a proteolytic-mediated process initiated by tPA, which activates the protein plasminogen, thereby forming plasmin. Plasmin in turn proteolytically degrades the fibrin strands of the blood clot, thereby effectively dissolving it (Figure 3.1). Inhibition of the fibrinolytic process may also be promoted by plasminogen activator inhibitors or by α_2-antiplasmin.

Initial reports of a tissue-derived factor (originally termed fibrinokinase) capable of activating plasminogen date back to the 1940s [2]. In the intervening years, tPA from various sources including human, pig, and bovine have been purified and characterized. Human tPA was first purified from uterine tissue in 1979 [3], and ensuing immunological studies illustrated that tissue, vascular, and blood-derived plasminogen activators are the same. Serum tPA is derived predominantly from vascular endothelial cells and is present in blood at concentrations approximating 5 ng/mL. tPA purified from a human (Bowes) melanoma cell line also facilitated early detailed characterization of this molecule [4]. The complementary DNA (cDNA) for human tPA has been cloned and expressed in a variety of systems, including *Escherichia coli* and various animal cell lines [5–7]. The human tPA gene is located on chromosome 8 and houses 14 exons [8]. The purified protein is generally a single-chain, 70 kDa, 527 amino-acid-glycosylated polypeptide. Limited plasma hydrolysis of the Arg275-Ile276 peptide bond generates a characteristic plasma 2 chain form of the molecule, held together by a single interchain disulfide bond (between cysteine residues 264 and 395). The molecule displays three actual glycosylation sites (asparagine residues 117, 184, and 448). In native tPA, a mixture of the fully glycosylated form and a variant devoid of a side chain at Asn184 predominate [6].

Structurally, tPA consists of five domains (Table 3.2). The F or "finger" domain resides toward the molecule's N terminus (residues 4 to 50) and mediates high-affinity binding to fibrin. The E or epidermal growth factor (EGF) domain (residues 51 to 87), binds hepatic

TABLE 3.1

Drugs Used for Thrombotic Therapy

Drug Name	Category
Aspirin	Antiplatelet
Dipyridamole	Antiplatelet
Ticlopidine	Antiplatelet
tPA/engineered tPA	Thrombolytic
Urokinase	Thrombolytic
Streptokinase	Thrombolytic
Heparin	Anticoagulant
Warfarin	Anticoagulant
Hirudin	Anticoagulant
Activated human protein C	Anticoagulant

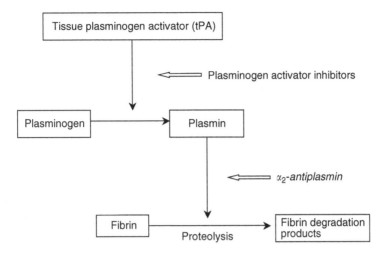

FIGURE 3.1   The fibrinolytic process.

TABLE 3.2

The Domain Structure of tPA

Domain	Function
Finger domain (F domain)	Promotes high-affinity binding to fibrin
Protease domain (P domain)	Plasminogen specific proteolytic activity
Epidermal growth factor domain (EGF domain)	Binds hepatic receptors, hence accelerating hepatic clearance
Kringle-1 domain (K_1 domain)	Associated with receptor binding
Kringle-2 domain (K_2 domain)	Allows stimulation by fibrin of proteolytic activity

receptors, thereby accelerating hepatic clearance from the plasma. The kringle-1 domain (residues 88 to 176) is associated with receptor binding, while the kringle-2 domain (residues 177 to 262) facilitates stimulation of activity by fibrin. The actual catalytic (proteolytic) domain resides toward the C terminus (residues 276 to 527), with His332, Asp371, and Ser478 constituting the active site [5,6]. The three-dimensional structure of three tPA domains are illustrated in Figure 3.2. The glycocomponent also plays a role in regulating the protein's serum half-life. The sugar side chain attached to Asn117 in particular is characterized by high mannose content, which is associated with the promotion of rapid plasma clearance [9,10]. An understanding of the biological functions of the various plasminogen activator domains has rendered possible the generation of various therapeutically important deletion product variants, as will be discussed later.

3.1.2   Mechanism of Action

As explained in Figure 3.1, tPA triggers the fibrinolytic process by catalyzing the proteolytic activation of plasminogen, yielding plasmin. Plasminogen is synthesized by the kidneys, from where it enters the bloodstream. It is a 90 kDa glycoprotein, stabilized by

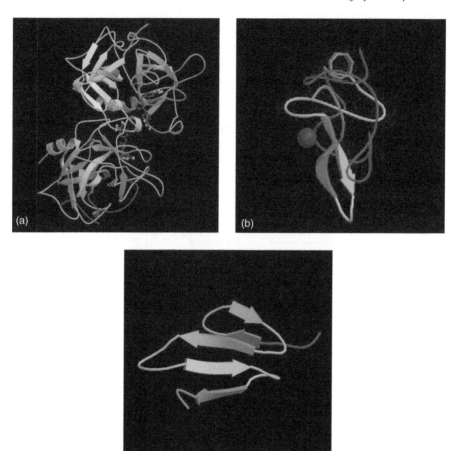

FIGURE 3.2
The three-dimensional structure of the (a) catalytic K2, (b) catalytic F1, and (c) domains of human tPA. (Courtesy of the Protein Databank, http://www.pdb.org. Entry ID numbers 1A5H, 1TPK, and 1TPM, respectively. With permission.)

several disulfide bonds. tPA cleaves a single peptide bond (Arg561-Val562) in the plasminogen backbone, yielding the active serine protease, plasmin. Plasmin contains several lysine-binding sites toward its N-terminal end, while the active site is found toward its C-terminal end. Plasmin lysine-binding sites help mediate binding of the molecule to fibrin (and hence effectively to the clot surface). They also play a role in facilitating plasmin inhibition by α_2-antiplasmin [11]. Fibrin contains binding sites for both plasminogen and tPA, thereby bringing these into close proximity. This facilitates activation of plasminogen by tPA directly at the clot surface (Figure 3.3). The activation process is potentiated by the fact that binding of tPA to fibrin (1) enhances subsequent binding of plasminogen and (2) increases tPA's activity toward plasminogen up to 600-fold. tPA itself displays very limited proteolytic activity in the absence of fibrin. This has physiological significance in that the substrate specificity of plasmin is poor. Activated plasmin, if free in the plasma, could degrade several coagulation factors. Free circulating plasmin displays a half-life of the order of 0.1 sec [11,12]. It is rapidly inactivated by yet another plasma protein, α_2-antiplasmin. This 70-kDa single-chain glycosylated polypeptide inactivates plasmin by binding to it in a tight 1:1 stoichiometric complex. In contrast to free plasmin, plasmin formed at the clot surface has both its active site and lysine-binding sites occupied,

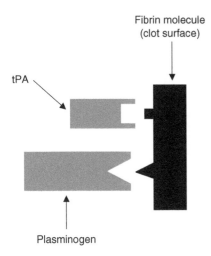

Fibrin molecule
(clot surface)

tPA

Plasminogen

FIGURE 3.3
Fibrin displays binding sites for both tPA and plasminogen, facilitating activation of the fibrinolytic process directly at the clot surface.

and in consequence is only slowly inactivated by α_2-antiplasmin. Such clot-bound plasmin displays an average half-life of approximately 1 min.

Overall, therefore, the thrombolytic system has evolved in a self-regulating fashion, which ensures efficient clot degradation while minimizing potential disruption of other elements of the hemostatic system.

3.1.3 Thrombolytic Therapy in Acute Myocardial Infarction

The beneficial effect of thrombolytic therapy in the treatment of acute myocardial infarction (AMI) is now well established [13–15]. Use of thrombolytic agents has become a standard emergency treatment in such situations to the extent that globally, such drugs are administered to over 500,000 patients each year. It has been estimated that three times that number could potentially benefit from such therapy [5,16]. Although effective, these products achieve complete reperfusion in, on an average, only 50% of patients, and side effects can include risk of hemorrhage (in particular intracranial bleeding) as well as hypertension.

The remainder of this chapter will focus upon the three tPA-based product variants now approved for general medical use: Alteplase, Reteplase, and Tenecteplase.

3.2 Alteplase

Alteplase (international nonproprietary name) is a first-generation recombinant human tPA approved for general medical use in the United States in 1987 (Table 3.3). Developed and manufactured by Genentech Inc. (San Francisco, CA) it is sold under the tradename Activase. It displays an amino acid sequence identical to native human tPA, and, like native tPA, is glycosylated. Alteplase is indicated in the United States for:

1. The management of AMI in adults for the improvement of ventricular function following AMI, the reduction of the incidence of congestive heart failure, and the reduction of mortality associated with AMI.
2. The management of acute ischemic stroke in adults for improving neurological recovery and reducing the incidence of disability.

TABLE 3.3

tPA Based Thrombolytic Agents Thus Far Approved in the USA and the EU

Product	Company	Therapeutic Indication	Approved
Activase (Alteplase) rh-tPA produced in CHO cells	Genentech	Acute myocardial infarction; Acute ischemic stroke and pulmonary embolism	1987 (USA)
Ecokinase (Reteplase) Domain deleted rtPA variant produced in *E. coli*	Galenus Mannheim	Acute myocardial infarction	1996 (EU), withdrawn in 1999 for commercial reasons
Retavase (Reteplase) See Ecokinase entry	Boehringer Mannheim/ Centocor	Acute myocardial infarction	1996 (USA)
Rapilysin (Reteplase) See Ecokinase entry	Boehringer Mannheim	Acute myocardial infarction	1996 (EU)
TNKase (tradename in USA) /**Metalyse** (tradename in EU) (Tenecteplase; modified rtPA produced in CHO cells	Genentech (USA) Boehringer Ingelheim (EU)	Myocardial infarction	2000 (USA) 2001 (EU)

Abbreviations: r = recombinant, rh = recombinant human, CHO = Chinese hamster ovary

3. The management of acute massive pulmonary embolism (PE) in adults: for the lysis of acute pulmonary emboli, defined as obstruction of blood flow to a lobe or multiple segments of the lung; and for the lysis of pulmonary emboli accompanied by unstable hemodynamics, e.g., failure to maintain blood pressure without support measures. The diagnosis should be confirmed by objective means such as pulmonary angiography or by noninvasive procedures such as lung scanning.

3.2.1 Manufacture and Composition

Alteplase is synthesized using the cDNA for native human tPA derived from a human melanoma cell line. The cDNA is cloned into a Chinese ovary cell (CHO) cell line, from which suitable master and working cell banks are produced. Product manufacture entails culture of the producer animal cell line in a nutrient medium containing the antibiotic gentamicin. The glycosylated protein is secreted by the producer cell line into the extracellular culture medium. While production protocols remain confidential, initial product recovery is likely to involve physical removal of the producer cells from the product-containing culture media by means of filtration or centrifugation. This is likely to be followed by initial product concentration via ultrafiltration. Product purification entails application of multiple high-resolution chromatographic purification steps, including anion-exchange, gel filtration, and lysine-affinity chromatography. The final product has been shown to be >99% pure by several analytical techniques, including high performance liquid chromatography (HPLC), sodium dodecyl sulfate-polyacrylamide gel electrophoresis (SDS–PAGE), tryptic mapping, and N-terminal sequencing. After excipient addition, the product is filter-sterilized, aseptically filled into vials, and freeze-dried. The final product is presented in single-dose vials containing either 50 or 100 mg active ingredient. It is a sterile white to off-white powder that must be reconstituted with water for injections (WFI) prior to intravenous (IV) administration. The final composition of the freeze-dried product is Alteplase (580,000 IU/mg), arginine, phosphoric acid, and polysorbate 80. Upon reconstitution, the product displays a pH of 7.3 [17].

3.2.2 Clinical Studies

Studies indicate that the plasma clearance displayed by Alteplase in AMI patients occurs with an initial half-life of under 5 min and a terminal half-life of 72 min [18]. Modes of product administration include infusion of a maximum of 100 mg over 90 min ("accelerated infusion"), infusion of a maximum of 100 mg over a period of 3 h ("3 h infusion") or, in the case of acute ischemic stroke, administration of a maximum of 90 mg by infusion over 1 h [17]. A number of trials have been undertaken in order to determine the safety and efficacy of the product [19–27]. For example, accelerated infusion of Activase was studied in a multicenter international trial (GUSTO) in which 41,000 patients presenting with AMI were randomized into one of four thrombolytic regimens: (1) accelerated infusion of Activase plus IV heparin ($n = 10,396$); (2) infusion of streptokinase (1.5 million units over 60 min) plus IV heparin ($n = 10,410$), (3) streptokinase plus heparin administered subcutaneously ($n = 9,841$), and (4) a combined Alteplase and streptokinase regimen. Endpoint measurements of 30 d mortality, 30 d mortality or nonfatal stroke, as well as 24 h mortality were all significantly better in the case of the accelerated Activase-treated group. However, the rate of intracerebral hemorrhage in this group was marginally higher than for the other treatments [10].

Two placebo-controlled, double-blind trials have also been carried out with acute ischemic stroke patients [24]. Patients were randomized and received either a placebo or 0.9 mg/kg

Activase, to a maximum of 90 mg total dose. The initial study ($n = 291$) evaluated neuro-logical improvement at 24 h after stroke onset, but revealed no significant difference between the two treatment groups. The second study ($n = 333$) assessed the clinical outcome 3 months after stroke occurrence; a favorable outcome was defined as minimal or no disability using four different stroke assessment scales (the Bartel index, modified Rankin scale, Glasgow outcome scale, and NIH stroke scale). In this study, a favorable outcome was recorded for 11 more patients per 100 in the Activase group than in the control group.

The effect of Activase in treating pulmonary embolism was also evaluated in a com-parative randomized trial [25]. Within 2 h of treatment initiation, 69% of patients experi-enced moderate or marked lysis of pulmonary emboli. Patients also experienced a significant reduction in embolism-induced pulmonary hypertension.

3.2.3   Adverse Reactions and Warnings

The most serious adverse event reported subsequent to Activase administration is bleeding. If serious intracranial, gastrointestinal, retroperitoneal, or pericardial bleeding occurs, treat-ment must be immediately discontinued. Allergic reactions, including anaphylactoid reac-tions, laryngeal edema, and urticaria have also been reported. The product should be used with extreme caution in pregnant women, for whom there are no well-controlled studies. Activase has an embryocidal effect in rabbits when administered in doses of twice the level used to treat AMI in humans. Caution should also be exercised with nursing mothers as it is not known if Activase is excreted into human milk. Negative results were recorded when the product was subjected to a mutagenicity test (the Ames test), chromosomal aberration assays in human lymphocytes, and short-term tumorigenicity studies. Long-term studies in animals to evaluate carcinogenic potential or effect on fertility have not been undertaken.

3.3   Reteplase

An understanding of the domain structure–function relationship of native tPA afforded researchers the possibility of developing engineered tPA variants displaying enhanced therapeutic properties. An ideal thrombolytic agent should (1) display fast action in order to minimize time to reperfusion, (2) display efficient clot lysis, (3) display a good safety profile, in particular, a reduced risk of intracranial bleeding, and (4) be quick and easy to administer.

Reteplase represents a second-generation engineered tPA which meets at least some of these requirements better than native tPA. It is marketed in the United States under the trade name Retavase and in Europe under the trade name Rapilysin. It also gained mar-keting approval in Europe under the trade name Ecokinase in 1996, but was later with-drawn from the market, apparently for commercial reasons (Table 3.3). Reteplase is an engineered tPA differing from the native molecule in two important respects: (1) it is a domain-deleted mutein, consisting only of the kringle 2 and protease domains of native tPA (i.e., residues 1 to 3 and 176 to 527 of the native tPA molecule), and (2) it is not glyco-sylated. Lack of glycosylation, as well as the absence of the EGF and K1 domains, confers a significantly extended half-life upon Reteplase, allowing its administration intrave-nously as discussed later. Moreover, absence of the F1 domain reduces the molecule's fibrin-binding affinity, allowing it to diffuse more extensively into the clot interior. This may facilitate accelerated clot lysis.

Reteplase is produced by recombinant DNA technology in *E. coli* (as described below) and displays a molecular mass of 39.57 kDa. It is indicated for the management of AMI in adults for the improvement of ventricular function following AMI, the reduction of the incidence of congestive heart failure, and the reduction of mortality associated with AMI [28].

3.3.1 Manufacture and Composition

During product development, a cDNA library from a Bowes melanoma cell line was screened and a full-length tPA cDNA clone produced. The sequence coding for the F, K1, and EGF domains were removed [29]. The Reteplase coding sequence was then introduced into the vector plasmid pKK223-3 and the resulting construct introduced into *E. coli* by transformation [30]. Master and working cell banks have been generated. An overview of the manufacturing procedure is presented in Figure 3.4. The product accumulates intracellularly in *E. coli* in the form of inclusion bodies [31,32]. Cell harvesting follows fermentation, with subsequent cellular disruption and inclusion body (IB) recovery. IBs are solubilized and denatured under reducing conditions, followed by *in vitro* product folding. Four primary steps characterize downstream processing: acidification and filtration, affinity chromatography using Erythrina trypsin inhibitor-Sepharose, and two ion-exchange steps. This is followed by a concentration step and removal of low molecular mass species via diafiltration. Excipient addition is followed by sterile filtration, aseptic filling, and lyophilization. Each 20-mL single-use glass vial contains Reteplase (active ingredient) as well as tranexamic acid, dipotassium hydrogen phosphate, phosphoric acid, and polysorbate as excipients. It appears as a white powder, which is reconstituted with WFI before administration. The solution pH following reconstitution is 6.0.

3.3.2 Clinical Studies

Reteplase displays favorable pharmacological profiles. Its plasma half-life in humans is approximately 14 min [33]. It therefore displays an activity half-life some 3.3-fold higher than native human tPA and a clearance rate 3.3-fold lower than the native molecule.

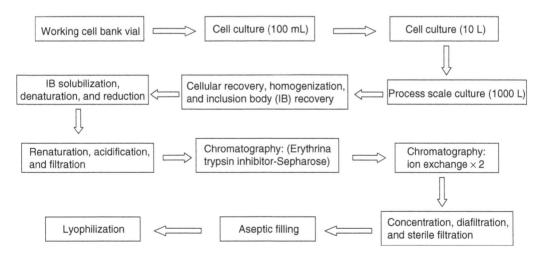

FIGURE 3.4 Overview of the likely method of manufacture of Reteplase.

Furthermore, the product appears to display only a modest effect upon hemostatic variables, suggesting a lowered potential for promoting bleeding [33,34].

Reteplase is indicated only for IV administration. It is usually administered as two separate 10-U bolus injections, each administered over 2 and 30 min apart.

The safety and efficacy of Reteplase has been evaluated in a number of trials [35–38]. The RAPID 1 clinical study [35] randomized 606 AMI patients into one of four groups: those receiving either (1) 100 mg native recombinant tPA (rtPA) intravenously over 3 h, (2) Reteplase administered as a single bolus dose, (3) Reteplase administered as a 10 and 5 U dose 30 min apart, or (4) Reteplase administered as a 10 U and 10 U double-bolus dose 30 min apart. The 10 U + 10 U Reteplase dosage regimen yielded the highest complete patency rates, 63% of patients after 90 min, compared with 49% of patients receiving the native tPA ($p = 0.019$).

The International Joint Efficacy Comparison of Thrombolytics trial [37] compared the efficacy of Reteplase and streptokinase in preventing mortality following AMI. A total of 6010 patients from nine different European countries were randomized and received either Reteplase administered as a 10 U + 10 U double-bolus dose (as described previously) or streptokinase, 1.5 MU, infused over 60 min. All patients also received adjunct aspirin and heparin. Average mortality after both 35 d and after 6 months was lower for the Reteplase group (8.9 vs. 9.4% and 11 vs. 12.1%).

A major trial (GUSTO-III, [38]) compared Reteplase and recombinant native tPA administration in 15,059 AMI patients from 20 different countries. Reteplase was administered as the 10 U + 10 U bolus dosage 30 min apart, whereas rtPA was administered as a 15 mg bolus IV dose followed by continuous infusion over a further 60 min. The results obtained for both groups were very similar across all endpoints measured. Thirty-day mortality rates, for example, stood at 7.47 and 7.24%, respectively. The combined rate of death or disabling stroke was 7.8 vs. 7.91%. While no difference in efficacy was recorded, the Reteplase dosage regime was recognized as being simpler and more convenient than that of the native rtPA.

3.3.3 Adverse Reactions and Warnings

Bleeding is the most common complication associated with Reteplase administration. Internal bleeding (intracranial, gastrointestinal, retroperitoneal, respiratory, and genitourinary) as well as superficial bleeding have been reported.

Long-term animal studies have not been carried out to evaluate the carcinogenic potential of Reteplase. Studies to determine mutagenicity, chromosomal aberrations, and micronuclear induction all proved negative. Reproduction toxicity studies in rodents revealed no effect, even when Reteplase was administered at 15 times the recommended human dose. Product administration at three times the recommended human dose did, however, promote hemorrhaging and midgestation abortions in pregnant rabbits. No well-controlled studies have been performed in pregnant women. It is not known if Reteplase is excreted in milk, so the product should be administered to nursing mothers only with great caution.

3.4 Tenecteplase

Tenecteplase is an engineered, second-generation tPA-derived thrombolytic produced in a CHO cell line [39]. The 527-amino acid glycoprotein differs from native tPA by (1) substitution of Thr103 with Asn, (2) substitution of Asn117 with Glu, and (3) replacement of residues 296 to 299 with four Ala residues. The first two modifications reside in the K1 domain whereas residues 296 to 299 reside in the protease domain. The changes have been introduced by site-directed mutagenesis of a cDNA coding for native tPA. The therapeutic rationale for developing Tenecteplase was the generation of a tPA variant that can be administered intravenously as a rapid single-dose bolus injection [40]. The product is manufactured by Genentech. It is marketed in the United States under the trade name TNKase and in Europe as Metalyse (Table 3.3).

Tenecteplase is indicated in the treatment of AMI. The indication wording in the United States is "for the reduction of mortality associated with AMI." The EU wording is "for the thrombolytic treatment of suspected myocardial infarction with persistent ST evaluation or recent left Bundle Branch Block within 6 h after the onset of AMI symptoms" [41]. A single-dose bolus based upon the patient's weight but not exceeding a total dose of 50 mg is generally administered over a 5 sec period.

3.4.1 Manufacture and Composition

Upstream processing (cell culture) is generally performed in three sequential stages; a lab-scale seed train, an inoculum train, and a production culture. The production-scale culture is normally undertaken in a 12,000 L fermenter. The product is exported by the CHO cells into the extracellular media. Downstream processing is initiated by removal of cells from the production media, followed by a combination of high-resolution chromatographic steps as well as a viral inactivation step and a number of filtration steps. After excipient adjustment and adjustment of potency, the product is filter sterilized, aseptically filled into glass vials, and lyophilized. The final product contains the active substance Tenecteplase as well as L-Arg, phosphoric acid, and polysorbate 80 as excipients. The product is reconstituted immediately before use in WFI, which is provided in a prefilled syringe for single bolus IV administration [40].

3.4.2 Clinical Trials

In vitro studies demonstrate that Tenecteplase displays at least a 10-fold higher fibrin specificity and an 80-fold higher resistance to inhibition by plasminogen activator inhibitor (PAI-1) than native tPA. The increased fibrin specificity reduces the propensity for causing peripheral bleeding and ameliorates the risk of cerebral hemorrhage in a rabbit model of embolic stroke. Tenecteplase is cleared from the plasma in humans with an initial half-life of 20 to 24 min and a terminal plasma half-life of 90 to 130 min. The molecule displays an altered glycosylation pattern as compared with native tPA. It does not contain high-mannose oligosaccharides and therefore the hepatic mannose receptor, which plays an important role in native tPA removal, is unlikely to be involved in Tenecteplase elimination. Instead, the hepatic low-density receptor-related protein (LRP) as well as the hepatic asialoglycoprotein receptor may mediate removal.

A number of clinical studies have investigated the safety and efficacy of Tenecteplase [42–45]. ASSENT-2 was a major ($n = 16,949$) international randomized double-blind trial that compared Tenecteplase and native tPA (Activase). All patients also received aspirin and heparin. Rates of 30-day mortality (6.2% in both), intracranial hemorrhage (0.9% in both), and stroke (1.8 vs. 1.7%) revealed no significant differences between products.

The TIMI 10B study [43] was an open-label dose ranging randomized angiography study in which patients ($n = 837$) were treated with fixed doses of 30, 40, or 50 mg Tenecteplase or accelerated infusion with Activase. The results revealed that 40- or 50-mg doses produced similar results to Activase in terms of restoring patency.

3.4.3   Adverse Reactions and Warnings

The most common complication associated with Tenecteplase administration is, predictably, bleeding, although the incidence of nonintracranial bleeding associated with the engineered product is significantly lower than that associated with native tPA use. (26.4 vs. 28.9%, $p = 0.0003$). As with other thrombolytics, the use of Tenecteplase may induce hypotension, angina pectoris, and heart rhythm or rate disorders.

No animal studies evaluating carcinogenic potential, mutagenicity, or effects upon fertility have been performed. The product, when administered at elevated doses, elicits vaginal hemorrhage and death in pregnant rabbits. It has not been determined if Tenecteplase is excreted in milk, so the product should be administered to nursing mothers with caution.

3.5   Conclusions

Innovations in the manufacture of tPA and, in particular, the development of engineered product variants, provide a fascinating insight into how technical advances have impacted upon the pharmaceutical biotechnology sector as a whole. Like many early biopharmaceuticals (e.g., blood factors and insulin), first-generation tPA was simply a recombinant version of a native human protein. In contrast, second-generation tPA-based products are engineered in order to tailor their therapeutic characteristics. tPA-based products command a not insignificant proportion of the total global biopharmaceutical market. Combined sales of Genentech's Activase and TNKase products alone reached US$185 million in 2003. Their therapeutic effectiveness, coupled with the significant and growing incidence of AMI worldwide, ensures that this group of therapeutic agents will remain a prominent category of biopharmaceutical for many years to come.

References

1. Kumar, P.J. and Clark, M.L., *Clinical Medicine*, 2nd ed., chap. 6, Bailliere Tindall, London, 1990.
2. Astrup, T. and Permin, P.M., Fibrinolysis in animal organisms, *Nature*, 159, 681–682, 1947.
3. Rijken, D.C., et al., Purification and partial characterization of plasminogen activator from human uterine tissue, *Biochim. Biophys. Acta*, 580, 140–153, 1979.
4. Rijken, D.C. and Collen, D., Purification and characterization of the plasminogen activator secreted by human melanoma cells in culture, *J. Biol. Chem.*, 256, 7035–7041, 1981.
5. Collen, D. and Lijnen, H.R., Tissue-type plasminogen activator: Helping patients with acute myocardial infarction, in *Recombinant Protein Drugs*, Buckel, P., Ed., Birkhauser Verlag, Berlin, 2001, pp. 107–128.
6. Pennica, D., et al., Cloning and expression of human tissue plasminogen activator cDNA in *E. coli.*, *Nature*, 301, 214–221, 1983.
7. Walsh, G., *Biopharmaceuticals: Biochemistry and Biotechnology*, John Wiley & Sons, Chichester, UK, 2002.
8. Rajput, B., et al., Chromosomal locations of human tissue plasminogen activator and urokinase genes, *Science*, 230, 672–674, 1985.
9. Smalling, R.W., Molecular biology of plasminogen activators: What are the clinical implications of drug design?, *Am. J. Cardiol.*, 78 (Suppl. 12A), 2–7, 1996.

10. Waller, M. and Kohnert, U., Reteplase, a recombinant plasminogen activator, in *Biopharmaceuticals, An Industrial Perspective*, Walsh, G. and Murphy, B., Eds., Kluwer Academic Publishers, Dordrecht, The Netherlands, 1999, pp. 185–314.

11. Wiman, B. and Collen, D., Molecular mechanism of physiological fibrinolysis, *Nature*, 272, 549–550, 1978.

12. Wiman, B. and Collen, D., On the kinetics of the reaction between human antiplasmin and plasmin, *Eur. J. Biochem.*, 84, 573–578, 1978.

13. Gruppo Italino per lo Studio della Streptochinasi nell'Infarto miocardico (GISSI), Effectiveness of intravenous thrombolytic treatment in acute myocardial infarction, *Lancet*, 1, 871–874, 1986.

14. ISIS-2 (second international study of infarct survival) Collaborative Group, Randomized trial on intravenous streptokinase, oral aspirin, both or neither 17,187 cases of suspected myocardial infarction: ISIS-2, *Lancet*, 2, 349–360, 1988.

15. ISAM study Group, A prospective trial of intravenous streptokinase in acute myocardial infarction (ISAM), *New Engl. J. Med.*, 314, 1465–1471, 1986.

16. Schlandt, R.C., Reperfusion in acute myocardial infarction, *Circulation*, 90, 2091–2102, 1994.

17. Activase (Alteplase) package insert leaflet, available at http://www.Activase.com

18. Tanswell, P., et al., Pharmacokinetics and fibrin specificity of Alteplase during accelerated infusions in acute myocardial infarction, *J. Am. Coll. Cardiol.*, 19, 1071–1075, 1992.

19. Mueller, H., et al., Thrombolysis in myocardial infarction (TMI): Comparative studies of coronary reperfusion and systemic fibrinogenolysis with two forms of recombinant tissue-type plasminogen activator, *J. Am. Coll. Cardiol.*, 10, 479–490, 1987.

20. Topol, E.J., et al. A multicentre, randomised, placebo controlled trial of a new form of intravenous recombinant tissue-type plasminogen activator (Activase) in acute myocardial infarction, *J. Am. Coll. Cardiol.* 9, 1205–1213, 1987.

21. Selfried, E., et al., Pharmacokinetics and haemostatic status during consecutive infusion of recombinant tissue-type plasminogen activator in patients with acute myocardial infarctions, *Thromb. Haemostas.*, 61, 497–501, 1989

22. Guerci, A.D., et al., A randomised trial of intravenous tissue plasminogen activator for acute myocardial infarction with subsequent randomisation to elective coronary angioplasty, *New Engl. J. Med.*, 317, 1613–1618, 1987.

23. Wilcox, R.G., et al., Trial of tissue plasminogen activator for mortality reduction in acute myocardial infarction: ASSET, *Lancet*, 2, 525–530, 1988.

24. The National Institute of Neurological Disorders and Stroke t-PA Stroke Study Group, Tissue plasminogen activator for acute ischemic stroke, *New Engl. J. Med.*, 333, 1581–1587, 1995.

25. Goldhaber, S.Z., et al., A randomised controlled trial of recombinant tissue plasminogen activator versus urokinase in the treatment of acute pulmonary embolism, *Lancet*, 2, 293–298, 1988.

26. Aylward, P., Relation of increased arterial blood pressure to mortality and stroke in the context of contemporary thrombolytic therapy for acute myocardial infarction: A randomised trial, *Ann. Int. Med.*, 125, 891–900, 1996.

27. National Heart Foundation of Australia Cornary Thrombolysis Group, Cornary thrombosis and myocardial infarction salvage by tissue plasminogen activator given upto 4 hours after onset of myocardial infarction, *Lancet*, 1, 203–207, 1988.

28. Retavase (Reteplase) package insert leaflet, available at http://www.retavase.com

29. Ny, T., et al., The structure of the human tissue-plasminogen activator gene: Correlation of intron and exon structures to functional and structural domains, *Proc. Natl. Acad. Sci.*, 81, 5355–5359, 1984.

30. Maniatis, T., et al., *Molecular cloning: A laboratory manual*, Cold Spring Harbor, NY, Cold Spring Harbor Laboratory Press, 1992.

31. Stern, A., et al., Gewebs-Plasminogenakativator-Derivat, European Patent Application 382174.

32. Rudolph R., et al., Verfahren zur Aktivierung von gentechnologisch hergestellten, heterologen, disulfidbrucken aufweisenden eukaryontischen Proteinen nach Expression in Prokaryonten, European Patent Application 219874.

33. Martin, U., et al., Dose-ranging study of the novel recombinant plasminogen activator BM 06.022 in healthy volunteers, *Clin. Pharmacol. Ther.*, 50, 429–436, 1991.

34. Martin, U., et al., Pharmacokinetic and hemostatic properties of the novel recombinant plasminogen activator BM 06.022 in healthy volunteers, *Thromb. Haemost.*, 66, 569–574, 1991.
35. Smalling, R.W., et al., More rapid, complete, and stable coronary thrombolysis with bolus administration of Reteplase compared with alteplase infusion in acute myocardial infarction, *Circulation*, 91, 2725–2732, 1995.
36. Bode, C., et al., Randomised comparison of coronary thrombolysis achieved with a double bolus Reteplase (recombinant plasminogen activator) and front-loaded, accelerated Alteplase (recombinant tissue plasminogen activator) in patients with acute myocardial infarction, *Circulation*, 94, 891–898, 1996.
37. International Joint Efficacy Comparison of Thrombolytics, Randomized double blind comparison of Reteplase double bolus administration with streptokinase in acute myocardial infarction (INJECT): Trial to investigate equivalence, *Lancet*, 346, 329–336, 1995.
38. The Global Use of Strategies to Open Occluded Coronary Arteries (GUSTO III) Investigators, A comparison of Reteplase with Alteplase for acute myocardial infarction, *New Engl. J. Med.*, 337, 1118–1123, 1997.
39. Van de Werf, F., et al., Incidence and predictors of bleeding events after fibrinolytic therapy with fibrin-specific agents: A comparison of TNK-tPA and rt-PA, *Eur. Heart J.*, 22, 2253–2261, 2001.
40. TNKase (Tenecteplase) package insert leaflet, available at http://www.tnkase.com
41. Methylase European Public Assessment Report (EPAR). Available at http://www.eudra.eu.org
42. ASSENT 2 Investigators, Single bolus Tenecteplase compared with front-loaded Alteplase in acute myocardial infarction: The ASSENT 2 double-blind randomised trial, *Lancet*, 354, 716–722, 1999.
43. Cannon, C.P., et al., TNK tissue plasminogen activator compared with front loaded Alteplase in acute myocardial infarction. Results of the TIMI 10B trial. *Circulation*, 98, 2805–2814, 1998.
44. Van de Werf, F., et al., Safety assessment of a single bolus administration of TNK-tPA in acute myocardial infarction: The ASSENT 1 trial, *Am. Heart J.*, 137, 786–791, 1999.
45. Angeia, B., et al., Safety of the weight-adjusted dosing regimen of Tenecteplase in the ASSENT trial, *Am. J. Cardiol.*, 88, 1240–1245, 2001.

4

Activated Protein C

Brian W. Grinnell, S. Betty Yan, and William L. Macias

CONTENTS

Protein C is a plasma protease that, when activated, plays a central role in the regulation of vascular function. As part of an integrated pathway, activated protein C (APC) aids in maintaining vascular patency, and in modulating the function of the vascular endothelium and its interface with the innate immune system. In this chapter, we will review the structure and function of protein C, its mechanistic biology and preclinical pharmacology, as well as the development of recombinant human activated protein C (rhAPC, nonproprietary name: drotrecogin alfa [activated]). Because protein C is an important component of the host response to severe infection, we will emphasize its clinical utility as a unique microvascular modulator for the treatment of severe sepsis.

4.1   Structure of APC

The complementary deoxyribonucleic acid (cDNA) sequence of human protein C (HPC) codes for a 461-amino acid protein [1] (Figure 4.1). The first 42 amino acids are a leader sequence consisting of a signal peptide (residues –42 to –25) and a propeptide (residues –24 to –1) that contains the recognition site for a vitamin K-dependent carboxylase [2].

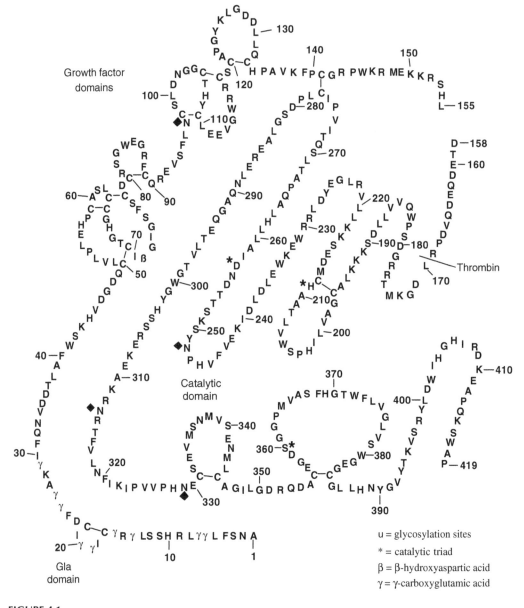

FIGURE 4.1
Schematic representation of human protein C precursor. Numbers refer to the amino acid position relative to the mature processed N terminus. Sequence 156 to 157 is removed during processing and the activation peptide is removed to convert PC zymogen into the activated enzyme (APC).

There are two proteolytic cleavage sites resulting in the removal of the propeptide and an internal Lys156-Arg157 dipeptide during cell secretion. Zymogen (90 to 95%) circulates as a heterodimer consisting of a light-chain (residues 1 to 155) disulfide linked to the heavy-chain serine protease domain (residues 157 to 419). The remaining 5 to 10% of the secreted, mature HPC zymogen circulates in a single-chain form, with the internal dibasic dipeptide Lys-Arg. The first nine glutamic acid residues in the light chain are sites of posttranslational modification to γ-carboxyglutamates (Gla) by the vitamin K-dependent carboxylase. The light chain also contains one residue (D71) posttranslationally modified to ε–β-hydroxyaspartate [3]. There are also four Asn-linked glycosylation sites for HPC (N97, N248, N313, and N329) [4,5], but there is no evidence of any O-linked glycosylation in the two epidermal growth factor-like domains in the light chain [6]. The processing of APC and the posttranslational modifications are shown schematically in Figure 4.2. The complete γ-carboxylation of the light chain, β-hydroxylation of N71 and correct propeptide processing are all required for full functional anticoagulant activity. Zymogen protein C can be converted into APC *in vitro* by either thrombin alone (in the absence of calcium ions) or by a thrombomodulin (TM)–thrombin complex (in the presence of calcium ions), both conditions resulting in the removal of a 12-amino-acid activation peptide (residues 158 to 169) from the N terminus of the heavy-chain HPC.

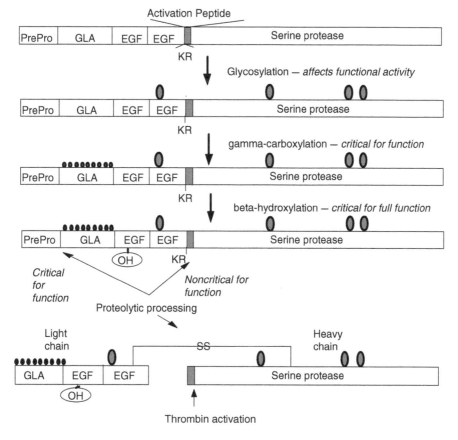

FIGURE 4.2
Summary of the posttranslational processing of human protein C to generate the circulating two-chain heterodimer (see text for details).

4.2   Development of rhAPC

As indicated above, protein C is a very complex and heavily processed protein that is challenging and difficult to produce. This section will describe the issues and challenges in the development of the recombinant protein C and APC. A more detailed overview of the development genetics, production, and formulation of commercial rhAPC (Xigris™) material can be found at the following websites: http://www.emea.eu.int/humandocs/ Humans/EPAR/xigris/xigris.htm and http://www.fda.gov/cder/biologics/products/ droteli112101.htm

Figure 4.3 shows a time line summarizing the key events in the history of the development of drotrecogin alfa (activated).

4.2.1   Cell Line Identification

In view of the complexity of the posttranslational modifications, identification of a mammalian cell line that expressed functionally active and correctly modified rHPC at a commercially viable level proved to be difficult. Although plasma-derived protein C is produced and secreted by the liver, commonly available liver cell lines such as HepG2 and FAZA cells failed to produce fully active rHPC. In the search for an appropriate host cell, the role of each of these posttranslational modifications in the functioning of recombinant protein C was studied extensively, using a variety of cell biology, biochemical, and molecular genetic approaches [4,7–12]. We demonstrated that the complete γ-carboxylation of the light chain was required for full functional anticoagulant activity. For example, the effect of reduced Gla content on the functional activity of rHPC, determined by Yan et al. [9], showed that the anticoagulant activity of recombinant protein C containing seven Gla residues instead of the full nine Gla, was only 20 to 30% of the anticoagulant activity of the purified human embryonic kidney 293 (HEK293)-cell-produced material, demonstrating the critical requirement for complete

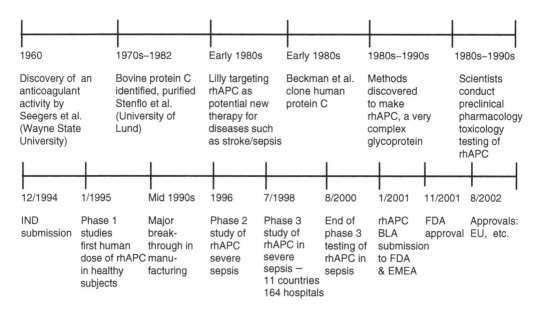

FIGURE 4.3   Summary of the development history of drotrecogin alpha (activated) (see text for details).

modification of the Gla domain. Point mutagenesis studies have shown that elimination of β-hydroxylation or incorrect processing of the propeptide essentially eliminated all the anticoagulant activity [10].

In the mid-1980s, we found that an engineered, adenovirus-transformed HEK293 cell line was capable of producing fully active rHPC [8,9,13,14]. There were substantial efforts both in academic and industrial laboratories to express and secrete active vitamin K-dependent proteins. However, with the exception of the HEK293 cell line, all cell lines thus far engineered secrete only partially active material at reasonable expression levels [8,13,15–20]. The human 293 parent cell line, into which the protein C expression vectors were introduced, is a permanent line of primary HEK. The cell line was isolated in 1973 by *in vitro* transfection of HEK cells with sheared human adenovirus type 5 (Ad5) DNA, as described by Graham et al. [21]. We found that the adenovirus transformation of a cell was critical for the secretion of highly functional, correctly modified protein in part because of the induction of the carboxylase enzyme [22]. In fact, it was possible to engineer improved γ-carboxylation in cells via viral transformation methods, although other important posttranslational processes such as correct proteolytic cleavage were not affected by transformation [22]. The inability to express correctly processed rHPC in commonly used cell lines such as Chinese hamster ovary (CHO), baby hamster kidney (BHK)-21, etc., required the development of new expression vectors and methods for the efficient secretion of rHPC in the HEK293 cells [23–28]. The vectors were designed with elements that could be transactivated by the endogenous E1A protein of adenovirus, which is constitutively expressed by the parent line. This eliminated the need for the commonly used method of gene amplification to drive high-level expression. Although the HEK293 cell line primarily secreted fully processed protein, the next challenge was to overcome a rate-limiting step in secretion, slow glycosyl processing in the endoplasmic reticulum [7]. To overcome this hurdle, a variant 293 line was developed by high-volume clonal selection, followed by reintroduction of a second strong E1A-dependent expression vector [11,26]. The resulting cell line showed no evidence of genetic instability or alterations, as determined by Southern-blot hybridization, RT–PCR analysis, and sequencing of the protein C mRNA by the RT–PCR in the original cell bank through postproduction cells. Extensive biosafety testing has failed to identify any evidence for the presence of adventitious agents in the recombinant derivative of this cell line.

4.2.2 Purification and Characterization of Recombinant-Produced Human APC

A novel method termed pseudo-affinity chromatography was developed for the purification of rHPC that took advantage of the conformational changes in HPC upon the addition or removal of calcium divalent ions [9,29]. This purification step proved to be economical, efficient, and highly selective, resulting in the recovery of only those molecules with full γ-carboxylation of the light chain following activation [22]. The process for the activation of the recombinant zymogen protein C utilized immobilized bovine thrombin and was followed by repurification steps. APC from HEK293 cells purified by this method had complete γ-carboxylation and displayed high functional activity comparable to or higher than that of plasma-derived HPC purified by amidolytic (protease) and anticoagulant assays. Plasma-derived HPC and the purified HEK293 cell-produced rHPCs both display apparent molecular masses from 62 to 66 kDa (as determined by SDS–PAGE). Like plasma-derived protein C, the HEK293 cell-derived rHPC was >90% two chain, and contained a similar pattern of the three heavy-chain α, β, γ glycoforms, but with HEK293 cell-derived rHPC being more enriched equally in both α, β glycoforms, and plasma-derived

HPC having more of the α glycoform. This similarity to plasma-derived material was not seen in rHPC produced from other cell lines, for example, BHK-21 cells [30]. The respective N-terminal sequences of the heavy and light chains of rHPC were identical to those previously reported for plasma-derived HPC [31]. Thus, the HEK293 cell line, unlike others such as the C127 and CHO cell lines [16], was capable of proper proteolytic processing of the propeptide, even at high expression levels. There was no significant difference in the amount of β-OH-Asp in the rHPC and plasma-derived HPC. Thus, with respect to the posttranslational modifications of proteolytic processing and the two types of amino acid modification, the rHPC from the HEK293 cell line appears to be processed in a manner similar to plasma-derived material, but more completely in the case of γ-carboxylation of the nine glutamate residues. γ-Carboxylation of glutamates is dependent on an adequate supplement of vitamin K in the diet, avoidance of medications interfering with the vitamin K-dependent pathway, and the normal liver function of the large number of blood donors from which the plasma APC is derived. One advantage of deriving rHPC from a culture of HEK293 cells is that there is more consistency in the optimum requirement for γ-carboxylation.

Unlike the other posttranslational modifications described above, the carbohydrates on rHPC differed from those on plasma-derived HPC. The structures of oligosaccharides on recombinant glycoproteins are determined to a large extent by the cell line used [32]. Oligosaccharides found on glycoproteins can influence parameters that are important to drug design, such as circulatory clearance, tissue targeting, immunogenicity, and efficacy [32]. In view of this, a detailed analysis of the oligosaccharide structures on rHPC from HEK293 cells was performed [9,33], and novel and rare Asn-linked oligosaccharides were identified (Figure 4.4). The novel trisaccharide epitope on rHPC was designated the PC293 determinant, and, along with the two rare disaccharide epitopes, GalNAcβ(1→4)GlcNAcβ(1→4) and NeuAcα(2→6)GalNAcβ(1→4), have been found in naturally occurring human glycoproteins [34–37]. Glycosyl composition analysis has shown that these GalNAc-containing rare oligosaccharides are not present in plasma-derived HPC. However, to date, clinical trial experience in healthy subjects and over 30,000 patients (both clinical trials and commercial use) suggests that these novel and rare oligosaccharides on HEK293-produced rhAPC probably do not pose any immunogenicity problem in humans. Studies in a primate arterial thrombotic model suggest that these rare Asn-linked oligosaccharides may slightly lessen the circulatory half-life and antithrombotic activity of rhAPC when compared with plasma-derived human APC for this model [38]. Because of the carbohydrate sequence homology of the PC293 determinant to the Lewis X determinant, Asn-linked oligosaccharides containing the PC293 determinants were

```
            Fucα(1→3)\
GalNAcβ(1→4)GlcNAcβ(1→2)Manα(1→6)\                 Fucα(1→6)\
                                    Manβ(1→4)GlcNAcβ(1→4)GlcNAc-Asn
  GalNAcβ(1→4)GlcNAcβ(1→2)Manα(1→3)/
        Fucα(1→3)/


            Fucα(1→3)\
GalNAcβ(1→4)GlcNAcβ(1→2)Manα(1→6)\                       Fucα(1→6)\
                                     Manβ(1→4)GlcNAcβ(1→4)GlcNAc-Asn
 NeuAcα(2→6)GalNAcβ(1→4)GlcNAcβ(1→2)Manα(1→3)/
```

FIGURE 4.4

Unique carbohydrates on recombinant human protein C [33, 43]. These determinants were shown to inhibit selectin-mediated adhesion [222].

tested for binding to E-selectin. Surprisingly, oligosaccharides containing the PC293 determinants had a higher affinity for E-selectin than the natural ligand sialyl Lewis X [12]. Thus, based on the *in vitro* study, the carbohydrate portion of rhAPC may impart some of the observed anti-inflammatory activity discussed below in section 4.3.2. These novel oligosaccharides, present on another natural human protein, were also shown to have immunomodulating effects [37,39,40]. While the structures of the carbohydrates on plasma-derived protein C are not known, this material does contain fucosylated oligosaccharides [9], suggesting that it could contain ligands for the selectin family. This is consistent with the fact that the site of normal biosynthesis for HPC is the liver, and it is known that fucosylated oligosaccharides, including sialyl Lewis X, are produced on glycoproteins synthesized by the liver [41,42].

Overall, the rhAPC, drotrecogin alfa (activated), produced in HEK293, has shown functional differences from plasma-derived APC in *in vitro* and *in vivo* nonclinical studies with respect to its antithrombotic activity, specific anticoagulant activity [43], and circulatory half-life in nonhuman primates [38,44,45]. Besides causing bleeding at high doses, no other adverse events have been observed for either recombinant or plasma-derived human APC. To date, only drotrecogin alfa (activated), and not plasma-derived APC, has been studied in pivotal phase 3 (PROWESS) and other clinical studies of severe sepsis described below [46,47].

4.2.3   rhAPC Derivatives

In the context of the structure–function relationships of protein C, it is illustrative to briefly review select protein C derivatives described in the literature. Although current clinical experience demonstrates that human APC is an effective agent, there are several approaches one might take to improve either the processing of the molecule for APC production or the molecule itself, by the creation of site-specific changes in the amino acid backbone. An effective method was reported for expressing recombinant APC directly from cells by replacing the thrombin-cleaved activation peptide with a sequence in the insulin receptor precursor (PRPSRKRR), a substrate for the cellular insulin receptor processing protease [48]. This derivative was secreted as APC, eliminating the activation and purification steps that were necessary with the secreted zymogen. It has also been possible to increase the functional anticoagulant activity of protein C by alterations in the sites for glycosylation [4]. For example, elimination of partial glycosylation at the unusual consensus sequence N329-X-Cys resulted in a high-activity β-form protein C molecule with twice the activity of the native molecule. Forms of protein C with increased activity through improved catalysis have been described [44,49], and by altering amino acids near the thrombin cleavage site, several protein C derivatives have been created that were much more sensitive to thrombin, less dependent on TM, and less sensitive to inhibition of activation by calcium ion [49–53]. This "prodrug" form of APC was more effective than native APC when administered as a zymogen in a hamster arteriovenous shunt model [54]. Alterations in the variable region one (VR1) region of the protein C serine protease domain have demonstrated interactions critical for heparin-stimulated inhibition by protein C inhibitor (PCI), the major plasma inhibitor of APC [55]. Using structure-based design, Berg et al. [56], identified and altered key residues that conferred resistance to plasma serpin inhibitors while simultaneously maintaining functional activity. This resulted in derivatives with longer functional half-lives in animal models. Finally, by altering the Gla domain, derivatives of protein C with enhanced interaction with phospholipid have been created that show increased potency in anticoagulant assays and in activity in an arteriovenous shunt model [57–59].

4.3   APC Mechanisms of Action

The protein C pathway was traditionally described as an endothelial-based complex, including TM–thrombin–protein C–protein S that generates the natural anticoagulant APC [60]. Many review articles have been published on the protein C anticoagulation pathway and its role in hemostasis and thrombosis [44,45,61–66]. However, more recently described anti-inflammatory and antiapoptotic properties of APC suggest a role for APC as an endothelial cell or microvascular modulator, with properties in opposition to thrombin and proinflammatory cytokines [67–71]. In this section, we will review anticoagulant–antithrombotic mechanism of APC, but focus on more recent data describing its role as a modulator of endothelial and leukocyte function (Figure 4.5).

4.3.1   Antithrombotic Mechanism

The major physiological control of thrombin generation occurs via the protein C anticoagulant pathway. This pathway maintains normal hemostasis by controlling the conversion of prothrombin into thrombin through a feedback-inhibition mechanism (Figure 4.5). Protein C itself is a serine protease that circulates in the blood as inactive zymogen. As thrombin is generated, it complexes with TM, an endothelial surface membrane protein [61], to form the physiological enzyme complex that converts zymogen protein C into its active form. APC, along with its cofactor protein S, functions to block thrombin generation

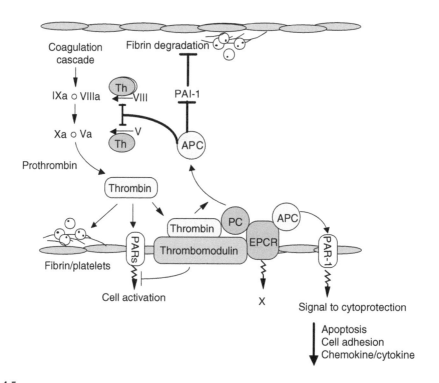

FIGURE 4.5
Mechanisms of action of activated protein C showing the feedback inhibition of thrombin generation and the signaling response mediated by interaction with the endothelial protein C receptor (EPCR) and protease activated receptor-1 (PAR-1).

by inactivating the activated forms of Factors V and VIII, thus inhibiting the prothrombinase and Factor Xase enzyme complexes, respectively. Therefore, it is the balance between thrombin's procoagulant activities (fibrin generation, platelet activation) and anticoagulant activity (APC generation) that determines a condition of either normal homeostasis or pathological thrombus formation. Because of the critical role played by the protein C pathway in maintaining normal hemostasis, factors that suppress the generation of APC or result in acquired deficiency in protein C can significantly shift this balance (discussed in detail below).

In addition to its ability to inhibit thrombin generation, APC also displays profibrinolytic activity. APC acts to enhance fibrinolysis by neutralizing plasminogen activator inhibitor one (PAI-1) [72], and possibly by preventing the activation of TAFI (thrombin-activatable fibrinolysis inhibitor) [73]. APC has also been shown to accelerate tPA-dependent clot lysis [74,75]. Studies in the canine coronary occlusion model [76] have demonstrated that rhAPC alone is capable of reperfusing occluded vessels, which was associated with suppression of PAI-1 [77]. APC has also been shown to remove PAI-1 from circulation [78], further exemplifying the potential importance of the profibrinolytic activity *in vivo*.

4.3.2 Anti-Inflammatory and Cytoprotective Mechanisms

The ability of protein C to inhibit thrombin generation could, in and of itself, reduce thrombin-mediated inflammatory effects resulting from decreased thrombin-receptor cleavage, and subsequently reduce platelet and endothelial cell activation (reviewed in [79]). However, there is growing evidence that APC has direct anti-inflammatory properties (reviewed in [44,45,64–66,80]), and modulatory effects on cellular functions. APC has been shown in supratherapeutic concentrations to inhibit the generation of cytokines such as tissue necrosis factor (TNF) and interleukin-1 (IL-1), to uncouple lipopolysaccharide (LPS) interactions with monocyte CD14, and has shown a selective inhibitory activity on the responses of human mononuclear phagocytes to LPS, interferon-γ, or phorbol ester [80–85]. However, these reported effects of APC on cytokine secretion with supratherapeutic concentrations of APC have not been demonstrated in human studies [86–88]. APC may also modulate macrophage migration inhibitory factor (MIF) [89] and, at relatively high concentrations, has been shown to inhibit LPS-induced translocation of nuclear factor κB (NF-κB) in monocytes *in vitro* [90]. Also, as indicated above, HPC can inhibit E-selectin-mediated cell adhesion via its unique carbohydrate structures [12]. Using broad transcriptional profiling, rhAPC with supratherapeutic concentrations has been shown to induce broad signaling changes in endothelial cells and to protect them from TNFα activation [69,70]. Specifically, it was found to directly modulate cell signaling and alter gene expression in two major pathways of inflammation, suppressing TNF induction of cell surface adhesion molecules (e.g., CX3C-fractalkine, ICAM-1, E-selectin, and VCAM-1), and pathways promoting antiapoptosis and cell survival [70]. Changes in these pathways have recently been confirmed in other cell systems and animal studies [91,92].

The cell-based activities of APC appear to require its interaction with the endothelial protein C receptor (EPCR) (Figure 4.5). EPCR, first identified as a receptor on the endothelium [93], plays an important role in the conversion of zymogen protein C into APC. However, in addition to its role in APC generation, mounting evidence suggests its role in the signaling responses of APC at the endothelium (Figure 4.6) [68–71,92]. In addition, EPCR-dependent cell signaling can function through the protease-activated receptors (PAR-1, PAR-2, and PAR-3) [71,94]. EPCR appears to be restricted to the endothelial–leukocyte interface of the innate immune system, and is expressed on monocytes, natural

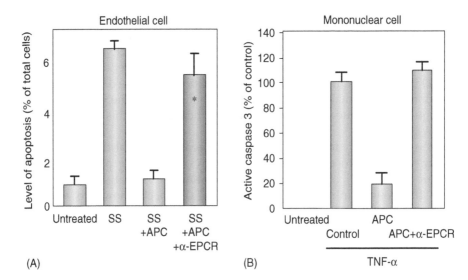

FIGURE 4.6
APC prevents the induction of apoptosis in endothelial cells (A) and the monocyte cell line U937 (B) and is dependent on interaction with the endothelial protein C receptor (EPCR) present on both cell types. Staurosporin (SS) was as described in [70] and blocking by pretreatment of U937 monocytes with 1 µg/mL antiEPCR monoclonal antibody JRT 1495. (Obtained from Dr Charles Esmon; Oklahoma Medical Research Foundation, Oklahoma City, USA.)

killer cells [95], neutrophils [96], and eosinophils [97]. The presence of EPCR on both human monocytes and cultured U937 cells appears to mediate the suppression of staurosporine-induced apoptosis by rhAPC (Figure 4.6) [69]. In addition, although the expression of EPCR on neutrophils is low, APC reduced response to certain chemotaxis agents in EPCR-expressing neutrophils as well as in eosinophils [97]. However, neither neutrophils nor eosinophils [97] were resistant to apoptosis with APC treatment, suggesting possible differences in response to EPCR signaling in different leukocyte populations or differences in APC dose response. The ability of APC to modulate both the endothelial and select leukocyte responses to inflammatory stimuli through the same receptor suggests a tight coupling at the vascular interface.

4.4   APC Pharmacology and Therapeutic Rationale

In this section, we will review the preclinical pharmacology of APC and the rationale for the clinical use of APC. However, in light of the approved use of drotrecogin alfa (activated), (Xigris), we will focus most of the discussion on severe sepsis.

4.4.1   Antithrombotic Activity of APC

APC (both plasma-derived and recombinant) has been shown to be an effective antithrombotic in a wide variety of venous and arterial thrombosis models (reviewed in [44,45,62]), and in a variety of species ranging from rodents to nonhuman primates [38,76,98–107]. Figure 4.7 provides an example of the antithrombotic activity of drotrecogin alfa (activated) and shows how it acts effects as a profibrinolytic agent by reducing PAI-1 levels.

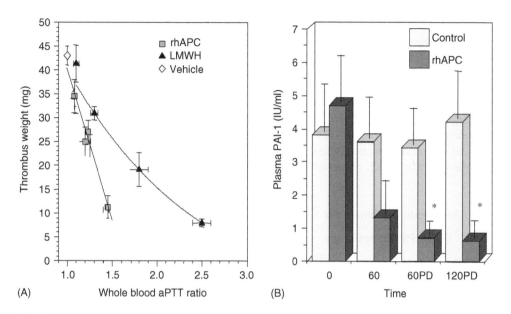

(A) Whole blood aPTT ratio

(B) Time

FIGURE 4.7

(A) Antithrombotic activity comparing drotrecogin alfa (activated) vs. low-molecular-weight heparin (LMWH) in a guinea-pig arteriovenous shunt model [57]. Data show that drotrecogin alfa (activated) reduces thrombus weight at lower systemic anticoagulant level relative to a traditional anticoagulant. (B) APC enhances fibrinolytic activity by suppressing plasminogen activator inhibitor-1 (PAI-1) in a canine coronary occlusion model [77].

Both plasma-derived APC and drotrecogin alfa (activated) have shown efficacy as an adjunctive therapy to thrombolytics [76,108–110].

In addition to these animal studies, the importance of protein C as a critical modulator of thrombin generation is clearly demonstrated by homozygous protein C-deficient individuals, who generally suffer from life-threatening neonatal purpura fulminans. While heterozygous protein C deficiency is generally not life threatening, many of these patients suffer from recurrent thrombotic episodes and, in those treated with coumadin, commonly present coumadin-induced skin necrosis [111]. Treatment of both of these genetically deficient patient groups with plasma concentrates containing HPC or APC as replacement therapy has been successful [62,112–122]. Dramatic treatment effects have been reported with plasma-derived human APC or rhAPC in congenital protein C-deficient patients with acute crisis purpura fulminans [123,124]. As added evidence for its role in microvascular thrombosis, APC has shown efficacy in the treatment of disseminated intravascular coagulopathy (DIC) in a phase 3 study, in a small number of cancer patients, and in patients with placental abruption [125–128]. In addition, plasma-derived human APC has also been used in the treatment of veno-occlusive disease of the liver after bone marrow transplantation, and as adjunctive therapy to thrombolytics in patients with acute myocardial infarction [129,130].

4.4.2 Efficacy in Models of Ischemic Injury

APC has been shown to be effective in models of ischemic stroke in both the rabbit [131] and mouse [92,132]. Reduced ICAM-1 expression and reduced tissue CD11b were observed in the murine model, indicating the likelihood of reduced neutrophil extravasation [132]. Moreover, efficacy was demonstrated to be dependent on both EPCR and PAR-1 or PAR-3

[94], suggesting that the cell-signaling mechanisms described above are required for APC's observed efficacy. Murakami et al. [133] showed in a rat model that APC could attenuate endotoxin-induced pulmonary vascular injury by inhibiting activated leukocytes. Moreover, APC was shown to reduce ischemia or reperfusion-induced renal injury in rats by inhibiting leukocyte activation [134]. Overall, these effects on leukocyte function *in vivo* are consistent with the mechanistic data of EPCR-dependent signaling and suppression of cell adhesion molecules from endothelial studies (Figure 4.8) [69,70]. APC has also shown efficacy in cardiac ischemic injury models [135]. These data suggest that APC, in addition to its effectiveness in severe sepsis (as discussed below), may be effective in reducing ischemic tissue damage in disorders such as stroke, cardiogenic shock, and acute renal failure.

4.4.3   Therapeutic Rationale for Sepsis

4.4.3.1   *Sepsis Pathophysiology*

Severe sepsis is a devastating disorder with high morbidity and mortality. Even with advances in supportive care, severe sepsis carries a mortality rate of 30 to 50% [136–142], and the incidence is expected to increase over the next decade [143,144]. In considering a role for protein C in sepsis pathogenesis and treatment, it is instructive to review briefly the pathophysiology of sepsis and septic shock. In-depth reviews on this topic can be found in many sources [72,145–153]. Severe sepsis results from a complex host response to insult following infection. Figure 4.9 depicts a simplified schematic representation of the series of events from insult (e.g., infection), through the release of various inflammatory and cytotoxic mediators, to vascular dysfunction, end-organ dysfunction, and death.

In the early events leading to severe sepsis, the host response results in the activation of a number of systems aimed at getting rid of the infection. The elucidation of cytokines such as TNFα following insult initiates cell surface activation, affecting a number of pathways (e.g., oxidation, adhesion, cytokine release, apoptosis, and nitric oxide production) as well as releasing a tissue factor that further contributes to inflammation through thrombin-induced activation of endothelium, platelets, and vascular smooth muscle [154]. These responses, however, can directly damage the vascular endothelium [146,155], resulting in neutrophil–endothelial cell adhesion, mononuclear cell adhesion, and tissue-factor-dependent activation of the coagulation cascade [150,156]. These responses can set in play a cycle

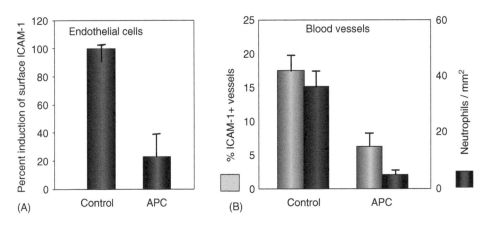

FIGURE 4.8
APC reduces the cell adhesion molecule ICAM in (A) cultured endothelial cells as described in [70] and (B) an ischemic stroke model. (Adapted from Shibata, et al., *Circulation*, 103, 1799–1805, 2001.)

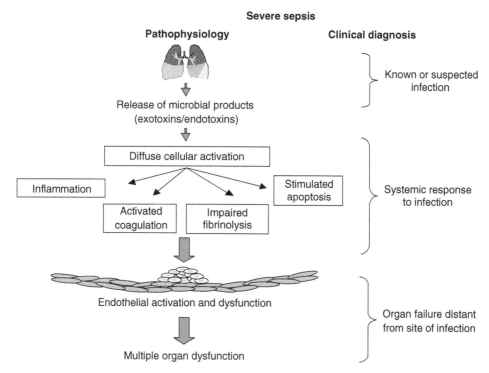

FIGURE 4.9

Schematic representation of the pathogenesis of sepsis leading to endothelial dysfunction, organ failure, and death (see text for details).

of further exacerbation of inflammation, proinflammatory mediator release, endothelial injury, tissue factor expression, and thrombin production, which leads to enhanced microvascular coagulation and endothelial cell dysfunction. Ultimately, microvascular function is compromised, which results in DIC and microvascular thrombosis, decreased tissue perfusion and hypoxemia, and resultant organ dysfunction and failure [145,148,157–161].

There is growing evidence for the role of apoptosis in systemic inflammatory response leading to severe sepsis. One may conclude that organ-specific cell death involving both parenchymal and microvascular endothelium underlies organ dysfunction, with increased apoptotic rates occurring in organ dysfunction [162–165]. Hematopoetic, hepatic, renal, pulmonary, and cardiac systems can each sustain some degree of apoptotic insult in sepsis [163]. The proinflammatory effects, including oxidation, nitric oxide production, enhanced adhesion, and TNF production, are intimately linked to endothelial apoptosis [164]. While apoptosis appears to be important in end-organ dysfunction, it also contributes to the amplification of the coagulation defect, as apoptotic endothelium is highly procoagulant [166].

4.4.3.2 Role of Protein C Pathway in Sepsis

The protein C pathway functions to maintain normal homeostasis, but following systemic inflammatory response, protein C is consumed and endothelial damage impairs both its activation and function via TM and EPCR [156,167]. The reduced endothelial expression of TM is likely due to both suppression of its expression by cytokines and its release from the endothelial surface by neutrophil elastase [168–170]. In addition to these procoagulant changes in sepsis, antifibrinolytic changes also come into play in response to endothelial damage [149,171,172]. Following an inflammatory insult, the initial fibrinolytic process is followed by profound and sustained inhibition [171], and this fibrinolytic deactivation appears to occur independent of the changes in coagulation [149]. The resulting deficiency in the function of the protein C pathway, along with suppressed fibrinolysis from increased levels of PAI-1 and TAFI [72,148,158,159,173,174], result in an inability to maintain normal homeostasis.

There have been a number of studies showing that a reduced protein C level is strongly correlated with mortality in both sepsis and septic shock [147,175–183]. Moreover, protein C deficiency appears to develop well before the onset of defined clinical parameters of severe sepsis or septic shock [148,158,184,185], and may be considered a prognostic indicator (reviewed in [151]). Reduction in protein C levels in sepsis patients has been suggested to be the cause of multiorgan failure [186] and low levels of protein C have been associated with multiorgan dysfunction and death in bone marrow transplant patients [187].

Considering its key role in maintaining normal hemostasis, a role for APC in sepsis therapy was further supported by suggestions that blocking DIC and the microthrombi that might promote end-organ dysfunction ought to be a target for clinical treatment in sepsis [150,171]. Work in model systems demonstrated that APC was in fact a key player in the pathogenesis of sepsis and that treatment with APC (or rhAPC) could inhibit DIC and reduce mortality in the baboon lethal *Escherichia coli* model [188,189]. Furthermore, anecdotal reports suggested success using protein C as an adjunct to aggressive conventional therapy in the management of numerous cases of coagulopathy and purpura fulminans in meningococcal sepsis [62,84,190–197] and Gram-positive sepsis [196,198]. A phase-2, placebo-controlled dose ranging study with plasma-derived HPC, not powered to show mortality outcome, has also been conducted [199,200].

4.4.3.3   APC Mechanism and Sepsis

As discussed above, homeostasis is lost in sepsis, resulting in an uncontrolled cascade of coagulation, inflammation, and endothelial cell dysfunction. APC functions by reducing thrombin generation and, via cell signaling, may modulate anti-inflammatory and cytoprotective mechanisms. Considering the prominent role of microvascular coagulation in sepsis and the major role of protein C in normal hemostasis, a major mechanism for the benefit of rhAPC is likely to be its direct antithrombotic activity, which prevents microvascular thrombosis, vascular congestion, and resulting organ failure. However, several animal studies with other antithrombotic/anticoagulants, while effective at inhibiting the DIC, did not reduce mortality [64,189,195]. Coupled with the failure of both tissue factor pathway inhibitor (TFPI) and antithrombin III (ATIII) in a large phase–III sepsis trial, it would appear that correcting the coagulation defect in sepsis, while probably necessary, may not be sufficient to provide a mortality benefit.

Given these data, the mechanism of APC's efficacy in the treatment of sepsis is also likely to require the EPCR-dependent effects that have been described in preclinical studies above, both suppressing endothelial activation and modulating the innate immune system. The ability of APC to suppress molecules such as ICAM, VCAM, and E-selectin may be important in light of the critical early role of cell adhesion in the inflammatory response and in sepsis [201–204]. Under normal circumstances, the vascular endothelium controls a number of regulatory mechanisms to modulate coagulation, inflammation, and vascular function to maintain homeostatic balance in the local environment [72,205]. During infection or inflammatory insult, the endothelium becomes activated, begins to initiate the expression of proinflammatory cytokines, chemokines, and cell surface adhesion molecules required for leukocyte adhesion and migration (reviewed in [67,206–208]). This adaptive response plays a critical role in host defense, protecting the endothelium from a variety of insults from toxins, sheer/oxidative stress, endotoxin, hypoxia, and various cytokines. However, in extreme inflammatory insult as it occurs in sepsis, this balance appears to be lost, resulting in unregulated endothelial activation that leads to an enhanced cascade of proinflammatory or procoagulant activity, and cell death. The possibility that APC can modulate endothelial function and protect it from inflammatory and apoptotic insult is an attractive hypothesis.

4.5 Clinical Development of Drotrecogin Alfa (Activated) for Severe Sepsis

Severe sepsis has been extremely challenging to dissect both in terms of defining its patho-physiology, and in defining targets for therapeutic intervention. Severe sepsis (sepsis associated with acute organ dysfunction) and septic shock (sepsis associated with hypo-tension) represent the more severe complications of an uncontrolled immune response to infection and are the most common causes of death in noncoronary intensive care units, with estimated mortality rates ranging between 30 and 50% [209]. The last decade has seen a significant advance in understanding this complex disorder, focused on the tight inter-play and coupling of inflammation, microvascular coagulation, and endothelial cell dys-function. In line with this changing view, studies with rhAPC were initiated, and early phase studies demonstrated a treatment benefit [210,211]. This prompted the initiation of the PROWESS trial, a phase III, placebo-controlled, international, blinded, randomized, 28-day all-cause mortality study, which showed reduced mortality among rhAPC-treated patients [47]. The following section will summarize the clinical development of drotrecogin alfa (activated) that led to its approval by global regulatory agencies. It is currently avail-able in over 50 countries for the treatment of severe sepsis. Details of the labeled indication for Xigris can be found at the following websites: http://www.emea.eu.int/humandocs/ Humans/EPAR/xigris/xigris.htm and http://www.fda.gov/cder/biologics/products/ droteli112101.htm

4.5.1 Clinical Experience with Drotrecogin Alfa (Activated)

Drotrecogin alfa (activated) was first tested in humans in 1995. At the time of the writing of this review, over 300 normal, healthy subjects have participated in multiple studies demon-strating the safety and pharmacokinetic profile of the protein. Regulatory approval of drotrecogin alfa (activated) was based on data from a single, randomized, placebo-con-trolled, phase III study [47] with supporting data from a single, randomized, placebo-con-trolled, phase II study [46]. The phase II study, completed in 1998, investigated multiple infusion rates and infusion durations of 48 and 96 h. Measures of coagulopathy (D-dimer, platelet count, fibrinogen level) was the primary endpoint of the effect of drotrecogin alfa (activated). In most patients, the platelet count and fibrinogen levels were normal and no effect of drotrecogin alfa (activated) therapy was observed [46]. However, concentrations of D-dimer were elevated in almost all patients. The decrease in D-dimer was only evident with infusion rates of 24 mcg/kg/h or higher and concentrations were maximally decreased following with 96 h infusions [46]. Mortality for all drotrecogin alfa (activated) patients ($n = 90$) was 28.9%, compared with 34.1% for placebo patients ($n = 41$). Based on the results of this study, the dose of 24 mcg/kg/h for 96 h was chosen for phase III testing.

The phase III study (PROWESS) was a randomized, placebo-controlled study of drotre-cogin alfa (activated) as well as a study of the best standard care for the treatment of adult patients with severe sepsis [47]. The study was discontinued in the summer of 2000 at its second interim analysis because the observed survival benefit in the drotrecogin alfa (acti-vated) group exceeded the predefined guidelines for stopping the study. In total, 1690 patients were randomized and received the study drug. Patients treated with drotrecogin alfa (activated) experienced a statistically significant reduction ($p = 0.005$) in 28-day all-cause mortality (Figure 4.10). The beneficial effect of drotrecogin alfa (activated) was observed in almost all subgroups examined [212]. Although relative reduction in the risk of death associated with drotrecogin alfa (activated) was similar across subgroups, absolute reductions in the risk of death were larger for more severely ill patients. Based on these subgroup analyses, regulatory agencies restricted the use of drotrecogin alfa (activated) to patients at high risk of death (in United States Package Insert [USPI]) or with multiple organ failure (in European Union Summary of Product Characteristics [EU SPC]). Analyses of serial measures of organ function demonstrated that drotrecogin alfa (activated)-treated patients experienced (1) more rapid resolution of cardiovascular organ dysfunction associated with more rapid withdrawal of vasopressor support [213]; (2) improvement in respiratory compared to placebo; and (3) reduced frequency of new hematologic dysfunction (as assessed by platelet count) [214]. The improvement in organ function and in survival resulted in drotrecogin alfa (activated) patients being discharged more rapidly from the study hospital. The mechanism by which drotrecogin alfa (activated) improved cardiovascular function in the phase III study is unknown. However, drotrecogin alfa (activated) was shown to prevent the rapid occurrence of hypotension in healthy subjects administered an intravenous dose of endotoxin [88].

For the safety assessment of drotrecogin alfa (activated), the only observed adverse drug reaction was an increase in the incidence of bleeding complications in treated patients. A higher percentage of drotrecogin alfa (activated) patients experienced a serious bleeding complication as compared with the placebo-treated patients (3.5% vs. 2.0%, $p = 0.06$) [47]. This difference was primarily related to events that occurred during the infusion period; 2.4% of drotrecogin alfa (activated) patients experienced a serious bleeding complication vs. 1.0% of placebo patients. Risk factors for a serious bleeding complication associated with drotrecogin alfa (activated) appeared to be invasive procedures and severe thrombocytopenia (platelet count <30,000/mL³). A subsequent review published in 2003 analyzed safety data from adult patients receiving drotrecogin alfa (activated) in clinical trials ($n = 2786$) and under commercial use (approximately 4000 patients) [215]. Serious bleeding complications occurred during the infusion period in 2.8% of the patients. Serious bleeding complications or central nervous system (CNS) bleeding events spontaneously reported from commercial use occurred in an estimated 0.9 and 0.2% of patients, respectively. Rates of CNS bleeding for placebo-treated patients in a number of severe sepsis studies ranged between 0.1 and 0.4% [47,216,217].

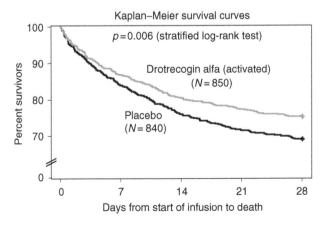

FIGURE 4.10
Effect of drotrecogin alfa (activated) on 28-day all-cause mortality in severe sepsis. (Adapted from Bernard, et al., *New Engl. J. Med.*, 344, 699–705, 2001.)

However, given its anticoagulant properties, the administration of drotrecogin alfa (activated) is associated with a small but definite risk of bleeding.

4.5.2 Mechanistic Observations from the Clinical Experience

As described above, preclinical studies have suggested several mechanisms by which APC might exert its efficacy in severe sepsis. Analysis of the clinical experience with drotrecogin alfa (activated) has brought about a reexamination of these mechanisms. Pharmacodynamic analyses of data obtained from the phase III study demonstrated that compared to placebo, the administration of drotrecogin alfa (activated) resulted in a significant increase in both prothrombin time (PT) and activated partial thromboplastin time (APTT) and a reduction in markers of thrombin generation, confirming both the anticoagulant and antithrombotic properties of the protein [86]. The anticoagulant effect was evident only during the infusion of drotrecogin alfa (activated), but given its short half-life, this effect would be likely to dissipate within 2 h of discontinuation of the infusion [218]. However, the profibrinolytic effect was less clearly demonstrated with only a statistical trend in lower PAI-1 levels observed in the drotrecogin alfa (activated) treatment arm. Furthermore, carriers of the prothrombotic single nucleotide polymorphism, factor V Leiden, who are known to be partially resistant to the anticoagulant activity of APC, derived similar treatment benefit from rhAPC as non-Leiden carriers in severe sepsis [219]. These clinical data from rhAPC studies strongly suggest that additional biological activities of rhAPC beyond its antithrombotic activity provide survival benefit in the treatment of severe sepsis [219,220].

Direct or indirect anti-inflammatory activity of drotrecogin alfa (activated) was less well demonstrated in clinical studies. Although a dose-dependent and statistically significant reduction in IL-6 levels was observed in the phase II study [46], only a slightly more rapid reduction in IL-6 levels was observed in drotrecogin alfa (activated)-treated patients as compared with placebo-treated patients in the phase III study. Exploratory analyses of other measured cytokines (TNF-α, IL-β, IL-8, and IL-10) did not show statistical differences between treatment groups in the latter study [86]. Additionally, studies in healthy volunteers who were administered a single dose of endotoxin with or without the concomitant administration of drotrecogin alfa (activated) failed to demonstrate any direct effect of therapy on the observed cytokine profile [87,88]. Taken together, these data suggest that drotrecogin alfa (activated) has minimal to no effect on the early response cytokines that characterize the acute response to infection. However, later-phase markers of immunomodulation were not assessed, and the current marker analysis would be unlikely to detect a direct impact by APC on endothelial or leukocyte function as described above. Although the exact mechanism by which drotrecogin alfa (activated) exerts its beneficial effects is unclear, it is highly likely that both the antithrombotic–profibrinolytic and the anti-inflammatory–cytoprotective properties (although less well understood) are important to the overall beneficial effect.

4.6 Summary and Conclusions

The critical nature of the protein C pathway in the control of normal hemostasis has intrigued investigators for decades, and has suggested the possibility of developing novel agents for the treatment of a variety of disorders, including sepsis. While we have long considered APC as an important antithrombotic modulator that provides feedback inhibition of coagulation, the emerging data suggests that APC is an agent that effectively modulates the complex network changes that occur during multisystem activation and

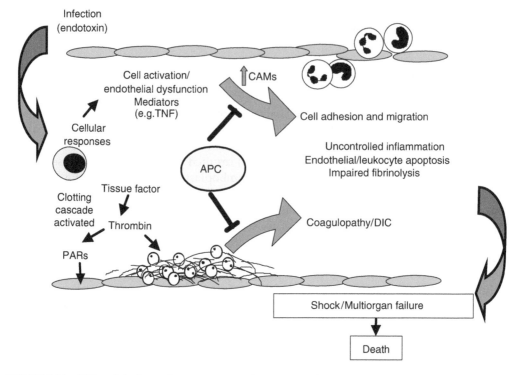

FIGURE 4.11 APC and the innate immune response in severe sepsis.

dysfunction in sepsis. In states of systemic inflammatory activation, loss of protein C results in a compromised ability to modulate coagulation, inflammatory, and cell survival functions, leading to vascular dysfunction, end-organ failure, and death (Figure 4.11). Drotrecogin alfa (activated), has been shown to reduce mortality in patients with severe sepsis. While the exact mechanism by which it improves survival is unknown, the data suggest that the pleripotent properties of the protein function at the endothelial interface to protect the organism from vascular insult and to prolong endothelial, cellular, and organ survival. Ongoing clinical trials of drotrecogin alfa (activated) will continue to refine the optimal use of this therapy, in conjunction with other therapies, to continue to improve outcomes in severe sepsis [221]. Moreover, the properties of drotrecogin alfa (activated) suggest that it will be useful in other disorders that result in microvascular coagulopathy, endothelial dysfunction, and vascular bed failure.

References

1. Beckmann, R.J., et al., The structure and evolution of a 461 amino acid human protein C precursor and its messenger RNA, based upon the DNA sequence of cloned human liver cDNAs, *Nucleic Acids Res.*, 13, 5233–5247, 1985.
2. Foster, D.C., et al., Propeptide of human protein C is necessary for gamma-carboxylation, *Biochemistry*, 26, 7003–7011, 1987.
3. Drakenberg, T., et al., β-Hydroxyaspartic acid in vitamin K-dependent protein C., *Proc. Natl. Acad. Sci. USA*, 80, 1802–1806, 1983.

4. Grinnell, B.W., Walls, J.D., and Gerlitz, B., Glycosylation of human protein C affects its secretion, processing, functional activities and activation by thrombin, *J. Biol. Chem.*, 226, 9778–9785, 1991.

5. Miletich, J.P. and Broze, G.J., Beta protein C is not glycosylated at asparagine 329, *J. Biol. Chem.*, 265, 11397–11404, 1990.

6. Harris, R.J. and Spellman, M.W., *O*-linked fucose and other post-translational modifications unique to EGF modules, *Glycobiology*, 3, 219–224, 1993.

7. McClure, D.B., Walls, J.D., and Grinnell, B.W., Post-translational processing events in the secretion pathway of human protein C, a complex vitamin K-dependent antithrombotic factor, *J. Biol. Chem.*, 267, 19710–19717, 1992.

8. Yan, S.C.B., Grinnell, B.W., and Wold, F., Post-translational modifications of protein: Some problems left to solve, *Trends Biochem. Sci.*, 14, 264–268, 1989.

9. Yan, S.B., et al., Characterization and novel purification of recombinant human protein C from three mammalian cell lines, *Bio/Technology*, 8, 655–661, 1990.

10. Gerlitz, B., et al., Effect of mutation of Asp71 on human protein C activation and function, *J. Cell. Biochem.*, 14E, 201, 1990.

11. Grinnell, B.W., et al., Native and modified recombinant human protein C: Function secretion and posttranslational modifications, in *Protein C and Related Anticoagulants*, Bruley, D. and Drohan, W., Eds., Gulf Publishing Co., Houston, 1990, pp. 13–46.

12. Grinnell, B.W., Hermann, R.B., and Yan, S.B., Human protein C inhibits selectin-mediated cell adhesion: Role of unique fucosylated oligosaccharide, *Glycobiology*, 4, 221–225, 1994.

13. Grinnell, B.W., et al., Trans-activated expression of fully gamma-carboxylated recombinant human protein C, an antithrombotic factor, *Bio/Technology*, 5, 1189–1192, 1987.

14. Grinnell, B.W., et al., Expression and characterization of fully functional recombinant human protein C from the human kidney cell line 293, in *Current Advances in Vitamin K Research*, Suttie, J.W., Ed., Elsevier, New York, 1988, pp. 191–198.

15. Fisher, B.E., and Will, H., Effects of intact fibrin and partially plasmin-degraded fibrin on kinetic properties of one-chain tissue plasminogen activator, *Biochem. Biophys. Acta*, 1041, 48–54, 1990.

16. Suttie, J.W., Report of workshop on expression of vitamin K-dependent proteins in bacterial and mammalian cells, *Thromb. Res.*, 44, 129–134, 1986.

17. Oppenheimer, C. and Wydro, R., *Cellular Processing of Vitamin K-Dependent Proteins*, Suttie, J.W., Ed., Elsevier, New York, 1988.

18. Anson, D.S., Austen, D.E.G., and Brownlee, G.G., Expression of active human clotting factor IX from recombinant DNA clones in mammalian cells, *Nature*, 315, 683–685, 1985.

19. de la Salle, H., et al., Active gamma-carboxylated human factor IX expressed using recombinant DNA techniques, *Nature*, 316, 268–270, 1985.

20. Busby, S., et al., Expression of active human factor IX in transfected cells, *Nature*, 316, 271–273, 1985.

21. Graham, F.L., *Transformation by and Oncogenicity of Human Adenoviruses*, Ginsberg, H.S., Ed., Plenum Press, New York, 1984, pp. 631–639.

22. Berg, D.T., et al., Viral transformation increases vitamin K-dependent gamma-carboxylation of glutamate, *Exp. Cell Res.*, 192, 32–40, 1991.

23. Berg, D.T., Walls, J., and Grinnell, B.W., A variant enhancer/regulatory region from a cloned human prototype BK virus genome, *Nucleic Acids Res.*, 16, 9057, 1988.

24. Berg, D.T., et al., E1A-induced enhancer activity of the poly(dG-dT).poly(dA-dC) element (GT element) and interactions with a GT-specific nuclear factor, *Mol. Cell. Biol.*, 9, 5248–5253, 1989.

25. Berg, D.T., McClure, D.B., and Grinnell, B.W., E1a-responsive mammalian host/vector system for the stable high-level expression of secreted proteins, *Nucleic Acids Res.*, 20, 5485–5486, 1992.

26. Berg, D.T., McClure, D.B., and Grinnell, B.W., High-level expression of secreted proteins from cell adapted to serum-free suspension culture, *Biotech.*, 6, 972–978, 1993.

27. Walls, J.D. and Grinnell, B.W., A rapid and versatile method for the detection and isolation of mammalian cell lines secreting recombinant proteins, *Biotechniques*, 8, 138–142, 1990.

28. Walls, J.D., et al., Amplification of multicistronic plasmids in the human 293 cell line and secretion of correctly processed recombinant human protein C, *Gene*, 81, 139–149, 1989.

29. Yan, S.B., Review of conformation-specific affinity purification methods for plasma vitamin K-dependent proteins, *J. Mol. Recognition*, 9, 211–218, 1996.

30. Foster, D.C., et al., Endoproteolytic processing of the dibasic cleavage site in the human protein C precursor in transfected mammalian cells: Effects of sequence alterations on efficiency of cleavage, *Biochemistry*, 29, 347–354, 1990.

31. Kisiel, W., Human plasma protein C: Isolation, characterization, and mechanism of activation by alpha-thrombin, *J. Clin. Invest.*, 64, 761–769, 1979.

32. Cumming, D.A., Glycosylation of recombinant protein therapeutics: Control and functional implications, *Glycobiology*, 1, 115–130, 1991.

33. Yan, S.B., Chao, Y.B., and van Halbeek, H., Novel Asn-linked oligosaccharides terminating in GalNAcβ(1-4)[Fucα(1-3)]GalNAcβ(1-2) are present in recombinant human protein C expressed in human kidney 293 cells, *Glycobiology*, 3, 597–608, 1993.

34. Chan, A.L., et al., A novel sialylated *N*-acetylgalactosamine-containing oligosaccharide is the major complex-type structure present in Bowes melanoma tissue plasminogen activator, *Glycobiology*, 1, 173–185, 1991.

35. Bergwerff, A.A., et al., Human urokinase contains GalNAcβ(1-4)[Fucα(1-3)]GlcNAcβ(1-2) as a novel terminal element in *N*-linked carbohydrate chains, *FEBS Lett.*, 314, 389–394, 1992.

36. Tomiya, N., et al., Structural elucidation of a variety of GalNAc-containing *N*-linked oligosaccharides from human urinary kallidinogenase, *J. Biol. Chem.*, 268, 113–126, 1993.

37. Dell, A., et al., Structural analysis of the oligosaccharide derived from glycodelin, a human glycoprotein with potent immunosuppresive and contraceptive activities, *J. Biol. Chem.*, 270, 24116–24126, 1995.

38. Gruber, A., et al., Inhibition of thrombus formation by activated recombinant protein C in a primate model of arterial athrombosis, *Circulation*, 82, 578–585, 1990.

39. Morris, H., et al., Gender-specific glycosylation of human glycodelin affects its contraceptive activity, *J. Biol. Chem.*, 271, 32159–32167, 1996.

40. van den Nieuwenhof, I., et al., Recombinant glycodelin carrying the same type of glycan structure as contraceptive glycodelin-A can be produced in human kidney 293 cells but not in Chinese hamster ovary cells, *Eur. J. Biochem.*, 267, 4753–4762, 2000.

41. De Graaf, T.W., et al., Inflammation-induced expression of sialyl Lewis X-containing Glycan structures on α1-acid glycoprotein (orosomucoid) in human sera, *J. Exp. Med.*, 177, 657–666, 1993.

42. Walz, G., et al., Recognition by ELAM-1 of the sialys-LeX determinant on myeloid and tumor cell, *Science*, 250, 1132–1135, 1990.

43. Yan, S.B., Chao, B.Y., and van Halbeek, H., Novel oligosaccharide structures on recombinant human protein C expressed in human kidney 293 cells, *J. Cell Biochem.*, 16D, 151, 1992.

44. Yan, S.B. and Grinnell, B.W., Recombinant human protein C, protein S and thrombomodulin as antithrombotics, *Perspective Drug Discovery Des.*, 1, 503–520, 1994.

45. Yan, S.B. and Grinnell, B.W., Antithrombotic and anti-inflammatory agents of the protein C anticoagulant pathway, *Ann. Rep. Med. Chem.*, 11, 103–112, 1994.

46. Bernard, G., et al., Safety and dose-relationship of recombinant human activated protein C (rhAPC) on coagulopathy in severe sepsis, *Crit. Care Med.*, 29, 2051–2059, 2001.

47. Bernard, G., et al., Efficacy and safety of recombinant human activated protein C for severe sepsis, *New Engl. J. Med.*, 344, 699–705, 2001.

48. Ehrlich, H.J., et al., Direct expression of recombinant activated human protein C, a serine protease, *J. Biol. Chem.*, 264, 14298–14304, 1989.

49. Richardson, M.A., Gerlitz, B., and Grinnell, B.W., Charge reversal at the P3′ position in protein C optimally enhances thrombin affinity and activation rate, *Protein Sci.*, 3, 711–712, 1994.

50. Ehrlich, H.J., et al., Recombinant human protein C derivatives: Altered response to calcium resulting in enhanced activation by thrombin, *EMBO J.*, 9, 2367–2373, 1990.

51. Richardson, M.A., Gerlitz, B., and Grinnell, B.W., Enhancing protein C interaction with thrombin results in a clot-activated antcoagulant, *Nature*, 360, 261–264, 1992.

52. Rezaie, A.R., et al., Mutation of Glu 80 to Lys results in a protein C mutant, that no longer requires Ca^{2+} for rapid activation by the thrombin-thrombomodulin complex, *J. Biol. Chem.*, 269, 3151–3154, 1994.

53. Rezaie, A.R. and Esmon, C.T., The function of calcium in protein C activation by thrombin and thrombin–thrombomodulin complex can be distinguished by mutational analysis of protein C derivatives, *J. Biol. Chem.*, 267, 26104–26109, 1992.

54. Kurz, K.D., et al., Antithrombotic efficacy in the guinea pig of a derivative of human protein C with enhanced activation by thrombin, *Blood*, 89, 534–540, 1997.

55. Glasscock, N.L., et al., Basic residues in the 37-loop of activated protein C modulate inhibition by protein C inhibitor but not by alpha (1) -antitrypsin, *Biochim. Biophys. Acta*, 1647, 106–117, 2003.

56. Berg, D.T., et al., Engineering the proteolytic specificity of activated protein C improves its pharmacological properties, *Proc. Natl. Acad. Sci. USA*, 100, 4423–4428, 2003.

57. Kurz, K.D., et al., Comparison in an arteriovenous (AV) shunt model of thrombosis in the guinea pig of the antithrombotic and anticoagulant activities of a gla-domain variant of human activated Protein C (APC) with native APC and with a low molecular weight heparin (LMWH), *Blood*, 100, 281a, 2002.

58. Shen, L., et al., Enhancement of human protein C function by site-directed mutagenesis of the gamma-carboxyglutamic acid domain, *J. Biol. Chem.*, 273, 31086–31091, 1998.

59. Nelsestuen, G., Enhancement of vitamin-K-dependent protein function by modification of the gamma-carboxyglutamic acid domain: Studies of protein C and factor VII, *Trends Cardiovasc. Med.*, 9, 162–167, 1999.

60. Esmon, C.T., The protein C anticoagulant pathway, *Arterioscler. Thromb.*, 12, 135–145, 1992.

61. Esmon, C.T., Molecular events that control the protein C anticoagulant pathway, *Thromb. Haemostas.*, 70, 29–35, 1993.

62. Esmon, C.T. and Schwarz, H.P., An update on clinical and basic aspects of the protein C anticoagulant pathway, *Trends Cardiovasc. Med.*, 5, 141–148, 1995.

63. Esmon, C.T., et al., The protein C pathway: New insights, *Thromb. Haemostas.*, 78, 70–74, 1997.

64. Esmon, C., The protein C pathway, *Crit. Care Med.*, 28 (Suppl. 9), S44–48, 2000.

65. Esmon, C.T., et al., Inflammation, sepsis, and coagulation, *Haematologica*, 84, 254–259, 1999.

66. Grinnell, B.W. and Yan, S.B., Novel antithrombotics based on modulation of the protein C pathway, *Coron. Artery Dis.*, 9, 89–97, 1998.

67. Horrevoets, A.J., et al., Vascular endothelial genes that are responsive to tumor necrosis factor-alpha *in vitro* are expressed in atherosclerotic lesions, including inhibitor of apoptosis protein-1, stannin, and two novel genes, *Blood*, 93, 3418–3431, 1999.

68. Grinnell, B. and Joyce, D.E., Recombinant human activated protein C: A system modulator of vascular function for treatment of severe sepsis, *Crit. Care Med.*, 29, S53–S61, 2001.

69. Joyce, D.E. and Grinnell, B.W., Recombinant human activated protein C attenuates the inflammatory response in endothelium and monocytes by modulating nuclear factor-kappaB, *Crit. Care Med.*, 30, S288–293, 2002.

70. Joyce, D.E., et al., Gene expression profile of antithrombotic protein C defines new mechanisms modulating inflammation and apoptosis, *J. Biol. Chem.*, 276, 11199–11203, 2001.

71. Riewald, M., et al., Activation of endothelial cell protease activated receptor 1 by the protein C pathway, *Science*, 296, 1880–1882, 2002.

72. Vervloet, M., Thijs, L., and Hack, C., Derangements of coagulation and fibrinolysis in critically ill patients with sepsis and septic shock, *Semin. Thromb. Hemostas.*, 24, 33–44., 1998.

73. Bajzar, L., Manuel, R., and Nesheim, M.E., Purification and characterization of TAFI, a thrombin-activatable fibrinolysis inhibitor, *J. Biol. Chem.*, 270, 14477–14484, 1995.

74. Bajzar, L., Fredenburgh, J.C., and Nesheim, M., The activated protein C-mediated enhancement of tissue-type plasminogen activator-induced fibrinolysis in a cell-free system, *J. Biol. Chem.*, 265, 16948–16954, 1990.

75. Bajzar, L., Nesheim, M., and Tracy, P.B., The profibrinolytic effect of activated protein C in clots formed from plasma is TAFI-dependent, *Blood*, 88, 2093–2100, 1996.

76. Jackson, C., Bailey, B., and Shetler, T., Pharmacological profile of recombinant, human activated protein C (LY203638) in a canine model of coronary artery thrombosis, *J. Pharmacol. Exp. Ther.*, 295, 967–971, 2000.

77. Jackson, C.V., et al., Recombinant human activated protein C (LY203638) induced reperfusion in a canine model of occlusive coronary artery thrombosis, *Circulation*, 98, I454, 1998.

78. Esmon, C.T., et al., Regulation and functions of the protein C anticoagulant pathway, *Haematologica*, 84, 363–368, 1999.

79. Coughlin, S.R., et al., Characterization of a functional thrombin receptor: Issues and opportunities, *J. Clin. Invest.*, 89, 351–355, 1992.

80. Hancock, W.W., and Bach, F.H., Immunobiology and therapeutic applications of protein C/protein S/thrombomodulin in human and experimental allotransplantation and xenotransplantation, *Trends Cardiovasc. Med.*, 7, 174–183, 1997.

81. Grey, S.T. and Hancock, W.W., Inhibition of LPS-induced activation of human monocytes by activated protein C (APC) occurs through a novel mechanism, *J. Leukocyte Biol.*, 114 A487, 1993.

82. Grey, S., et al., Selective effects of protein C on activation of human monocytes by lipopolysaccharide, interferon-gamma or PMA: Modulation of effects on CD11b and CD14 but not CD25 or CD54 induction, *Transplant. Proc.*, 25, 2913–2914, 1993.

83. Grey, S.T., et al., Selective inhibitory effects of the anticoagulant activated protein C on the responses of human monocuclear phagocytes to LPS, IFN-γ, or phorbol ester, *J. Immunol.*, 153, 3664–3672, 1994.

84. Taylor, F.B., et al., Protein C prevents the coagulopathic and lethal effects of *E. coli* infusion in the baboon, *J. Clin. Invest.*, 79, 918–925, 1987.

85. Hancock, W.W., et al., The anticoagulants protein C and protein S display potent antiinflammatory and immunosuppressive effects relevant to transplant biology and therapy, *Transplantation Proc.*, 24, 2302–2303, 1992.

86. Dhainaut, J.F., et al., Drotrecogin alfa (activated) (recombinant human activated protein C) reduces host coagulopathy response in patients with severe sepsis, *Thromb. Haemostas.*, 90 (4), 642–653, 2003.

87. Derhaschnig, U., et al., Recombinant human activated protein C (rhAPC; drotrecogin alfa [activated]) has minimal effect on markers of coagulation, fibrinolysis, and inflammation in acute human endotoxemia, *Blood*, 102, 2093–2098, 2003.

88. Kalil, A., et al., Effects of drotrecogin alfa (activated) in human endotoxemia, *Shock*, 21, 222–229, 2004.

89. Schmide-Supprian, M., et al., Activated protein C inhibits tumor necrosis factor and macrophage migration inhibitory factor production in monocytes, *Eur. Cytokine Network*, 11, 407–413, 2000.

90. White, B., et al., Activated protein C inhibits lipopolysaccharide-induced nuclear translocation of nuclear factor kappaB (NF-kappaB) and tumour necrosis factor alpha (TNF-alpha) production in the THP-1 monocytic cell line, *Br. J. Haematol.*, 110, 130–134, 2000.

91. Mosnier, L.O. and Griffin, J.H., Inhibition of staurosporine-induced apoptosis of endothelial cells by activated protein C requires protease activated receptor-1 and endothelial cell protein C receptor, *Biochem. J.*, 8, 65–70, 2003.

92. Cheng, T., et al., Activated protein C blocks p53-mediated apoptosis in ischemic human brain endothelium and is neuroprotective, *Nat. Med.*, 9, 338–342, 2003.

93. Laszik, Z., et al., Human protein C receptor is present primarily on endothelium of large blood vessels: Implications for the control of the protein C pathway, *Circulation*, 96, 3633–3640, 1997.

94. Guo, H., et al., Activated protein C prevents neuronal apoptosis via protease activated receptors 1 and 3, *Neuron*, 41, 563–572, 2004.

95. Joyce, D.E., Nelson, D.R., and Grinnell, B.W., Leukocyte and endothelial interactions in sepsis: Relevance of the Protein C pathway, *Crit. Care Med.*, 32 (Suppl.5), S280–S286, 2004.

96. Sturn, D.H., et al., Expression and function of the endothelial protein C receptor in human neutrophils, *Blood*, 102, 1499–1505, 2003.

97. Feistritzer, C., et al., Endothelial protein C receptor-dependent inhibition of human eosinophil chemotaxis by protein C, *J. Allergy Clin. Immunol.*, 112, 375–381, 2003.

98. Gruber, A., et al., Inhibition of platelet-dependent thrombus formation by human activated protein C in a primate model, *Blood*, 73, 639–642, 1989.

99. Hanson, S.R., et al., Antithrombotic effects of thrombin-induced activation of endogenous protein C in primates, *J. Clin. Invest.*, 92, 2003–2012, 1993.

100. Araki, H., et al., Inhibitory effects of activated protein C and heparin on thrombotic arterial occlusion in rat mesenteric arteries, *Thromb. Res.*, 62, 209–216, 1991.

101. Arnlijots, B., Bergqvist, D., and Dahlback, B., Inhibition of microarterial thrombosis by bovine activated protein C in a rabbit model, *Thromb. Haemostas.*, 69, (Abstr.), 589, 1993.

102. Emerick, S.C., et al., Preclinical pharmacology of activated protein C, in *The Pharmacology and Toxicology of Proteins*, J.S. Holcenberg and J.L. Winkelhake, Eds., Anal R. Liss, Inc., New York, 1987, pp. 351–367.

103. Wakefield, T.W., et al., Deep venous thrombosis in the baboon: An experimental model, *J. Vasc. Surg.*, 14, 588–598, 1991.

104. McBane, R., et al., Antithrombotic action of endogenous porcine protein C activated with a latent porcine thrombin preparation, *Thromb. Haemostas.*, 74, 879–885, 1995.

105. Sakamoto, T., et al., Prevention of arterial reocclusion after thrombolysis with activated protein C: Comparison with heparin in a canine model of coronary artery thrombosis, *Circulation*, 90, 427–432, 1994.

106. Yamashita, T., et al., The antithrombotic effect of human activated protein C on He–Ne laser-induced thrombosis in rat mesenteric microvessels, *Thromb. Res.*, 75, 33–40, 1994.

107. Smirnov, M., et al., Low doses of activated protein C delay arterial thrombosis in rats, *Thromb. Res.*, 57, 645–650, 1991.

108. Romisch, J., et al., Activated protein C : Antithrombotic properties and influence on fibrinolysis in an animal model, *Fibrinolysis*, 5, 191–196, 1991.

109. Krishnamurti, C., et al., Enhancement of tissue plasminogen activator-induced fibrinolysis by activated protein C in endotoxin-treated rabbits, *J. Lab. Clin. Med.*, 118, 523–530, 1991.

110. Gruber, A., et al., Antithrombotic effects of combining activated protein C and urokinase in nonhuman primates, *Circulation*, 84, 2454–2462, 1991.

111. Clouse, L.H. and Comp, P.C., The regulation of hemostasis: The protein C system, *New Engl. J. Med.*, 314, 1298-1304, 1986.

112. Auberger, K., Evaluation of a new protein C concentrate and comparison of protein C assays in a child with congenital protein C deficiency, *Ann. Hematol.*, 64, 146–151, 1992.

113. De Stefano, V., et al., Replacement therapy with a purified protein C concentrate during initiation of oral anticoagulation in severe protein C congenital deficiency, *Thromb. Haemostas.*, 70, 247–249, 1993.

114. Dreyfus, M., et al., Treatment of homozygous protein C deficiency and neonatal purpura fulminans with purified protein C concentrate, *New Engl. J. Med.*, 325, 1565–1568, 1991.

115. Lewandowski, K. and Zawilska, K., New approach to the treatment of warfarin-induced skin necrosis in the protein C deficiency, *Thromb. Haemostas.*, 69, (Abstr.), 725, 1993.

116. Manco-Johnson, M. and Nuss, R., Protein C concentrate prevents peripartum thrombosis, *Am. J. Hematol.*, 40, 69–70, 1992.

117. Schramm, W., et al., Treatment of coumarin-induced skin necrosis with a monoclonal antibody purified Protein C concentrate, *Arch. Dermatol.*, 129, 753–759, 1993.

118. Schwarz, H.P., et al., Acute and long-term treatment of severe congenital protein C deficiency with protein C concentrate, *Thromb. Haemostas.*, 69, (Abstr.), 1020, 1993.

119. Dreyfus, M., et al., Replacement therapy with a monoclonal antibody purified protein C concentrate in newborns with severe congenital Protein C deficiency, *Semin. Thromb. Haemostas.*, 21, 371–381, 1995.

120. Muller, F.M., et al., Purpura fulminans in severe congenital protein C deficiency: Monitoring of treatment with protein C concentrate, *Eur. J. Pediatr.*, 155, 20–25, 1996.

121. Wada, H., Deguch, K., and Shirakawa, S., Successful treatment of deep vein thrombosis in homozygous protein C deficiency with activated protein C, *Am. J. Hematol.*, 44, 218–219, 1993.

122. Wada, H., Shirakawa, S., and Shiku, H., Multicenter trail of plasma-derived activated protein C concentrate (CTC-111) in patients with venous thrombosis associated with inherited protein C deficiency, *Blood*, 94, 111, 1999.

123. Nakayama, T., et al., A case of purpura fulminans is caused by homozygous 8857 mutation (protein C-Nagoya) and successfully treated with activated protein C concentrate, *Br. J. Haematol.*, 110, 727–730, 2000.

124. Manco-Johnson, M. and Knapp-Clevenger, R., Activated protein C concentrate reverses purpura fulminans in severe genetic protein C deficiency, *J. Pediatric Hematology/Oncology*, 26 (1), 25–27, 2004.

125. Aoki, N., A phase III clinical study of a plasma derived human activated protein C for the treatment of DIC, *J. New Remedies Clinics*, 47, 448–482, 1998.
126. Kobayashi, T., et al., Activated protein C is effective for disseminated intravascular coagulation associated with placental abruption, *Thromb. Haemostas.*, 82, 1363, 1999.
127. Okajima, K., et al., Treatment of patients with disseminated intravascular coagulation by protein C, *Am. J. Hematol.*, 33, 277–278, 1990.
128. Okajima, K., et al., Effect of protein C and activated protein C on coagulation and fibrinolysis in normal human subjects, *Thromb. Haemostas.*, 63, 48–53, 1990.
129. Sakamoto, T., et al., Effect of activated protein C on plasma plasminogen activator inhibitor activity in patients with acute myocardial infarction treated with alteplase, *J. Am. Coll. Cardiol.*, 42, 1389–1394, 2003.
130. Oh, H., et al., Activated protein C (APC) for the prevention and treatment of veno-occlusive disease (VOD) of the liver after bone marrow transplantation (BMT), *Blood*, 92, 325b, 1998.
131. Oda, Y., Tsumoto, K., and Mizokami, H., Inhibitory effect of activated protein C on the experimental cerebral infarction in rabbits, *Thromb. Haemostas.*, 69, (Abstr.), 724, 1993.
132. Shibata, M., et al., Anti-inflammatory, antithrombotic, and neuroprotective effects of activated protein C in a murine model of focal ischemic stroke, *Circulation*, 103, 1799–1805, 2001.
133. Murakami, K., et al., Activated protein C attenuates endotoxin-induced pulmonary vascular injury by inhibiting activated leukocytes in rats, *Blood*, 87, 642–647, 1996.
134. Mizutani, A., et al., Activated protein C reduces ischemia/reperfusion-induced renal injury in rats by inhibiting leukocyte activation, *Blood*, 95, 3781–3787, 2000.
135. Snow, T.R., et al., Protein C activation following coronary artery occlusion in the *in situ* porcine heart, *Circulation*, 84, 293–299, 1991.
136. Natanson, C., Anti-inflammatory therapies to treat sepsis and septic shock: A reassessment, *Crit. Care Med.*, 25, 1095–1100, 1997.
137. Zeni, F., Freeman, B., and Natanson, C., Anti-inflammatory therapies to treat sepsis and septic shock: A reassessment, *Crit. Care Med.*, 25, 1095–1100, 1997.
138. Brun-Buisson, C., et al., Incidence, risk factors and outcome of severe sepsis and septic shock in adults, *JAMA*, 274, 968–974, 1995.
139. Abraham, E., Therapies for sepsis emerging therapies for sepsis and septic shock, *West J. Med.*, 166, 195–200, 1997.
140. Sands, K., et al., Epidemiology of sepsis syndrome in 8 academic medical centers, *JAMA*, 278, 234–240, 1997.
141. Friedman, G., Silva, E., and Vincent, J.-L., Has the mortality of septic shock changed with time?, *Crit. Care Med.*, 26, 2078–2086., 1998.
142. Natanson, C., Esposito, C., and Banks, S., The sirens' songs of confirmatory sepsis trials: Selection bias and sampling error, *Crit. Care Med.*, 26, 1927–1931, 1998.
143. Linde-Zwirble, W., et al., Age-specific incidence and outcome of sepsis in the US, *Crit. Care. Med.*, 27, 33, 1999.
144. Opal, S. and Cohen, J., Clinical Gram-positive sepsis: Does it fundamentally differ from Gram-negative bacterial sepsis?, *Crit. Care Med.*, 27, 1608–1616, 1999.
145. Bone, R.C., The pathogenesis of sepsis, *Ann. Intern. Med.*, 115, 457–469, 1991.
146. Wheeler, A.P. and Bernard, G.R., Treating patients with severe sepsis, *New Engl. J. Med.*, 340, 207–214, 1999.
147. Hesselvik, J.F., et al., Protein C, protein S and C4b-binding protein in severe infection and septic shock, *Thromb. Haemostas.*, 65, 126–129, 1991.
148. Kidokoro, A., et al., Alterations in coagulation and fibrinolysis during sepsis, *Shock*, 5, 223–228, 1996.
149. Levi, M., et al., The cytokine-mediated imbalance between coagulant and anticoagulant mechanisms in sepsis and endotoxaemia, *Eur. J. Clin. Invest.*, 27, 3–9, 1997.
150. Carvalho, A.C. and Freeman, N.J., How coagulation defects alter outcome in sepsis: Survival may depend on reversing procoagulant conditions, *J. Crit. Illness*, 9, 51–75, 1994.
151. Fisher, C.J. and Yan, S.B., Protein C levels as a prognostic indicator of outcome in sepsis and related diseases, *Crit.Care Med.*, 28, S49–S56, 2000.
152. Matthay, M., Severe sepsis — a new treatment with both anticoagulant and antiinflammatory properties, *New Engl. J. Med.*, 344, 759–762, 2001.

153. Hotchkiss, R. and Karl, I.E., The pathophysiology and treament of sepsis, *New Engl. J. Med.*, 348, 138–150, 2003.
154. Coughlin, S.R., Sol Sherry lecture in thrombosis: How thrombin 'talks' to cells: Molecular mechanisms and roles *in vivo*, *Arterioscler. Thromb. Vasc. Biol.*, 18, 514–518, 1998.
155. Aird, W.C., The role of the endothelium in severe sepsis and multiple organ dysfunction syndrome, *Blood*, 101, 3765–3777, 2003.
156. Esmon, C., Inflammation and thrombosis. Mutual regulation by protein C, *Immunologist*, 6, 84–89, 1998.
157. Astiz, M. and Rackow, E., Septic shock, *Lancet*, 351, 1501-1505, 1998.
158. Lorente, J., et al., Time course of hemostatic abnormalities in sepsis and its relation to outcome, *Chest*, 103, 1536–1542, 1993.
159. Iba, T., Kidokoro, A., and Yagi, Y., The role of the endothelium in changes in procoagulant activity in sepsis, *J. Am. Coll. Surg.*, 187, 321–329, 1998.
160. Levi, M. and ten Cate, H., Disseminated intravascular coagulation, *New Engl. J. Med.*, 341, 586–592, 1999.
161. McGilvray, I.D. and Rotstein, O.D., Role of the coagulation system in the local and systemic inflammatory response, *World J. Surg.*, 22, 179–186, 1998.
162. Hotchkiss, R., et al., Sepsis-induced apoptosis causes progressive profound depletion of B and CD4+ T lymphocytes in humans, *J. Immunol.*, 166, 6952–6963, 2001.
163. Papathanassoglou, E.D., Moynihan, J.A., and Ackerman, M.H., Does programmed cell death (apoptosis) play a role in the development of multiple organ dysfunction in critically ill patients? A review and a theoretical framework, *Crit. Care Med.*, 28 (2), 537–549, 2000.
164. Stefanec, T., Endothelial apoptosis: Could it have a role in the pathogenesis and treatment of disease?, *Chest*, 117, 841–854, 2000.
165. Mahidhara, R. and Billiar, T.R., Apoptosis in sepsis, *Crit. Care Med.*, 28 (Suppl. 4), N105–113, 2000.
166. Bombeli, T., et al., Apoptotic vascular endothelial cells become procoagulant, *Blood*, 89, 2429–2442, 1997.
167. Faust, S., et al., Dysfunction of endothelial protein C activation in severe meningococcal sepsis, *New Engl. J. Med.*, 345, 408–416, 2001.
168. Conway, E.M. and Rosenberg, R.D., Tumor necrosis factor suppresses transcription of the thrombomodulin gene in endothelial cells, *Mol. Cell. Biol.*, 8, 5588–5592, 1988.
169. Takano, S., et al., Plasma thrombomodulin in health and diseases, *Blood*, 76, 2024–2029, 1990.
170. Moore, K.L., Esmon, C.T., and Esmon, N.L., Tumor necrosis factor leads to the internalization and degradation of thrombomodulin from the surface of bovine aortic endothelial cells in culture, *Blood*, 73, 159–165, 1989.
171. Levi, M., et al., Pathogenesis of disseminated intravascular coagulation in sepsis, *JAMA*, 270, 975–979, 1993.
172. Mesters, R.M., et al., Increase of plasminogen activator inhibitor levels predicts outcome of leukocytopenic patients with sepsis, *Thromb. Haemostas.*, 75, 902–907, 1996.
173. Bajzar, L., Nesheim, M.E., and Tracy, P.B., The profibrinolytic effect of activated protein C in clots formed from plasma is TAFI-dependent, *Blood*, 88, 2093–2100, 1996.
174. Bajzar, L., Morser, J., and Nesheim, M., TAFI, or plasma procarboxypeptidase B, couples the coagulation and fibrinolytic cascades through the thrombin-thromobmodulin complex, *J. Biol. Chem.*, 271, 16603–16608, 1996.
175. Roman, J., et al., Protein C, protein S and C4b-binding protein in neonatal severe infection and septic shock, *J. Perinat. Med.*, 20, 111–116, 1992.
176. Fourrier, F., et al., Septic shock, multiple organ failure and disseminated intravascular coagulation: Compared patterns of antithrombin III, protein C and protein S deficiencies, *Chest*, 101, 816–823, 1992.
177. Leclerc, F., et al., Protein C and S deficiency in severe infectious purpura of children: A collaborative study of 40 cases, *Intensive Care Med.*, 18, 202–205, 1992.
178. Alcaraz, A., et al., Activation of the protein C pathway in acute sepsis, *Thromb. Res.*, 79, 83–93, 1995.
179. Fijnvandraat, K., et al., Coagulation activation and tissue necrosis in meningococcal septic shock: Severely reduced protein C levels predict a high mortality, *Thromb. Haemostas.*, 73, 15–20, 1995.

180. Massignon, D., et al., Coagulation/fibrinolysis balance in septic shock related to cytokines and clinical state, *Haemostas.*, 24, 36–48, 1994.
181. Wuillemin, W.A., et al., Activation of the intrinsic pathway of coagulation in children with meningococcal septic shock, *Thromb. Haemostas.*, 74, 1436–1441, 1995.
182. Mesters, R., et al., Prognostic value of protein C levels in Neutropenic patients at high risk of severe septic complications, *Crit. Care Med.*, 28, 2209–2216, 2000.
183. Yan, S., et al., Low levels of protein C are associated with poor outcome in severe sepsis, *Chest*, 120, 915–922, 2001.
184. Mesters, R., et al., Factor VIIa and antithrombin III activity during severe sepsis and septic shock in neutropenic patients, *Blood*, 88, 881–886, 1996.
185. Mammen, E., The haematological manifestations of sepsis, *J. Antimicrob. Chemother.*, 41 (Suppl. A), 17–24, 1998.
186. Mesters, R.M., et al., Factor VIIa and antithrombin III activity during severe sepsis and septic shock in neutropenic patients, *Blood*, 88, 881–886, 1996.
187. Hairo, W.D., et al., Multiple organ dysfunction syndrome in bone marrow transplantation, *JAMA*, 274, 1289–1295, 1995.
188. Taylor, F.B. Jr., et al., Protein C prevents the coagulopathic and lethal effects of *Escherichia coli* infusion in the baboon, *J. Clin. Invest.*, 79, 918–925, 1987.
189. Taylor, F.B., et al., DEFR-Factor Xa blocks disseminated intravascular coagulation initiated by *E. coli* without preventing shock or organ damage, *Blood*, 78, 364–368, 1991.
190. Rivard, G.E., et al., Treatment of purpura fulminans in meningococcemia with protein C concentrate, *J. Pediatr.*, 126, 646–652, 1995.
191. Rintala, E., et al., Protein C in the treatment of coagulopathy in meningococcal disease, *Lancet*, 347, 1767, 1996.
192. Smith, O.P., White, B., and Rafferty, M., Successful treatment of meningococcal induced protein C deficiency/purpura fulminans in children with protein C concentrate and heparin, *Thromb. Haemostas.*, 97, 419, 1997.
193. Powars, D., et al., Epidemic meningococcemia and purpura fulminans with induced protein C deficiency, *Clin. Infectious Disease*, 17, 254–261, 1993.
194. Rintala, E., et al., Protein C in the treatment of coagulopathy in meningococcal disease, *Crit. Care Med.*, 26, 965–968, 1998.
195. Esmon, C.T., Introduction: Are natural anticoagulants candidates for modulating the inflammatory response to endotoxin?, *Blood*, 95, 1113–1116, 2000.
196. Smith, K., et al., Purpura fulminans and *S. pneumonia* sepsis with severe acquired protein C deficiency successfully treated with recombinant human activated protein C, *Thromb. Hemostas.* (Suppl.82), 731, 1999.
197. Rintala, E., et al., Protein C substitution in sepsis-associated purpura fulminans, *Crit. Care Med.*, 28, 2373–2378, 2000.
198. Gerson, W.T., et al., Severe acquired protein C deficiency in purpura fulminans associated with disseminated intravascular coagulation: Treatment with protein C concentrate, *Pediatrics*, 91, 418–422, 1993.
199. deKleijn, E., et al., Activation of protein C following infusion of protein C concentrate in children with severe meningococcal sepsis and purpura fulminans: A randomized, double-blinded, placebo-controlled, dose-finding study, *Crit. Care Med.*, 31, 1839–1847, 2003.
200. Yan, S. and Dhainaut, J.F., Only activated protein C treatment and not protein C has demonstrated an improvement in survival in severe sepsis, *Crit Care Med*, 32, 2004.
201. Redl, H., et al., Expression of endothelial leukocyte adhesion molecule-1 in septic but not traumatic/hypovolemic shock in the baboon, *Am. J. Pathol.*, 139, 461–466, 1991.
202. Newman, W., et al., Soluble E-selectin is found in supernatants of activated endothelial cells and is elevated in the serum of patients with septic shock, *J. Immunol.*, 150, 644–654, 1993.
203. Bevilacqua, M.P. and Nelson, R.M., Selectins, *J. Clin. Invest.*, 91, 379–387, 1993.
204. Kukielka, G.L., et al., Induction of myocardial ELAM-1 by ischemia and reperfusion, *FASEB J.*, 6, 1060A, 1992.
205. Rosenberg, R. and Aird, W., Vascular-bed-specific hemostasis and hypercoagulable states, *New Engl. J. Med.*, 340, 1555–1564, 1999.

206. Krishnaswamy, G., et al., Human endothelium as a source of multifunctional cytokines: Molecular regulation and possible role in human disease, *J. Interferon Cytokine Res.*, 19, 91–104, 1999.

207. Gonzalez-Amaro, A. and Sanchez-Madrid, F., Cell adhesion molecules: Selectins and integrens, *Crit. Reviews Immunol.*, 19, 389–429, 1999.

208. Pohlman, T. and Harlan, J., Adaptive response of the endothelium to stress, *J. Surg. Res.*, 89, 85–119, 2000.

209. Angus, D., et al., Epidemiology of severe sepsis in the United States: Analysis of incidence, outcome, and associated costs of care, *Crit. Care Med.*, 29, 1303–1310, 2001.

210. Bernard, G.R., et al., Recombinant human activated protein C (rhAPC) produces a trend toward improvement in morbidity and 28 day survival in patients with severe sepsis, *Crit. Care Med.*, 27, S4, 1999.

211. Fisher, C.J., et al., Recombinant human activated protein C (rhAPC) improves coagulation abnormalities, morbidity and 28 day mortality in patients with severe sepsis, *J. Antimicrob. Chemother.*, 44 (Suppl. A), 10, 1999.

212. Ely, E.W., et al., Drotrecogin alfa (activated) administration across clinically important subgroups of patients with severe sepsis, *Crit. Care Med.*, 31, 12–19, 2003.

213. Vincent, J.L., et al., Effects of drotrecogin alfa (activated) on organ dysfunction in the PROWESS trial, *Crit. Care Med.*, 31, 834–840, 2003.

214. Macias, W.L., Yan, S.B., and Grinnell, B.W., The development of drotrecogin alfa (activated) for the treatment of severe sepsis, *Int. J. Artificial Organs*, 27, 360–370, 2004.

215. Bernard, G.R., et al., Safety assessment of drotrecogin alfa (activated) in the treatment of adult patients with severe sepsis, *Crit. Care (London)*, 7, 155–163, 2003.

216. Warren, B.L., et al., Caring for the critically ill patient. High-dose antithrombin III in severe sepsis: A randomized controlled trial, *JAMA*, 286, 1869–1878, 2001.

217. Abraham, E., Reinhart, K., and Opal, S., Efficacy and safety of tifacogin (recombinant tissue factor pathway inhibitor) in severe sepsis; A randomized controlled trial, *JAMA*, 290, 238–247, 2003.

218. Macias, W.L., et al., Pharmacokinetic-pharmacodynamic analysis of drotrecogin alfa (activated) in patients with severe sepsis, *Clin. Pharmacol. Therapeut.*, 72, 391–402, 2002.

219. Kerlin, B., et al., Survival advantage associated with heterozygous factor V Leiden mutation in patients with severe sepsis and in mouse endotoxemia, *Blood*, 102, 3085–3092, 2003.

220. Aird, W., Thrombin paradox redux, *Blood*, 102, 3077–3078, 2003.

221. Dellinger, R., et al., Surviving sepsis campaign guidelines for management of severe sepsis and septic shock, *Crit. Care Med.*, 32, 858–873, 2004.

222. Grinnell, B.W., Hermann, R.B., and Yan, S.B., Human protein C inhibits selectin-mediated cell adhesion: Role of unique fucosylated oligosaccharide, *Glycobiology*, 4, 221–225, 1994.

5

Deoxyribonuclease I

Niek N. Sanders, Stefaan C. De Smedt, and Joseph Demeester

CONTENTS

5.1 Introduction

Deoxyribonucleases (DNases) are phosphodiesterases that catalyze the hydrolysis of deoxyribonucleic acid (DNA). Human DNases have been divided into two classes: DNase I and DNase II [1]. In recent years, many new human DNases such as caspase-activated Dnase (CAD) and liver-spleen DNase (LS-DNase), resembling either DNase I or DNase II, have been discovered [2,3]. The ability of these human DNases to degrade DNA extensively and nonspecifically distinguishes them from other endonucleases. Mammalian DNase I (E.C.3.1.21.1), also called Dornase, has been studied extensively. DNase I cleaves DNA through the hydrolysis of P–O$_3'$ bonds, producing 5′-phosphate oligonucleotides (Figure 5.1). Dornase is found mainly in the pancreas and has been primarily regarded as a digestive enzyme contributing to the supply of oligonucleotides in parallel with their *de novo* synthesis. DNase I is also produced by other organs (e.g., salivary glands, stomach, and small intestine) and is present in many biological fluids such as urine, serum, and amniotic and cerebral fluid [1,4–6]. In 1945, McCarty [7] purified DNase I for the first time from bovine

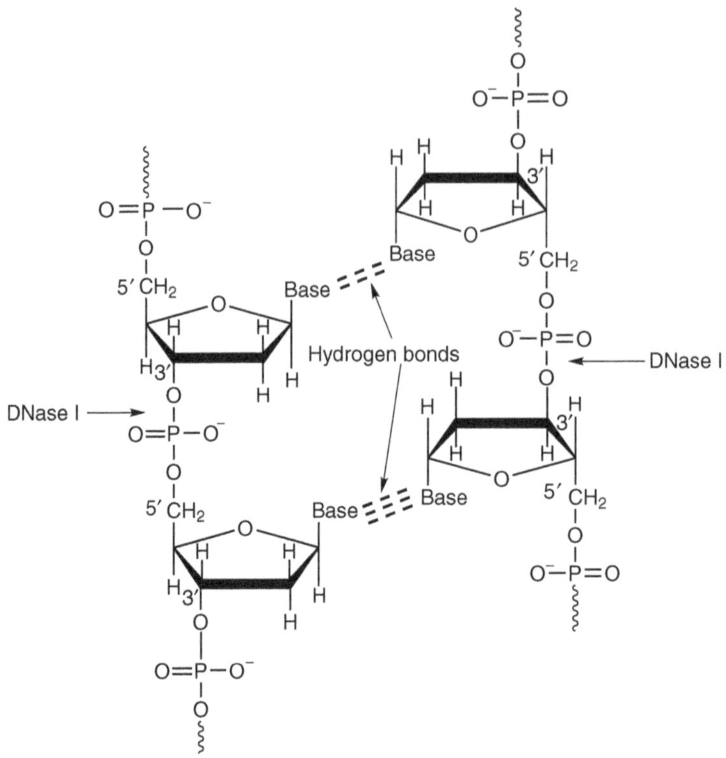

FIGURE 5.1
Schematic representation of double-stranded DNA. DNase I can generate single-chain nicks in both DNA strands at the indicated phosphate–oxygen bonds. The obtained oligonucleotides, which are at least two nucleotides long, bear a 5′-phosphate and a 3′-hydroxyl termini.

pancreas. This drastically intensified the biochemical investigations on and with DNase I. In 1950, Armstrong, et al., reported that partially purified bovine pancreatic DNase I reduced the viscosity of purulent cystic fibrosis (CF) lung secretions [8]. Clinical trials with inhaled bovine DNase I followed soon after and showed clinical improvements in CF patients and patients with purulent secretions [9–11]. In 1958, bovine pancreatic DNase I (Dornavac) was approved in the United States as a mucolytic agent for human use [12]. However, in the early 1960s, severe adverse reactions like bronchospasms and asthmatic attacks led to the withdrawal of bovine pancreatic DNase I from the market [13,14]. During the following decades, clinical interest in DNase I diminished, but DNase I received much attention once again when Shak, et al. [12] cloned the human version of it in 1990. In 1993, this led to the marketing of recombinant human (rh) DNase I under the trade name Pulmozyme® (Genentech Inc., San Francisco, CA) for use in CF patients. In this chapter, we will focus on the biochemical properties, clinical use, pharmacological aspects, and production of rhDNase I.

5.2 Biochemical Aspects

In the late 1980s, after screening the human pancreatic complementary DNA (cDNA) library, Shak, et al. [12] found the cDNA encoding human DNase I. This cDNA was subsequently sequenced and expressed in human embryonic kidney 293 cells (HEK293), yielding rhDNase I, also called dornase alfa. The recombinant enzyme contains, as does purified human pancreatic DNase I, 260 amino acids, shows a 77% homology with bovine DNase I, and contains at its N terminus a 22–amino-acid-long sequence encoding a secretion signal [12,15] (Figure 5.2). The rhDNase I purified from the supernatant of transfected cells is a mixture of various glycosylated species with a pI between 3 and 4 and an average molecular mass of approximately 35 kDa [16]. Like bovine DNase I, rhDNase I contains four cysteine residues (amino acids 101, 104, 173, and 209) and two potential N-linked glycosylation sites, N18 and N106 [15,17,18]. Depending on the expressing cell type, one or both sites become glycosylated [19]. The carbohydrate chains, which are not essential for enzymatic activity, contain *N*-acetylglucosamine, sialic acid, mannose, fucose, and mannose-6-phosphate [20]. Similar to its bovine counterpart, rhDNase I contains two disulfide bridges [21]. The first one (C101–C104) is not essential for enzyme activity, while the second one (C173–C209) is essential for the structure and activity of the enzyme [17]. Close to this essential disulfide bridge, a strong binding site for Ca^{2+} is present in the loop formed by residues 201 to 207. Binding of Ca^{2+} to this site is mediated by the negatively charged side chain of D201, by the hydroxyl group of T203, and by the amide oxygens of T203, T205, and T207. A second strong binding site for Ca^{2+} is located near the flexible loop region (residues 100 to 105) that contains the nonessential disulphide bridge. The negatively charged side chains of D99, D107, E112, and the amide oxygen of F109 form this binding site. Mg^{2+} and Mn^{2+} can compete with Ca^{2+} for binding to one of these strong binding sites [22]. The affinity of these binding sites for Ca^{2+} decreases with pH; at pH 5.5, DNase I binds only one Ca^{2+} ion with high affinity. Upon heating, rhDNase I (10 mg/mL,

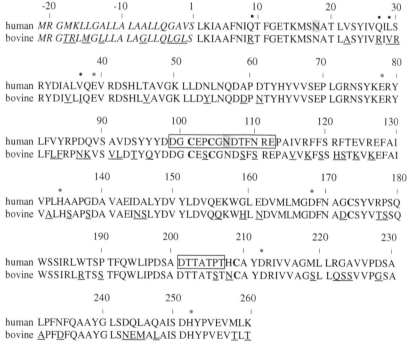

FIGURE 5.2

The amino acid sequences of human and bovine DNase I (Swiss-Prot P24855 and P00639) [170]. The first 22 amino acids shown in italics form a secretion signal sequence. The shaded residues, N18 and N106, indicate the possible glycosylation sites. The four cysteine residues are in bold print. Amino acids marked with an asterisk (*) are involved in the catalysis. Residues that differ between human and bovine DNase I are underlined. Conserved differences are indicated by a dot. The Ca^{2+} binding regions are outlined.

pH 6.8, and in the absence of divalent cations) is irreversibly denaturized at a melting temperature of 67.4°C. Binding of the two Ca^{2+} ions to their aforementioned sites increases the melting temperature of the enzyme, and makes the enzyme more resistant to proteolysis, pH-induced structural alterations, reduction, and denaturants such as urea [21,23,24]. Indeed, the Ca^{2+} ions are known to enhance the structural and chemical stability of rhD-Nase I by stabilization of the disulfide bridges [25]. However, in contrast to bovine DNase I, rhDNase I shows fewer overall changes in its secondary and tertiary structures after removal of these Ca^{2+} ions [21]. Recently, it has also been proposed that binding of Ca^{2+} to the aforementioned sites results in a fine-tuning of the DNase I activity [26]. Two other metal ion (Mg^{2+}) binding sites, which play a critical role in the enzymatic cleavage of DNA, exist at the active center of the enzyme. The carboxyl side chains of E39, D168, and possibly also D251 form these binding sites. A strong binding of these divalent cations to these sites requires the presence of DNA [17,27,28].

The three-dimensional X-ray crystallographic structure of rhDNase I is very similar to the bovine form of DNase I. Figure 5.3 shows a schematic representation of the three-dimensional structure of DNase I. The enzyme has a mixed α/β composition, with a hydro-phobic core of two six-stranded β-pleated sheets flanked by eight α-helices and six extensive loop regions. Except for one region in the β-sheet structure, almost all of the differences

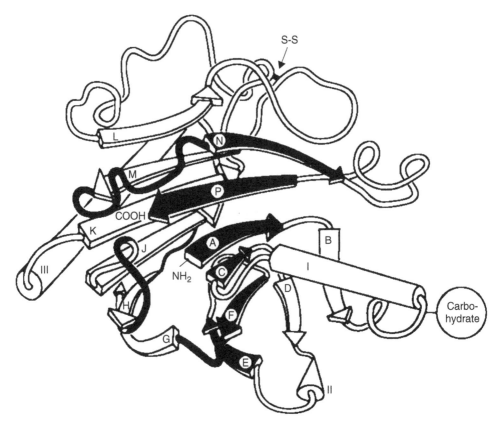

FIGURE 5.3
The three-dimensional structure of DNase I. β-Strands (capital letters) are represented by arrows and α-helices by cylinders. Two six-stranded β-pleated sheets consisting of strands E, F, C, A, P, N (sheet 1) and strands G, H, J, K, M, L (sheet 2) are packed against each other forming the core of the enzyme. The flexible loop region connects β-strands H and G. The carbohydrate side chain is attached to N18 at the beginning of helix I. The disulfide bridge between Cl73 and C209 is indicated. (From Suck, D., Oefner, C., and Kabsch, W., *EMBO J.*, 3, 2423–2430, 1984. With permission.)

between the human and bovine enzyme are located in the hydrophilic regions on the surface of the molecule. Consequently, the gathering of almost all the differences between human and bovine DNase I on the surface may explain the development of antiDNase I bodies in half of the patients who received multiple doses of bovine DNase I [12,29].

In recent years, hyperactive variants of human DNase I have been created by introducing basic amino acids at selected positions on the DNA-binding interface to generate attractive interactions with the negatively charged phosphates on the DNA backbone. These variants digest DNA more efficiently under physiological saline conditions and show a >10,000-fold higher activity than wild-type rhDNase I [30].

5.3   Catalytic Mechanism

DNase I shows a strong preference for double-stranded DNA, and it degrades DNA in the presence of divalent cations by introducing single-stranded nicks through hydrolysis of $P–O_3'$-bonds (Figure 5.1). It has been shown that Mn^{2+} and Co^{2+} also change the structure of DNA to a form in which bovine DNase can introduce double-stranded breaks [31]. The enzyme shows an optimal activity at neutral pH in the presence of Ca^{2+} and Mg^{2+} or Ca^{2+} and Mn^{2+}. DNase I also cleaves single-stranded DNA, but this occurs at a 10,000-fold slower rate. Although the enzyme is neither base nor sequence-specific, its cutting rate is strongly sequence-dependent. This indicates that DNase I recognizes variations in the geometry of the DNA backbone [27,28,31–33], as discussed below.

The first step in the cleavage of DNA by DNase I involves the binding of the exposed loop between R73 and K77 of DNase I to the minor groove of B-type DNA [34] (Figure 5.4). Upon binding, the DNA is bent away from the enzyme toward the major groove, widening the minor groove by 3 Å. This is mainly due to an unusual stacking-type interaction of Y76 with the deoxyribose of a thymidine nucleoside [35,36]. No significant conformational changes take place in DNase I during binding [35]. Only one side of the DNA double helix is in contact with the DNase I over approximately 8 base pairs (bp), i.e., over almost a complete turn [17]. Therefore, DNase I cannot efficiently bind and cut pieces of DNA shorter than 8 bp. The binding of DNA to bovine DNase I involves several hydrogen bonds between either backbone NH groups (E13, T14, S43) or side chains (R9, E39, N74, Y175, S206, Y211) of DNase I and the sugar–phosphate backbones of both DNA strands [32,34]. Additionally, an ionic bond is formed between R111 of DNase I and the phosphate adjacent to the cleavage site. The side chain of R41 forms hydrogen bonds with the oxygen atoms of two successive pyrimidines [36,37]. In human DNase I, seven of these interacting residues, namely, Q9, R41, Y76, R111, N170, Y175, and Y211, are located around the catalytic center, and make contacts with the DNA that are critical for the activity of human DNase I [28].

The fit of the exposed loop between R73 to K77 in the minor groove is rather tight. Optimal binding of DNase I occurs when the width of this groove is 12 to 13Å, a value occurring only in B-DNA near mixed bp sequences. This may explain the lower cleavage probabilities in regions of B-DNA consisting of runs of consecutive adenosines or thymidines, which cause a narrowing of the minor groove. The lower cutting rates in guanosine—cytidine (GC)-rich regions and polyadenosine stretches are related to their lower flexibility, which complicates the widening of the minor groove upon DNase I binding. Additionally, steric hindrance of the interaction of R41 in the minor groove by two NH2 groups of guanine bases may also account for the lower average cleavage rates in GC-rich regions [32,36,38].

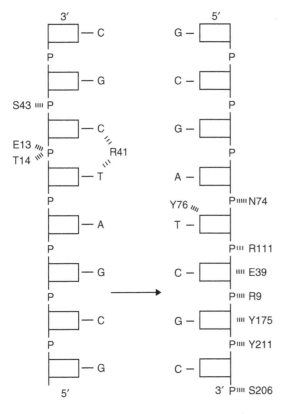

FIGURE 5.4
Schematic diagram of the DNase I–DNA contacts. Phosphate groups are represented by the letter P, deoxyribose moieties by a square, and bases by their one letter code. A, T, C, and G correspond to adenine, thymine, cytosine and guanine, respectively. (Adapted from Weston, S.A., Lahm, A., and Suck, D., *J. Mol. Biol.*, 226, 1237–1256, 1992. With permission.)

The width of the minor groove and the helical stiffness cannot, however, explain the rather drastic differences in cutting rates at neighboring phosphodiester bonds. It is likely that the orientation of the scissile phosphate group determines the local cleavage rates. Nuclear magnetic resonance (NMR) studies showed that cleavage of the P–O$_3$' bonds in DNA by DNase I are accompanied by an inversion of the configuration at the phosphorous atom [17]. This is brought about by the unusual stacking-type interaction of Y76 with a deoxyribose, which suggests that the hydrolysis of the P–O$_3$' bonds occurs through an in-line nucleophilic attack by a water molecule. From crystallographic data [17,35,38] and especially site-directed mutagenesis studies [27,28,37], it is known that E39, E78, H134, D168, D212, and H252 of bovine and human DNase I are directly involved in catalysis. Figure 5.5 shows how these DNase I residues are involved in the acid–base-catalyzed hydrolysis of DNA [27]. The first step in the mechanism is the abstraction of a proton from a water molecule by H252 (step 1). The obtained hydroxyl ion subsequently attacks the phosphodiester, generating a pentacovalent transition state (steps 2 and 3). The magnesium (or zinc, manganese) ions, which are coordinated to the scissile phosphate group, E39 and D168, stabilize this pentacovalent transition state. They are also required for a correct positioning of the phosphate group relative to the enzyme. The second histine residue (H134) functions as a general acid, protonating the O3' as it leaves (steps 4–6). The strong hydrogen bonds between the N1 of H134 and E78, and between H252 and D212 increase the pK_a values of the histidine residues and consequently favor the acid–base-catalyzed nucleophilic attack of water. Finally, E78 is not only hydrogen-bound to H134 but also to the phenolic OH of Y76. Thus, E78 serves as a link between a DNA-binding (Y76), and a DNA-cutting amino acid (H134).

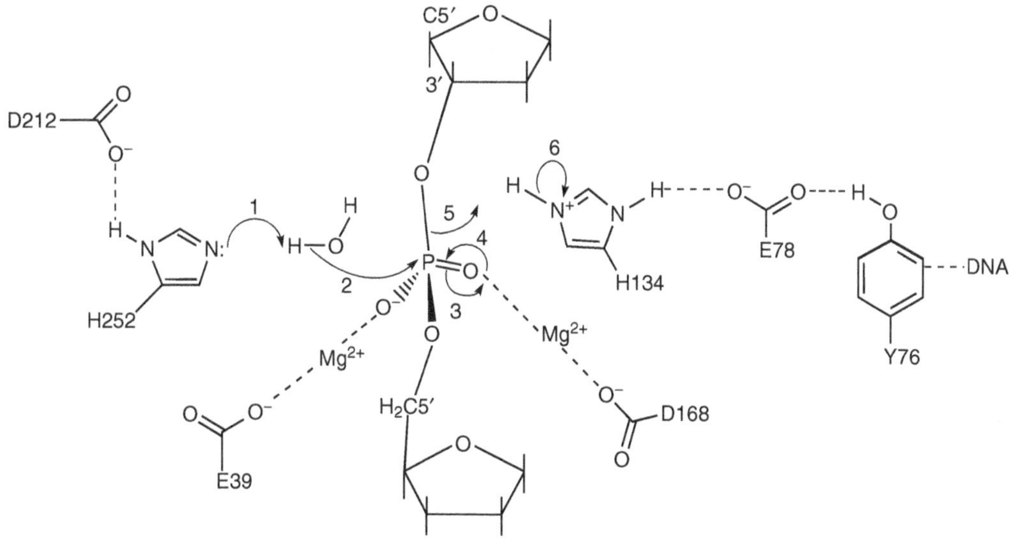

FIGURE 5.5
Mechanism of the acid–base catalyzed hydrolysis of DNA by DNase I. (From Jones, S.J., Worrall, A.F., and Connolly, B.A., *J. Mol. Biol.*, 264, 1154–1163, 1996. With permission.)

5.4   Determination of Activity

Various types of assays based on, e.g., viscosimetry, electrophoresis, production of acid-soluble radio-labeled DNA, DNA aggregation, and *p*-nitrophenyl phosphate-labeled substrates, have been developed for quantification of DNase I activity [39–41]. However, the most used assay is based on the "hyperchromicity" method, initially developed by Kunitz, and determines the increase in absorbance at 260 nm upon cleavage of DNA [42]. One Kunitz unit was originally defined as the amount of DNase I that causes at 25°C and pH 5.0, an optical density increase of 1unit/min of a solution containing 0.03 mg/mL calf thymus DNA, 3.75 mM $MgSO_4$, and 75 mM acetate buffer [42]. However, one should be cautious when comparing DNase I activities expressed in Kunitz units, as the reaction conditions are not always the same. Additionally, to quantify DNase I activity, most methods do not give well-defined units owing to poor substrate definition or the use of unnatural low-molecular-mass substrates.

To characterize the enzymatic activity of the commercially available rhDNase I, Sinicropi, et al. [43] adapted a method developed by Kurnick [44]. The assay is based on the hydrolysis of a highly polymerized native DNA complexed with methyl green. Hydrolysis of the DNA liberates free methyl green, which fades away, leading to a decrease in the absorbance at 620 nm. The method enables quantification of rhDNase I activity over a 10,000-fold concentration range. To overcome the variability in DNA properties, a relative assay against an internal rhDNase I standard with a purity >99% is used. No stability data on this standard preparation is available. This causes difficulties in a worldwide comparison of different assay results. For example, the "methyl green" unit is defined as the amount of activity equivalent to 1 µg of a rhDNase I internal standard used by Sinicropi, et al. [43].

Extremely sensitive DNase I assays have been developed using fluorescent DNA and fluorescent probes [45]. Using oligonucleotides with two different fluorescent molecules at their ends and FRET-FCS (fluorescence resonance energy transfer-fluorescence correlation spectroscopy), we developed recently a technique that allows us to characterize DNase activities in native CF sputum and even in living cells (unpublished data).

5.5   Therapeutic Applications

5.5.1   DNase I in CF

5.5.1.1   Rationale and Clinical Results

CF is the most common autosomal-recessive lethal disease in Caucasians. About 1 in 2500 newborns has CF. The disease is characterized by the presence of highly viscous and elastic mucus, especially in the lungs and intestinal system [46,47]. The origin of this pathological mucus is a mutation in the CF transmembrane conductance regulator (CFTR) gene. This gene codes for a protein that functions as a chloride channel in the apical membrane of epithelial cells of the lung, sweat glands, and the intestinal and genital tracts [46]. In the lung, the defective CFTR protein is thought to lead to a decreased chloride flux from the epithelial cells into the respiratory mucus and an increased sodium flux from the mucus into the cells. These disturbances in ion fluxes result in water absorption from the mucus into the cells, which enhances mucus viscosity and elasticity, and consequently impedes the clearance of the mucus, where inhaled pathogens are captured [48]. The impaired clearance of airway secretions promotes infection and inflammation. The inflammation response is characterized by a massive migration of serum proteins and neutrophils into the mucus [49]. The neutrophils, together with the pathogens and epithelial cells, degenerate, and their nuclear DNA and actin are released within the mucus [50]. These biopolymers, especially DNA, enhance the viscosity and elasticity of the mucus and further impede its clearance from the airways [51–53]. The DNA concentration in mucus of CF patients typically ranges between 1 and 14 mg/mL [54–56]. As mentioned in the introduction, bovine DNase I was used with success in the 1950s as a mucolytic agent in humans with purulent lung secretions. However, following reports of a severe adverse respiratory reaction, bovine DNase I fell into disuse.But the availability of rhDNase I in 1990 gave rise to many *in vitro* studies with rhDNase I on CF sputum and clinical trials in CF patients. Indeed, the capability of rhDNase I to reduce the viscosity, elasticity, adhesiveness, and spinability of CF sputum *in vitro* [57–60] and *in vivo* [54,61] as well as its safety and efficacy in CF patients, has been extensively demonstrated [16,62–68]. This section presents a short summary of the outcomes of the major clinical trials.

The first short-term (<14 d) clinical trials (phases 1 and 2), which primarily aimed to assess optimal dose and evaluate safety, showed that inhalation of 2.5 mg rhDNase I twice daily for up to 10 days improved the forced expiratory volume in 1 sec (FEV_1) and forced vital capacity (FVC) by ~10%, reduced the number of bacteria in the sputum, and increased the overall well-being of CF patients with moderate disease (i.e., FVC > 40% of predicted value based on sex, age, and height) [69–71]. Improvements were evident within 3 d of initiating therapy. However, short-term studies [72,73] of patients with severe pulmonary disease (FVC < 40% of predicted value) or with acute pulmonary exacerbations did not, relative to placebo, reveal improvements in lung function.

Long-term (6–24 months) randomized placebo-controlled trials (phase 3) involving the daily inhalation of 2.5 mg rhDNase I by adults and children (≥5 years) with moderate disease (FVC > 40% of predicted value) showed a significant improvement in FEV_1 and FVC during the first weeks, which then dropped and stabilized at values around 6 and 4%, respectively, relative to baseline [74,75] (Figure 5.6). Additionally, reduced relative risk of

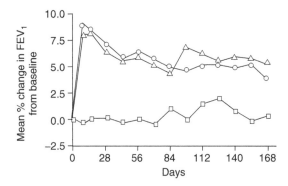

FIGURE 5.6
Mean percentage change from baseline in FEV_1 after long-term inhalation of 2.5 mg rhDNase I twice daily (circles), once daily (up triangles), and placebo (squares). (From Fuchs, et al., *New Engl. J. Med.*, 331, 637–642, 1994. With permission.)

respiratory exacerbations by 22 to 34% and an increase in the well-being of the patient were observed. With placebo, neither increase in lung function nor decrease in exacerbations was observed. The long-term inhalation of rhDNase I was found to improve, or at least maintain, lung function in patients with advanced [76] and mild lung disease[77–79]. This is a striking and important observation, as the former are at a greater risk of losing lung function [76], while the latter can hardly improve their lung functions as the baseline values are close to 100% of the predicted values [79]. Many other nonrandomized placebo-controlled studies have revealed similar data [80–83]. Additionally, Suri, et al. [84] showed in a randomized trial that inhalation of rhDNase I on alternate days is as effective as daily inhalation. Recently, a long-term trial over a period of 3 years revealed that inhalation of rhDNase I also had a positive impact on airway inflammation in CF patients [85].

In 1998, inhalation of rhDNase I was demonstrated to be safe in children younger than five years. This led to the approval of rhDNase I for the treatment of CF patients under the age of 5 [86]. Later on, studies showed that, over a long term, younger patients appear to benefit more from rhDNase I therapy than older, and often more sickly patients [68,78].

5.5.1.2   *Adverse Effects, Interactions, and Pharmacokinetics*

Dosages of up to 30 mg rhDNase I per day were well tolerated in healthy volunteers and CF patients [69,87]. Severe bronchospasms or anaphylactic reactions, as seen after inhalation of bovine DNase I, have never been observed with rhDNase I. The most common adverse effects reported after daily inhalation of 2.5 mg rhDNase I were voice alterations (hoarseness), pharyngitis, rash, laryngitis, and conjunctivitis [74,76,78]. All these events are generally mild and transient. In patients with severe pulmonary disease (FVC < 40%), rhinitis, fever, dyspepsia, dyspnea, and an FVC decrease of ≥ 10% have also been reported [76,88]. Facial edema has been reported to an exceptional degree in patients receiving 2.5 or 10 mg rhDNase I twice daily [70]. It has also been shown that rhDNase I may increase airway inflammation by releasing elastase and proinflammatory cytokines that are bound to DNA in the airway secretions [89–91]. However, other studies did not confirm this observation [92–94]. Antibodies against rhDNase I have been found in the serum of 3% of CF patients receiving 2.5 mg rhDNase I once daily for 6 months [74]. Whether these antibodies decrease the efficacy of rhDNase I is not known. Experiments on cell cultures and animals showed that rhDNase I did not have teratogenic, mutagenic, or carcinogenic activity, and that it did not affect the fertility and reproductive performance of either male or female rats at doses much higher (>29-fold) than recommended [88].

rhDNase I can be used in conjunction with standard CF therapies, but it should not be used in patients with known hypersensitivity to rhDNase I and Chinese hamster ovary (CHO) products. Caution is also indicated in pregnant women and nursing mothers, since it is not known whether rhDNase I is excreted in human milk [62,88]. Patients are advised not to take rhDNase I shortly before going to bed, as clearance of their mucus will be ineffective in their sleep [62,65,88].

Pharmacokinetic studies on animals have been reviewed by Green [95]. In animal studies, inhalation of a single high dose of rhDNase I revealed a low bioavailability of <15% in rats and <2% in monkeys. Estimation of the bioavailability of rhDNase I in animals following repeated inhalation was confounded by the development of serum antibodies against rhDNase I. The half-life of rhDNase I in the lungs of rats is about 11 h [62,95]. In human studies, neither short-term nor long-term inhalation of rhDNase I at doses of 30 and 5 mg per d resulted in a significant increase of the DNase I concentration in serum [74,87]. The half-life of rhDNase I in the lungs of CF patients is much shorter than in animals and is estimated to be between 2 and 5 h [96,97]. An rhDNase I binding protein has been identified in the serum of rats, which may modulate the activity of rhDNase I [98].

5.5.1.3   *Formulation and Administration Aspects*

A sterile solution of rhDNase I for inhalation is on the market under the trade name Pulmozyme. It contains 1000 Genentech Units rhDNase I /mL (equivalent to 1 mg/mL), 150 mM sodium chloride as a tonicity modifier, 1.35 mM calcium chloride as a stabilizer, and water for injection [88]. The pH of this solution is 6.3. The enzyme solution should be protected from intense light and stored at 2 to 8°C. The recommended dose is 2500 Genentech Units (one ampoule of 2.5 mL, i.e., 2.5 mg) once daily. However, some patients may benefit from a twice-daily administration of this dose. It is preferable that the drug be inhaled via compressed air-driven nebulizers. Ultrasonic nebulizers are not recommended [16]. For an optimal deposition in the lower airways, the mass median aerodynamic diameter (MMAD) of the droplets generated by the nebulizers should be between 1 and 6 μm [99]. However, according to Shah, et al. [100] and Geller, et al. [77], higher improvements in lung function can, especially in patients with advanced lung disease, be obtained when rhDNase I is administered by nebulizers that generate smaller droplets (~2 μm). Besides the MMAD of the droplets, aerosol deposition also strongly varies in CF patients due to fluctuations in airway calibre. An increased lung disposition of rhDNase I is observed with increasing pulmonary obstruction [101]. An average deposition in the lungs of 0.5 mg after administration of a 2.5 mg dose of rhDNase I has been reported [101]. From this value and the rhDNase I concentration measured in mucus (3 μg/mL) after inhalation of 2.5 mg rhDNase I [96], we can estimate that the volume of mucus in the lungs of CF patients must be around 165 mL. Finally, mixing rhDNase I in the nebulizer with other drugs commonly used in CF patients may decrease the functionality of both drugs due to, for example, complexation or aggregation [16,88]. The latter may also increase the risk of an immune reaction against rhDNase I.

The relative low efficiency and in convenience associated with the use of nebulizers have urged research groups to develop dry powders of rhDNase I for inhalation via dry powder inhalers [102–105].

5.5.1.4   *Nonresponders and Inhibition of DNase I by Actin*

Although clinical trials have shown that rhDNase I significantly improves lung function and decreases exacerbations in CF patients, not all patients respond to this therapy. Moreover different studies claim that there is a wide variation in clinical response to rhDNase I; about 50% of CF patients do not benefit from rhDNase I therapy [67,106–109]. The individual response to rhDNase I cannot be predicted from baseline lung function or other clinical parameters [67,110]. But the response to rhDNase I after 6 weeks is highly predictive of the response over a longer term [110]. The reason why rhDNase I fails in certain CF patients is not known. We have, however, recently discovered that a magnesium deficiency in CF mucus of nonresponders may increase the inhibition of rhDNase I by G-actin [111], a known

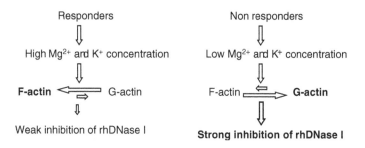

FIGURE 5.7

Schematic representation of the influence of magnesium and potassium on the degradation of DNA in CF mucus by rhDNase I. CF mucus contains actin, which can be in the globular (G-actin, M_r 42,000) or in the polymer, i.e., filamentous (F) form. G-actin is a potent inhibitor (K_i~1 nM) of DNase I and magnesium is known to promote the polymerization of G-actin into F-actin, which does not inhibit DNase I.

inhibitor of DNase I [112] (Figure 5.7). Although the amount of G-actin in CF mucus is not well defined, filamentous actin (F-actin), which is in equilibrium with G-actin, is present in CF mucus at concentrations ranging from 0.06 to 5 mg/mL [52,111].

On the basis of ternary model of the DNase I–actin–DNA complex, Ulmer, et al. [113] showed that actin binds DNase I near the DNA-binding site [113]. Consequently, the inhibition of DNase I by actin is most likely due to a steric blockage of the active site of DNase I [113,114]. Binding of G-actin to DNase I involves hydrogen bonds and electrostatic interactions between E13, H44, D53, Y65, V67, E69, A114 of DNase I and T203, E207/G63, R39, Q41/V43, V45, K61, V45 of G-actin [113,115,116]. Additionally, the actin residues G42, V43, and M44 are incorporated as a parallel strand of a β-pleated sheet in DNase I with partners Y65, V66, and V67. The DNase I–actin complex (binding constant $5 \times 10^8 \text{ M}^{-1}$) can be separated by 5′-nucleotidase, resulting in a reactivation of DNase I [117,118]. In CF mucus, the inhibition of rhDNase I by actin has also been overcome by actin-binding proteins (gelsolin), and by actin-resistant variants of human DNase I [113,119]. The latter were created by substitution of the amino acids of rhDNase I involved in actin binding by charged, oppositely charged, or bulky amino acids [113]. These actin-resistant variants are 10- to 50-fold more potent in CF mucus than in wild-type rhDNase I [120]. Additionally, different naturally occurring actin-resistant forms of human DNases I and II, such as LS-DNase, and DNase II-like acid DNase (DLAD), have been discovered and proposed as suitable candidates to substitute the actin-sensitive rhDNase I in the treatment of CF [121–123]. Moreover, the finding that DLAD is a secreted enzyme that is also expressed in the human lung led to the speculation that DLAD is responsible for normal DNA clearance in the airways and that the CF defect may result in reduced secretion or activity of the endogenous DLAD [123].

5.5.2   DNase I in Non-CF Respiratory Diseases

Highly viscoelastic lung mucus causes many other respiratory disorders like atelectasis, bronchiectasis, bronchiolitis, bronchitis, and primary ciliary dyskinesia (PCD), giving rise to suffering and even morbidity. Under these conditions, the high viscosity of the lung secretions is often also due to high DNA concentrations, a result of a neutrophil-dominated airway inflammation. Consequently, rhDNase I may be of benefit to these patients. However, unlike the situation in CF, only a few controlled clinical trials have evaluated the efficacy of rhDNase I in these non-CF respiratory diseases. Most of the evidence of benefits are based on case reports or the experience of small groups of patients [124]. In summary, rhDNase I has been applied with success in the treatment of atelectasis [125–131], PCD [132,133], bronchiolitis [134], and empyema thoracis [135]. On the other hand, non-CF patients with bronchiectasis or bronchitis do not benefit from rhDNase I [136–139].

5.5.3   DNase I in Systemic Lupus Erythematosus

Systemic lupus erythematosus (SLE) is an autoimmune disease that affects over one million people in the United States alone [140]. SLE is characterized by the presence of antinuclear antibodies (ANA) directed against naked DNA and nucleosomes. The resulting immune complexes are deposited in the kidney, joints, and blood vessels, causing glomerulonephritis, arthritis, and vasculitis, respectively. The underlying cause of this disease is linked with deficiencies in serum amyloid P (SAP) component [141], certain complement proteins [142,143], and a decreased serum DNase I activity [144–146]. These proteins are all known to be involved in the clearance of apoptotic bodies in extracellular fluids like serum. The decreased activity of DNase I in SLE has originally been associated with increased concentrations of actin in serum of SLE patients [146]. Later on, however, a mutation of the gene encoding DNase I [147] and antiDNase I antibodies were found in certain SLE patients [148,149]. Considering the pathophysiology of SLE, degradation of extracellular DNA, nucleosomes, or DNA-containing immune complexes by DNase I may reduce the production of ANA and the deposition of immune complexes. In the 1960s, Lachmann [150] reported that subcutaneous (s.c.) bovine DNase I in SLE patients resulted in a reduction of ANA and improvements in systemic symptoms. However, after 4–6 weeks of treatment, the positive effects were lost due to the development of antibodies against bovine DNase I. The availability of rhDNase I and recombinant murine (rMu) DNase I in the 1990s led to several trials with DNase I in mice and humans. Intraperitoneal injection of rMuDNase I in young SLE mice delayed the development of antiDNA antibodies (Figure 5.8) and lupus symptoms by about one month [151,152]. In one placebo-controlled study, rMuDNase I even reduced nephritis in older SLE mice with established renal disease [151]. A phase I clinical trial in humans with SLE showed that rhDNase I is well tolerated in SLE patients after a single intravenous dose of up to 125 µg/kg, and five consecutive daily s.c. administrations of up to 125 µg/kg rhDNase I [153]. Antibodies against rhDNase I were

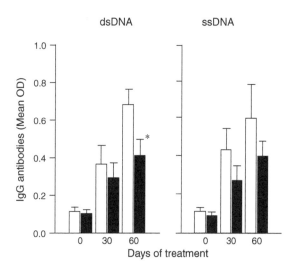

FIGURE 5.8
Serum IgG antibodies to dsDNA, and ssDNA before (0 d), 30 and 60 days after treatment of 4 month old female SLE mice with 0 µg/g (placebo, white bars) or 15 µg/g (black bars) of rMuDNase I ($n = 10$ mice/group, $*p < 0.05$). (Adapted from Verthelyi, et al., *Lupus*, 7, 223–230, 1998. With permission.)

not detected. However, rhDNase I obtained in the serum after s.c. injections was too low to guarantee degradation of DNA and nucleosomes [153,154]. To some extent, this also explains the lack of clinical efficacy of rhDNase I in this study. Therefore, higher doses of rhDNase I, or actin-resistant variants of it, should be injected subcutaneously in further clinical trials. Alternatively, intravenous administration of these enzymes should also be considered.

5.5.4   DNase I in Wound Healing and Cancer

An ointment (Elase® or Fibrolan®) containing bovine DNase I and bovine fibrinolysin has been used clinically as a debriding agent in a variety of inflammatory and infected lesions [155]. The combination of these two enzymes was based on the observation that purulent exudates of infected lesions consist largely of fibrinous material and DNA. The ointment improved the healing of infected accidental or surgical wounds [156], ulcerative lesions [157,158], and second- and third-degree burns [159]. However, in the late 1990s, *in vitro* and placebo-controlled studies clearly showed that Elase was not significantly more effective than a placebo ointment [160–162]. This led to the withdrawal of the ointment from the American market in 1999.

DNases have also been evaluated in the treatment of cancer. Linardou, et al. [163] made a fusion protein by combining bovine DNase I and a single-chain Fv fragment of an antibody directed to tumor-specific antigens. The obtained chimeric protein was highly cytotoxic *in vitro* in tumor cells expressing the antigen [163]. Recently, a more potent and human-based chimeric protein comprising gonadotropin-releasing hormone as a tumor-targeting moiety and CAD as a cytotoxic moiety caused a targeted killing of adenocarcinoma cells *in vitro* and in mice [164].

5.6   Production and Stability of rhDNase I

The first step in the production of rhDNase I is the construction of a eukaryotic expression vector comprising the rhDNase I gene and a selection gene, dihydrofolate reductase (DHFR). Subsequently, CHO cells lacking the DHFR gene are transfected with this vector and put into a selection medium lacking essential nucleotides. This leads to the selection of transformed cells [165]. These transformed cells are further grown in an optimized medium and in conditions that guarantee a maximal expression and secretion of rhDNase I [166]. The rhDNase I secreted by the CHO cells is a mixture of nondeamidated and deamidated forms of rhDNase I [167]. Deamidation of proteins is a common phenomenon and occurs in asparagine and glutamine residues. The deamidated form of rhDNase I has a twofold lower activity, and about 50 to 80% of the secreted rhDNase I is deamidated. Therefore, only the nondeamidated rhDNase I is purified from the medium using tangential flow filtration, affinity and tentacle ion-exchange chromatography [88,168]. A gradual deamidation of rhDNase I also occurs during storage in vials and is the major cause of its short shelf life [21]. Decreasing the pH can slow down deamidation of proteins. However, at lower pH values, rhDNase I tends to aggregate. The current pH (6.3) of the clinically used rhDNase I solution warrants a minimal deamidation and aggregation of the enzyme. However, it has recently been shown that the pH-induced aggregation of rhDNase I can be slowed down by high concentrations of calcium (>10 mM Ca^{2+}) [167].

5.7 Prospects

Different, well-designed clinical trials have demonstrated the effectiveness of rhDNase I in CF patients. However, the response shows a large interindividual variability; about 50% of CF patients do not benefit from rhDNase I therapy [109]. It has recently been discovered that globular actin may be involved in the failure of rhDNase I in these nonresponders [111]. Therefore, clinical trials are required to elucidate whether actin-resistant variants of human DNases can overcome the inhibition of actin in CF patients who do not respond to rhDNase I.

Small trials and case reports have demonstrated the clinical efficacy of rhDNase I in certain non-CF respiratory diseases and SLE [124,146]. However, these observations have to be confirmed further by detailed, long-term studies. Moreover, the promising hyperactive and actin-resistant variants of human DNases also await clinical investigations in these diseases. Treatment of SLE with DNase will probably require an enduring or prolonged presence of DNase in the serum. This can be achieved via a controlled release of DNase or by introducing in these patients, via gene therapy, a gene encoding DNase.

The recent discovery of the involvement of DNases in apoptosis and cancer has focused the spotlight on these enzymes even more [169]. More anticancer agents based on DNases (especially CAD) or on agents that influence these enzymes will probably emerge in the near future.

References

1. Kreuder, V., et al., Isolation, characterization and crystallization of deoxyribonuclease-I from bovine and rat parotid-gland and its interaction with rabbit skeletal-muscle actin, *Eur. J. Biochem.*, 139, 389–400, 1984.
2. Shiokawa, D. and Tanuma, S., Characterization of human DNase I family endonucleases and activation of DNase gamma during apoptosis, *Biochemistry*, 40, 143–152, 2001.
3. Evans, C.J. and Aguilera, R.J., DNase II: Genes, enzymes and function, *Gene*, 322, 1–15, 2003.
4. Nadano, D., Yasuda, T., and Kishi, K., Measurement of deoxyribonuclease I activity in human tissues and body fluids by a single radial enzyme-diffusion method, *Clin. Chem.*, 39, 448–452, 1993.
5. Zanotti, S., et al., Localization of deoxyribonuclease-I gene transcripts and protein in rat-tissues and its correlation with apoptotic cell elimination, *Histochem. Cell Biol.*, 103, 369–377, 1995.
6. Napirei, M., et al., Expression pattern of the deoxyribonuclease 1 gene: Lessons from the Dnase 1 knockout mouse, *Biochem. J.*, 380, 929–937, 2004.
7. McCarty, M., Purification and properties of deoxyribonuclease isolated from beef pancreas, *J. Gen. Physiol.*, 29, 123–139, 1946.
8. Armstrong, J.B. and White, J.C., Liquefaction of viscous purulent exudates by deoxyribonuclease, *Lancet*, 259, 739–742, 1950.
9. Salomon, A., Herchfus, J.A., and Segal, M.S., Aerosols of pancreatic dornase in bronchopulmonary disease, *Ann. Allergy*, 12, 71, 1954.
10. Elmes, P.C. and White, J.C., Deoxyribonuclease in the treatment of purulent bronchitis, *Thorax*, 8, 295–300, 1953.
11. Spier, R., Witebsky, E., and Paine, J., Aerosolized pancreatic dornase and antibiotics in pulmonary infections: Use in patients with postoperative and nonoperative infections, *JAMA*, 178, 878, 1961.
12. Shak, S., et al., Recombinant human DNase I reduces the viscosity of cystic fibrosis sputum, *Proc. Natl. Acad. Sci. USA*, 87, 9188–9192, 1990.

13. Parker, R.H., Wilcox, W.D., and Dietrich, T.S., Toxicity of intrathecally administered pancreatic dornase, *JAMA*, 192, 169, 1965.

14. Raskin, P., Bronchospasm after inhalation of pancreatic dornase, *Am. Rev. Respir. Dis.*, 98, 697–698, 1968.

15. Liao, T.H., et al., Bovine pancreatic deoxyribonuclease-A. Isolation of cyanogen bromide peptides — Complete covalent structure of polypeptide-chain, *J. Biol. Chem.*, 248, 1489–1495, 1973.

16. Gonda, I., Inhalation therapy with recombinant human deoxyribonuclease I, *Adv. Drug Deliv. Rev.*, 19, 37–46, 1996.

17. Oefner, C. and Suck, D., Crystallographic refinement and structure of DNase-I at 2Å resolution, *J. Mol. Biol.*, 192, 605–632, 1986.

18. Lazarus, R.A., Deoxyribonucleases, in *Wiley Encyclopedia of Molecular Medicine*, T.E. Creighton, Ed., Wiley, New York, 2002, pp. 1025–1028.

19. Nishikawa, A. and Mizuno, S., The efficiency of *N*-linked glycosylation of bovine DNase I depends on the Asn-Xaa-Ser/Thr sequence and the tissue of origin, *Biochem. J.*, 355, 245–248, 2001.

20. Cacia, J., et al., Human DNase I contains mannose 6-phosphate and binds the cation-independent mannose 6-phosphate receptor, *Biochemistry*, 37, 15154–15161, 1998.

21. Chen, B., et al., Influence of calcium ions on the structure and stability of recombinant human deoxyribonuclease I in the aqueous and lyophilized states, *J. Pharm. Sci.*, 88, 477–482, 1999.

22. Price, P.A., Characterization of Ca^{++} and Mg^{++} binding to bovine pancreatic deoxyribonuclease A, *J. Biol. Chem.*, 247, 2895–2899, 1972.

23. Poulos, T.L. and Price, P.A., Some effects of calcium ions on structure of bovine pancreatic deoxyribonuclease A, *J. Biol. Chem.*, 247, 2900–2904, 1972.

24. Chan, H.K., Au-Yeung, K.L., and Gonda, I., Effects of additives on heat denaturation of rhDNase in solutions, *Pharm. Res.*, 13, 756–761, 1996.

25. Price, P.A., Stein, W.H., and Moore, S., Effect of divalent cations on the reduction and re-formation of the disulfide bonds of deoxyribonuclease, *J. Biol. Chem.*, 244, 929–932, 1969.

26. Chen, C.Y., Lu, S.C., and Liao, T.H., The distinctive functions of the two structural calcium atoms in bovine pancreatic deoxyribonuclease, *Protein Sci.*, 11, 659–668, 2002.

27. Jones, S.J., Worrall, A.F., and Connolly, B.A., Site-directed mutagenesis of the catalytic residues of bovine pancreatic deoxyribonuclease I, *J. Mol. Biol.*, 264, 1154–1163, 1996.

28. Pan, C.Q., et al., Mutational analysis of human DNase I at the DNA binding interface: Implications for DNA recognition, catalysis, and metal ion dependence, *Protein Sci.*, 7, 628–636, 1998.

29. Suck, D., Oefner, C., and Kabsch, W., Three-Dimensional structure of bovine pancreatic DNase I at 2.5 Å resolution, *EMBO J.*, 3, 2423–2430, 1984.

30. Pan, C.Q. and Lazarus, R.A., Hyperactivity of human DNase I variants — Dependence on the number of positively charged residues and concentration, length, and environment of DNA, *J. Biol. Chem.*, 273, 11701–11708, 1998.

31. Campbell, V.W. and Jackson, D.A., The effect of divalent cations on the mode of action of DNase I — The initial reaction products produced from covalently closed circular DNA, *J. Biol. Chem.*, 255, 3726–3735, 1980.

32. Suck, D., DNA recognition by DNase I, *J. Mol. Recognit.*, 7, 65–70, 1994.

33. Funakoshi, A., et al., Purification and properties of human pancreatic deoxyribonuclease I, *J. Biochem.*, 82, 1771–1777, 1977.

34. Weston, S.A., Lahm, A., and Suck, D., X-ray structure of the DNase I-d(GGTATACC)$_2$ complex at 2.3 Å resolution, *J. Mol. Biol.*, 226, 1237–1256, 1992.

35. Lahm, A. and Suck, D., DNase I-induced DNA conformation 2 Å structure of a DNase I-octamer complex, *J. Mol. Biol.*, 222, 645–667, 1991.

36. Doherty, A.J., Worrall, A.F., and Connolly, B.A., The roles of arginine 41 and tyrosine 76 in the coupling of DNA recognition to phosphodiester bond-cleavage by DNase I: A study using site-directed mutagenesis, *J. Mol. Biol.*, 251, 366–377, 1995.

37. Worrall, A.F. and Connolly, B.A., The chemical synthesis of a gene coding for bovine pancreatic DNase I and its cloning and expression in *Escherichia coli*, *J. Biol. Chem.*, 265, 21889–21895, 1990.

38. Suck, D. and Oefner, C., Structure of DNase I at 2.0 Å resolution suggests a mechanism for binding to and cutting DNA, *Nature*, 321, 620–625, 1986.

39. Liao, T.H. and Hsieh, J.C., Hydrolysis of para-nitrophenyl phenylphosphonate catalyzed by bovine pancreatic deoxyribonuclease, *Biochem. J.*, 255, 781–787, 1988.

40. Pan, C.Q., Sinicropi, D.V., and Lazarus, R.A., Engineered properties and assays for human DNase I mutants, in *Methods in Molecular Biology*, Vol. 160, Shein, C.H., Ed., Humana Press Inc., Totowa, 2001, pp. 309–321.

41. Sinicropi, D.V. and Lazarus, R.A., Assays for human DNase I activity in biological matrices, in *Methods in Molecular Biology*, Vol. 160, Shein, C.H., Ed., Humana Press Inc., Totowa, 2001, pp. 325–333.

42. Kunitz, M., Crystalline desoxyribonuclease. 1. Isolation and general properties; spectrophotometric method for the measurement of desoxyribonuclease activity, *J. Gen. Physiol.*, 33, 349–362, 1950.

43. Sinicropi, D., et al., Colorimetric determination of DNase I activity with a DNA-methyl green substrate, *Anal. Biochem.*, 222, 351–358, 1994.

44. Kurnick, N.B., The determination of deoxyribonuclease activity by methyl green; Application to serum, *Arch. Biochem.*, 29, 41–53, 1950.

45. Choi, S.J. and Szoka, F.C., Fluorometric determination of deoxyribonuclease I activity with PicoGreen, *Anal. Biochem.*, 281, 95–97, 2000.

46. Wine, J.J., The genesis of cystic fibrosis lung disease, *J. Clin. Invest.*, 103, 309–312, 1999.

47. Ratjen, F. and Doring, G., Cystic fibrosis, *Lancet*, 361, 681–689, 2003.

48. Sheppard, D.N. and Welsh, M.J., Structure and function of the CFTR chloride channel, *Physiol. Rev.*, 79, S23–S45, 1999.

49. Konstan, M.W. and Berger, M., Current understanding of the inflammatory process in cystic fibrosis: Onset and etiology, *Pediatr. Pulmonol.*, 24, 137–142, 1997.

50. Lethem, M.I., et al., The origin of DNA associated with mucus glycoproteins in cystic fibrosis sputum, *Eur. Respir. J.*, 3, 19–23, 1990.

51. Picot, R., Das, I., and Reid, L., Pus, deoxyribonucleic acid, and sputum viscosity, *Thorax*, 33, 235–242, 1978.

52. Vasconcellos, C.A., et al., Reduction in viscosity of cystic fibrosis sputum *in vitro* by gelsolin, *Science*, 263, 969–971, 1994.

53. Robinson, M. and Bye, P.T.B., Mucociliary clearance in cystic fibrosis, *Pediatr. Pulmonol.*, 33, 293–306, 2002.

54. Shah, P.L., et al., *In vivo* effects of recombinant human DNase I on sputum in patients with cystic fibrosis, *Thorax*, 51, 119–125, 1996.

55. Puchelle, E., et al., Effects of rhDNase on purulent airways secretions in chronic bronchitis, *Eur. Respir. J.*, 9, 765–769, 1996.

56. Sanders, N.N., et al., Structural alterations of gene complexes by cystic fibrosis sputum, *Am. J. Respir. Crit. Care Med.*, 164, 486–493, 2001.

57. Zahm, J.M., et al., Dose dependent *in vitro* effect of recombinant human DNase on rheological and transport properties of cystic fibrosis respiratory mucus, *Eur. Respir. J.*, 8, 381–386, 1995.

58. Deneuville, E., et al., Revisited physicochemical and transport properties of respiratory mucus in genotyped cystic fibrosis patients, *Am. J. Respir. Crit. Care Med.*, 156, 166–172, 1997.

59. King, M., et al., Rheology of cystic fibrosis sputum after *in vitro* treatment with hypertonic saline alone and in combination with recombinant human deoxyribonuclease I, *Am. J. Respir. Crit. Care Med.*, 156, 173–177, 1997.

60. Zahm, J.M., et al., Improvement of cystic fibrosis airway mucus transportability by recombinant human DNase is related to changes in phospholipid profile, *Am. J. Respir. Crit. Care Med.*, 157, 1779–1784, 1998.

61. Ratjen, F. and Tummler, B., Comparison of the *in vitro* and *in vivo* response to inhaled DNase in patients with cystic fibrosis, *Thorax*, 54, 91, 1999.

62. Bryson, H.M. and Sorkin, E.M., Dornase alfa — A review of its pharmacological properties and therapeutic potential in cystic fibrosis, *Drugs*, 48, 894–896, 1994.

63. Shak, S., Aerosolized recombinant human DNase I for the treatment of cystic fibrosis, *Chest*, 107, 65S–70S, 1995.

64. Hodson, M.E. and Shah, P.L., DNase trials in cystic fibrosis, *Eur. Respir. J.*, 8, 1786–1791, 1995.

65. Shah, P.L. and Hodson, M.E., Dornase alfa — A practical guide to patient selection and drug use in cystic fibrosis, *Biodrugs*, 8, 439–445, 1997.

66. Davies, J., et al., Retrospective review of the effects of rhDNase in children with cystic fibrosis, *Pediatr. Pulmonol.*, 23, 243–248, 1997.

67. Christopher, F., et al., rhDNase therapy for the treatment of cystic fibrosis patients with mild to moderate lung disease, *J. Clin. Pharm. Ther.*, 24, 415–426, 1999.

68. Hodson, M.E., et al., Dornase alfa in the treatment of cystic fibrosis in Europe: A report from the Epidemiologic Registry of Cystic Fibrosis, *Pediatr. Pulmonol.*, 36, 427–432, 2003.

69. Hubbard, R.C., et al., A preliminary study of aerosolized recombinant human deoxyribonuclease I in the treatment of cystic fibrosis, *New Engl. J. Med.*, 326, 812–815, 1992.

70. Ramsey, B.W., et al., Efficacy and safety of short-term administration of aerosolized recombinant human deoxyribonuclease in patients with cystic fibrosis, *Am. Rev. Respir. Dis.*, 148, 145–151, 1993.

71. Ranasinha, C., et al., Efficacy and safety of short-term administration of aerosolized recombinant human DNaseI in adults with stable stage cystic fibrosis, *Lancet*, 342, 199–202, 1993.

72. Shah, P.I., et al., Recombinant human DNase I in cystic fibrosis patients with severe pulmonary disease — A short-term, double-blind study followed by 6 months open-label treatment, *Eur. Resp. J.*, 8, 954–958, 1995.

73. Wilmott, R.W., et al., Aerosolized recombinant human DNase in hospitalized cystic fibrosis patients with acute pulmonary exacerbations, *Am. J. Respir. Crit. Care Med.*, 153, 1914–1917, 1996.

74. Fuchs, H.J., et al., Effect of aerosolized recombinant human DNase on exacerbations of respiratory symptoms and on pulmonary function in patients with cystic fibrosis, *New Engl. J. Med.*, 331, 637–642, 1994.

75. Shah, P.L., et al., 2 Years Experience with recombinant human DNase-I in the treatment of pulmonary disease in cystic fibrosis, *Respir. Med.*, 89, 499–502, 1995.

76. McCoy, K., Hamilton, S., and Johnson, C., Effects of 12-week administration of dornase alfa in patients with advanced cystic fibrosis lung disease, *Chest*, 110, 889–895, 1996.

77. Geller, D.E., et al., Effect of smaller droplet size of dornase alfa on lung function in mild cystic fibrosis, *Pediatr. Pulmonol.*, 25, 83–87, 1998.

78. Quan, J.M., et al., A two-year randomized, placebo-controlled trial of dornase alfa in young patients with cystic fibrosis with mild lung function abnormalities, *J. Pediatr.*, 139, 813–820, 2001.

79. Robinson, P.J., Dornase alfa in early cystic fibrosis lung disease, *Pediatr. Pulmonol.*, 34, 237–241, 2002.

80. Harms, H.K., et al., Multicenter, open-label study of recombinant human DNase in cystic fibrosis patients with moderate lung disease, *Pediatr. Pulmonol.*, 26, 155–161, 1998.

81. Johnson, C.A., et al., Estimating effectiveness in an observational study: A case study of dornase alfa in cystic fibrosis, *J. Pediatr.*, 134, 734–739, 1999.

82. Furuya, M.E.Y., et al., Efficacy of human recombinant DNase in pediatric patients with cystic fibrosis, *Arch. Med. Res.*, 32, 30–34, 2001.

83. Shah, P.L., et al., A case-controlled study with dornase alfa to evaluate impact on disease progression over a 4-year period, *Respiration*, 68, 160–164, 2001.

84. Suri, R., et al., Comparison of hypertonic saline and alternate day or daily recombinant human deoxyribonuclease in children with cystic fibrosis: A randomised trial, *Lancet*, 358, 1316–1321, 2001.

85. Paul, K., et al., Effect of treatment with dornase alpha on airway inflammation in patients with cystic fibrosis, *Am. J. Respir. Crit. Care Med.*, 169, 719–725, 2004.

86. Wagener, J.S., et al., Aerosol delivery and safety of recombinant human deoxyribonuclease in young children with cystic fibrosis: A bronchoscopic study, *J. Pediatr.*, 133, 486–491, 1998.

87. Aitken, M.L., et al., Recombinant human DNase inhalation in normal subjects and patients with cystic fibrosis — A phase 1 study, *JAMA*, 267, 1947–1951, 1992.

88. Pulmozyme® Product monograph Genentech Inc., South San Franscisco, 2001.

89. Shah, P.L., et al., The effects of recombinant human DNase on neutrophil elastase activity and interleukin-8 levels in the sputum of patients with cystic fibrosis, *Eur. Resp. J.*, 9, 531–534, 1996.

90. Cantin, A.M., DNase I acutely increases cystic fibrosis sputum elastase activity and its potential to induce lung hemorrhage in mice, *Am. J. Respir. Crit. Care Med.*, 157, 464–469, 1998.

91. Perks, B. and Shute, J.K., DNA and actin bind and inhibit interleukin-8 function in cystic fibrosis sputa — *In vitro* effects of mucolytics, *Am. J. Respir. Crit. Care Med.*, 162, 1767–1772, 2000.

92. Paul, K., et al., Effect of treatment with dornase alpha on airway inflammation in patients with cystic fibrosis, *Am. J. Respir. Crit. Care Med.*, 169, 719–725, 2004.

93. Henry, R.L., et al., Airway inflammation after treatment with aerosolized deoxyribonuclease in cystic fibrosis, *Pediatr. Pulmonol.*, 26, 97–100, 1998.

94. Suri, R., et al., Effects of recombinant human DNase and hypertonic saline on airway inflammation in children with cystic fibrosis, *Am. J. Respir. Crit. Care Med.*, 166, 352–355, 2002.

95. Green, J.D., Pharmacotoxicological Expert Report — Pulmozyme™ rhDNase Genentech, Inc., *Hum. Exp. Toxicol.*, 13, S1–42, 1994.

96. Sinicropi, M.W., et al., Sputum pharmacodynamics and pharmacokinetics of recombinant DNase I in cystic fibrosis, *Am. J. Respir. Crit. Care Med.*, 149, A671, 1994.

97. Robinson, M., et al., Effect of a short course of rhDNase on cough and mucociliary clearance in patients with cystic fibrosis, *Pediatr. Pulmonol.*, 30, 16–24, 2000.

98. Mohler, M., et al., Altered pharmacokinetics of recombinant human deoxyribonuclease in rats due to the presence of a binding protein, *Drug Metab. Dispos.*, 21, 71–75, 1993.

99. Fiel, S.B., et al., Comparison of 3 jet nebulizer aerosol delivery systems used to administer recombinant human DNase-I to patients with cystic fibrosis, *Chest*, 108, 153–156, 1995.

100. Shah, P.L., et al., An evaluation of two aerosol delivery systems for rhDNase, *Eur. Respir. J.*, 10, 1261–1266, 1997.

101. Diot, P., et al., RhDNase I aerosol deposition and related factors in cystic fibrosis, *Am. J. Respir. Crit. Care Med.*, 156, 1662–1668, 1997.

102. Chan, H.K., et al., Spray dried powders and powder blends of recombinant human deoxyribonuclease (rhDNase) for aerosol delivery, *Pharm. Res.*, 14, 431–437, 1997.

103. Chan, H.K. and Gonda, I., Solid state characterization of spray-dried powders of recombinant human deoxyribonuclease (RhDNase), *J. Pharm. Sci.*, 87, 647–654, 1998.

104. Bustami, R.T., et al., Generation of fine powders of recombinant human deoxyribonuclease using the aerosol solvent extraction system, *Pharm. Res.*, 20, 2028–2035, 2003.

105. Zijlstra, G.S., et al., Pharmacoeconomic review of recombinant human DNase in the management of cystic fibrosis, *Expert Rev. Pharmacoeconomics Outcomes Res.*, 4, 49–59, 2004.

106. Davis, P.B., Evolution of therapy for cystic fibrosis, *New Engl. J. Med.*, 331, 672–673, 1994.

107. Davies, J., et al., Retrospective review of the effects of rhDNase in children with cystic fibrosis, *Pediatr. Pulmonol.*, 23, 243–248, 1997.

108. Milla, C.E., Long term effects of aerosolised rhDNase on pulmonary disease progression in patients with cystic fibrosis, *Thorax*, 53, 1014–1017, 1998.

109. Cobos, N., et al., DNase use in the daily care of cystic fibrosis: Who benefits from it and to what extent? Results of a cohort study of 199 patients in 13 centres, *Eur. J. Pediatr.*, 159, 176–181, 2000.

110. Suri, R., et al., Predicting response to rhDNase and hypertonic saline in children with cystic fibrosis, *Pediatr. Pulmonol.*, 37, 305–310, 2004.

111. Sanders, N.N., De Smedt, S.C., and Demeester, J., Therapeutic Compositions for the Treatment of a Respiratory Tract Disease, Universiteit Gent, Patent WO02083167, 2002.

112. Lazarides, E. and Lindberg, U., Actin is the naturally occurring inhibitor of deoxyribonuclease I, *Proc. Natl. Acad. Sci., USA*, 71, 4742–4746, 1974.

113. Ulmer, J.S., et al., Engineering actin-resistant human DNase I for treatment of cystic fibrosis, *Proc. Natl. Acad. Sci., USA*, 93, 8225–8229, 1996.

114. Mannherz, H.G., et al., The interaction of bovine pancreatic deoxyribonuclease I and skeletal muscle actin, *Eur. J. Biochem.*, 104, 367–379, 1980.

115. Kabsch, W., et al., Atomic structure of the actin: DNase I complex, *Nature*, 347, 37–44, 1990.

116. McLaughlin, P.J. and Weeds, A.G., Actin binding protein complexes at atomic resolution, *Annu. Rev. Biophys. Biomol. Struct.*, 24, 643–675, 1995.

117. Mannherz, H.G. and Rohr, G., 5'-Nucleotidase reverses the inhibitory action of actin on pancreatic deoxyribonuclease I, *FEBS Lett.*, 95, 284–289, 1978.

118. Rohr, G. and Mannherz, H.G., The activation of actin: DNase I complex with rat liver plasma membranes. The possible role of 5'-nucleotidase, *FEBS Lett.*, 99, 351–356, 1979.

119. Davoodian, K., et al., Gelsolin activates DNase I *in vitro* and in cystic fibrosis sputum, *Biochemistry*, 36, 9637–9641, 1997.

120. Zahm, J.M., et al., Improved activity of an actin-resistant DNase I variant on the cystic fibrosis airway secretions, *Am. J. Respir. Crit. Care Med.*, 163, 1153–1157, 2001.

121. Baron, W.F., et al., Cloning and characterization of an actin-resistant DNase I-like endonuclease secreted by macrophages, *Gene*, 215, 291–301, 1998.

122. Shiokawa, D. and Tanuma, S., DLAD, a novel mammalian divalent cation-independent endonuclease with homology to DNase II, *Nucleic Acids Res.*, 27, 4083–4089, 1999.

123. Krieser, R.J., et al., The cloning, genomic structure, localization, and expression of human deoxyribonuclease IIβ, *Gene*, 269, 205–216, 2001.

124. Ratjen, F., Dornase in non-CF, *Pediatr. Pulmonol.*, 26 (Suppl.), 154–155, 2004.

125. Gershan, W.M., et al., Resolution of chronic atelectasis in a child with asthma after aerosolized recombinant human DNase, *Pediatr. Pulmonol.*, 18, 268–269, 1994.

126. Touleimat, B.A., Conoscenti, C.S., and Fine, J.M., Recombinant human DNase in management of lobar atelectasis due to retained secretions, *Thorax*, 50, 1319–1321, 1995.

127. Voelker, K.G., Chetty, K.G., and Mahutte, C.K., Resolution of recurrent atelectasis in spinal cord injury patients with administration of recombinant human DNase, *Intensive Care Med.*, 22, 582–584, 1996.

128. Greally, P., Human recombinant DNase for mucus plugging in status asthmaticus, *Lancet*, 346, 1423–1424, 1995.

129. Durward, A., Forte, V., and Shemie, S.D., Resolution of mucus plugging and atelectasis after intratracheal rhDNase therapy in a mechanically ventilated child with refractory status asthmaticus, *Crit. Care Med.*, 28, 560–562, 2000.

130. El-Hassan, N.O., et al., Rescue use of DNase in critical lung atelectasis and mucus retention in premature neonates, *Pediatrics*, 108, 468–470, 2001.

131. Merkus, P.J.F.M., et al., DNase treatment for atelectasis in infants with severe respiratory syncytial virus bronchiolitis, *Eur. Respir. J.*, 18, 734–737, 2001.

132. Desai, M., Weller, P.H., and Spencer, D.A., Clinical benefit from nebulized human recombinant DNase in Kartagener's syndrome, *Pediatr. Pulmonol.*, 20, 307–308, 1995.

133. ten Berge, M., et al., DNase treatment in primary ciliary dyskinesia — Assessment by nocturnal pulse oximetry, *Pediatr. Pulmonol.*, 27, 59–61, 1999.

134. Nasr, S.Z., et al., Efficacy of recombinant human deoxyribonuclease I in the hospital management of respiratory syncytial virus bronchiolitis, *Chest*, 120, 203–208, 2001.

135. Simpson, G., Roomes, D., and Reeves, B., Successful treatment of empyema thoracis with human recombinant deoxyribonuclease, *Thorax*, 58, 365–366, 2003.

136. Wills, P.J., et al., Short-term recombinant human DNase in bronchiectasis. Effect on clinical state and *in vitro* sputum transportability, *Am. J. Respir. Crit. Care Med.*, 154, 413–417, 1996.

137. Hudson, T.J., Dornase in treatment of chronic bronchitis, *Ann. Pharmacother.*, 30, 674–675, 1996.

138. O'Donnell, A.E., et al., Treatment of idiopathic bronchiectasis with aerosolized recombinant human DNase I, rhDNase Study Group, *Chest*, 113, 1329–1334, 1998.

139. Rubin, B.K., Who will benefit from DNase? *Pediatr. Pulmonol.*, 27, 3–4, 1999.

140. Vanholder, R., et al., The pathophysiology of lupus erythematosus, *Eur. J. Dermatol.*, 8, 4–7, 1998.

141. Bickerstaff, M.C.M., et al., Serum amyloid P component controls chromatin degradation and prevents antinuclear autoimmunity, *Nat. Med.*, 5, 694–697, 1999.

142. Botto, M., et al., Homozygous C1q deficiency causes glomerulonephritis associated with multiple apoptotic bodies, *Nat. Genet.*, 19, 56–59, 1998.

143. Manderson, A.P., Botto, M., and Walport, M.J., The role of complement in the development of systemic lupus erythematosus, *Annu. Rev. Immunol.*, 22, 431–456, 2004.

144. Macanovic, M. and Lachmann, P.J., Measurement of deoxyribonuclease I (DNase) in the serum and urine of systemic lupus erythematosus (SLE)-prone NZB/NZW mice by a new radial enzyme diffusion assay, *Clin. Exp. Immunol.*, 108, 220–226, 1997.

145. Napirei, M., et al., Features of systemic lupus erythematosus in Dnase1-deficient mice, *Nat. Genet.*, 25, 177–181, 2000.

146. Lachmann, P.J., Lupus and desoxyribonuclease, *Lupus*, 12, 202–206, 2003.

147. Yasutomo, K., et al., Mutation of DNASE1 in people with systemic lupus erythematosus, *Nat. Genet.*, 28, 313–314, 2001.

148. Puccetti, A., et al., Anti-DNA antibodies bind to DNase I, *J. Exp. Med.*, 181, 1797–1804, 1995.

149. Yeh, T.M., et al., Deoxyribonuclease-inhibitory antibodies in systemic lupus erythematosus, *J. Biomed. Sci.*, 10, 544–551, 2003.
150. Lachmann, P.J., Allergic reactions, connective tissue, and disease, *Sci. Basis Med. Annu. Rev.*, 36–58, 1967.
151. Macanovic, M., et al., The treatment of systemic lupus erythematosus (SLE) in NZB/W F_1 hybrid mice; studies with recombinant murine DNase and with dexamethasone, *Clin. Exp. Immunol.*, 106, 243–252, 1996.
152. Verthelyi, D., et al., DNAse treatment does not improve the survival of lupus prone (NZB × NZW) F_1 mice, *Lupus*, 7, 223–230, 1998.
153. Davis, J.C., et al., Recombinant human Dnase I (rhDNase) in patients with lupus nephritis, *Lupus*, 8, 68–76, 1999.
154. Prince, W.S., et al., Pharmacodynamics of recombinant human DNase I in serum, *Clin. Exp. Immunol.*, 113, 289–296, 1998.
155. Clark, M.G., Topical Ointment Composition, U.S. Patent 4005191, 1977.
156. Schwarz, N., Wound cleansing with the enzyme combination fibrinolysin/deoxy-ribonuclease, *Fortschr. Med.*, 99, 978–980, 1981.
157. Westerhof, W., et al., Controlled double-blind trial of fibrinolysin-deoxyribonuclease (Elase) solution in patients with chronic leg ulcers who are treated before autologous skin-grafting, *J. Am. Acad. Dermatol.*, 17, 32–39, 1987.
158. Toriyabe, S., Saito, H., and Sakurai, R., Use of a food wrap as a dressing material, *Adv. Skin Wound Care*, 6, 405–406, 1999.
159. Romancalderon, J., Treatment of 2nd and 3rd degree burns — Comparison of effects of proteolytic-enzyme combination and silver-nitrate, *Curr. Ther. Res.*, 32, 305–311, 1982.
160. Mekkes, J.R., et al., *In vitro* tissue digesting properties of krill enzymes compared with fibrinolysin/DNAse, papain and placebo, *Int. J. Biochem. Cell Biol.*, 29, 703–706, 1997.
161. Falabella, A.F., et al., The safety and efficacy of a proteolytic ointment in the treatment of chronic ulcers of the lower extremity, *J. Am. Acad. Dermatol.*, 39, 737–740, 1998.
162. Mekkes, J.R., Zeegelaar, J.E., and Westerhof, W., Quantitative and objective evaluation of wound debriding properties of collagenase and fibrinolysin/desoxyribonuclease in a necrotic ulcer animal model, *Arch. Dermatol. Res.*, 290, 152–157, 1998.
163. Linardou, H., Epenetos, A.A., and Deonarain, M.P., A recombinant cytotoxic chimera based on mammalian deoxyribonuclease I, *Int. J. Cancer*, 86, 561–569, 2000.
164. Ben-Yehudah, A., et al., Using apoptosis for targeted cancer therapy by a new gonadotropin releasing hormone-DNA fragmentation factor 40 chimeric protein, *Clin. Cancer Res.*, 9, 1179–1190, 2003.
165. Shak, S., Human DNase, Genentech, Patent WO9007572, 1989.
166. Mather, J.P. and Tsao, M.C., Method for Culturing Chinese Hamster Ovary Cells to Improve Production of Recombinant Proteins, Genentech, U.S. Patent 5122469, 1992.
167. Chan, H.K., et al., DNase Liquid Solutions, Genentech, U.S. Patent Application 20030054532, 2003.
168. Frenz, J., Steven, J., and Sliwkowski, M.B., Purified Forms of DNase, Genentech, Patent WO9325670, 1993.
169. Hsieh, S.Y., et al., Aberrant caspase-activated DNase (CAD) transcripts in human hepatoma cells, *Br. J. Cancer*, 88, 210–216, 2003.
170. Bairoch A., et al., Swiss-Prot: Juggling between evolution and stability, *Brief. Bioinform.*, 5, 39–55, 2004.

6

β-*Glucocerebrosidase Ceredase® and Cerezyme®*

Tim Edmunds

CONTENTS

6.1   Introduction

Glucocerebrosidase (acid β-glucosidase, β-D-glucosyl-*n*-acylsphingosine glucohydrolase, EC 3.2.1.45) is a lysosomal hydrolase that catalyzes the hydrolysis of glucosylceramide to glucose and ceramide (Figure 6.1). Deficiency of the enzyme results in the accumulation of glucosylceramide in macrophages of the reticular endothelial system, giving rise to the lysosomal storage disease known as Gaucher Disease. Gaucher Disease was the first of the lysosomal storage diseases to be successfully treated by enzyme replacement therapy (ERT), first using the natural enzyme isolated from human placenta (Ceredase®) and then a recombinant enzyme produced in a Chinese hamster ovary (CHO) cell line (Cerezyme®). Ceredase was also the first therapeutic protein to utilize carbohydrate engineering to target a specific cell type in order to improve efficacy. This chapter will outline the development of Ceredase and Cerezyme from the initial discovery of the enzymatic defect in Gaucher Disease to the approval of Cerezyme.

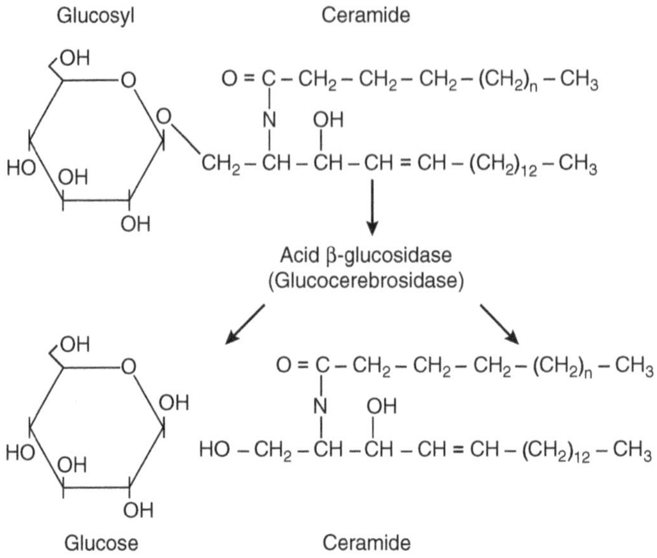

Glucosyl Ceramide

$$O = C - CH_2 - CH_2 - CH_2 - (CH_2)_n - CH_3$$

$$CH_2 - CH - CH - CH = CH - (CH_2)_{12} - CH_3$$

Acid β-glucosidase
(Glucocerebrosidase)

$$O = C - CH_2 - CH_2 - CH_2 - (CH_2)_n - CH_3$$

$$HO - CH_2 - CH - CH - CH = CH - (CH_2)_{12} - CH_3$$

Glucose Ceramide

FIGURE 6.1 Glucosylceramide cleavage by β-glucocerebrosidase.

6.2 Gaucher Disease

Gaucher Disease is named after its discoverer, Philippe Gaucher, who first described the disease in 1882. Gaucher Disease is a member of the family of disorders known as lysosomal storage diseases [1]. These diseases are characterized by the accumulation of various substrates within the lysosome due to a deficiency in the activity of one or more catabolic enzymes. The pathology of the lysosomal storage diseases is varied and depends on the organ and cell type in which the substrate accumulation occurs. In the case of Gaucher Disease, it is characterized by the accumulation of the glycolipid glucocerebroside (glucosylceramide) in the cells of the reticuloendothelial system, in particular, the macrophages of the liver, spleen, and bone marrow [2–6]. The accumulation of glucocerebroside results in a gross enlargement of the macrophages, giving rise to cells with a very distinct appearance, termed "Gaucher's cells". The presence of these large Gaucher's cells, which in turn give rise to hepatosplenomegaly, is characteristic of the disease. Other manifestations of the disease include hematological and skeletal abnormalities.

Gaucher Disease is an autosomal-recessive genetic disorder and is the most common of the lysosomal storage diseases. Even so, it is still very rare (~6000 cases worldwide), with the highest disease prevalence (1 in 855) found in the Ashkenazi Jewish population [7]. Historically, Gaucher Disease has been classified into three types based on the time of onset and the severity of the disease (Table 6.1). Type I disease is most common of the three forms and is distinguished from Types II and III by the lack of neurological involvement [7]. Since Types II and III are now considered to present a continuum of disease severity, the current classification refers to nonneuronopathic (Type I) and neuronopathic (Type II and III) Gaucher Disease [8]. Type I disease is the least severe of the three forms, with patients displaying a wide phenotype ranging from mildly symptomatic to fatal. The most common genetic defect found in the Type I patients is a point mutation resulting in an asparagine to serine substitution at amino acid residue 370

TABLE 6.1

Gaucher Disease Variants

Clinical Features	Nonneuronopathic	Neuronopathic	
	Type I	Type II	Type III
Age at onset	Childhood/adulthood	Infancy	Childhood
Lifespan	Infancy to 80+ years	Infancy	Childhood–middle age
Hepatosplenomegaly	Yes	Yes	Yes
Skeletal disease	Yes	No	Yes
Primary CNS disease	No	Yes	Yes
Predominant ethnic group	Ashkenazi Jewish	Panethnic	Panethnic

(N370S). The N370S mutation accounts for ~70% of the mutant alleles in the Ashkenazi Jewish population and ~45% of the mutant alleles in the nonJewish population. The presence of the N370S mutation is associated with less severe forms of the disease and has never been associated with the Type II or Type III disease. In contrast, the substitution of a proline for leucine at amino acid residue 444 (L444P) leads to severe forms of the disease, accompanied by neurological impairment. The mutations giving rise to the disease have been identified in the majority of patients, and it is clear from these studies that, within a given genotype, there is considerable phenotypic variation both with respect to the age of onset and severity of the disease [9].

6.3 Biochemistry

Early research identified glucosylceramide as the compound that accumulated in Gaucher's cells but it was not until 1965 that the pioneering efforts of Brady, et al. [10,11] in the United States and Patrick [12] in the United Kingdom, revealed that a deficiency of the lysosomal enzyme β-glucocerebrosidase was the defect leading to the accumulation of glucosylceramide in Gaucher Disease. Following the identification of the defective enzyme, it was suggested, as early as 1966 [13] that the disease may be treated by ERT. Several groups put a great deal of effort over the following years into purifying and characterizing the enzyme. Since we now know that β-glucocerebrosidase is hydrophobic in nature, unstable at neutral pH, and requires the presence of detergents for solubility and full activity [14–16], it is not surprising that these early attempts to produce a pure preparation of the enzyme met with varying degrees of success [17–23].

Initial characterization of the enzyme was carried out on material purified from human placenta, liver, and spleen. These early purification attempts gave poor yields and produced proteins with different physical and biochemical properties. After several years, an efficient procedure for the extraction and purification of material from human placentas was developed based on lessons learned from the early purification schemes. This improved purification process incorporated detergent and organic solvent extractions as well as hydrophobic interaction chromatography [18,19,22], and the use of ethylene glycol-containing buffers maintained enzyme activity. The purified protein resulting from this procedure had a molecular mass of 67 kDa and ~ 7% carbohydrate content. As would be expected for a lysosomal protein, β-glucocerebrosidase has an acidic pH optimum of ~5.5. Due to the insolubility of the natural substrate, glucosylceramide, β-glucocerebrosidase activity is normally measured using soluble artificial substrates such as 4-methylumbelliferyl-β-D-glucopyranoside or *p*-nitrophenyl-β-D-glucopyranoside.

The presence of a heat-stable activating factor of β-glucocerebrosidase was identified in early crude preparations of the enzyme by several investigators [24–32]. The stabilizing factor was isolated and characterized from normal and Gaucher patient's spleens, and is now known as saposin C. Saposin C is a small (9 kDa) acidic glycoprotein containing three disulfide bonds and is generated by proteolytic processing of prosaposin, a larger precursor protein. It is believed that *in vivo* β-glucocerebrosidase is activated by the formation of a complex with saposin C and the lysosomal membrane [33,34]. The interaction with saposin C is essential for the *in vivo* activity of β-glucocerebrosidase. Genetic deficiency of saposin C leads to accumulation of glucosylceramide and to a very rare variant of Gaucher Disease [35].

In vitro studies have demonstrated that β-glucocerebrosidase activation by saposin C is dependent on the presence of acidic phospholipids. Although acidic phospholipids alone will activate β-glucocerebrosidase, this activation is significantly enhanced in he presence of saposin C [29,36]. In contrast, no activation by saposin C alone is observed. β-Glucocerebrosidase is also activated by detergents such as taurocholate and Triton X-100, so for convenience these are the preferred activators for routine enzyme assays [15].

The protein sequence of β-glucocerebrosidase was predicted from the complementary deoxyribonucleic acid (cDNA) sequence independently by two groups in 1985 [37,38]. The two published sequences differed at two locations. The Sorge sequence contained a phenylalanine at residue 259 and a histidine at residue 495, whereas the Tsuji sequence contained leucine and arginine residues, respectively, at these positions. Afterwards, however, Tsuji reported that phenylalanine was the residue identified at position 259 by protein sequence analysis, and Sorge, et al. [39] published a correction identifying arginine as the true amino acid encoded at residue 495.

The β-glucocerebrosidase cDNA sequence encodes a 516-amino-acid protein that includes a 19-amino-acid leader sequence. The mature protein is monomeric and contains seven cysteine residues which form two intrachain disulfide bonds. X-ray crystallographic studies show that the disulfide bonds are located between C4 to C16 and C18 to C23 with C126, C248, and C342 being free thiols [40]. The significance of the three thiol groups has not been determined, but mutagenesis studies suggest that C126 and C248 are not essential for catalytic activity [9]. The X-ray structure indicates that β-glucocerebrosidase contains three distinct domains, with the catalytic site residues located in the third domain consisting of residues 30 to 75 and 431 to 497. X-ray data also confirms earlier biochemical analysis suggesting that the active-site residues are E235 and E340.

Based on amino acid sequence, β-glucocerebrosidase contains five potential N-linked glycosylation sites at N19, N59, N146, N270, and N462, but only the first four of these sites are occupied [41,42]. The enzyme isolated from human placenta was shown to contain a mixture of bi- and triantennary complex oligosaccharides as well as oligomannose-type chains [43]. This glycosylation pattern is unusual for a lysosomal enzyme because the oligomannose chains of β-glucocerebrosidase do not contain mannose-6-phosphate [43,44]. This observation is significant since the trafficking of most lysosomal glycoproteins is mediated through the binding of mannose-6-phosphate to the cation-independent mannose-6-phosphate receptor. In the case of endogenous β-glucocerebrosidase, the means by which it is targeted to the lysosome is unknown.

6.4   Early Attempts at Therapy

Following the identification of β-glucocerebrosidase as the defective enzyme in Gaucher Disease and the proposal that the disease could be treated by replacing the defective enzyme, it took several years until sufficient material of optimum purity was available for clinical studies. Brady, et al. [45] performed an initial clinical study on two patients in 1974 using this highly purified material from human placenta. Despite a relatively low single dose of enzyme in each case, a reduction of glucocerebroside was observed in the liver of both patients. This early clinical study demonstrated the feasibility of ERT but also highlighted the need for much larger quantities of enzyme. Subsequent clinical studies using enzyme purified by a modified and scaled-up procedure resulted in both a more modest and more variable reduction in glucocerebroside levels [46].

When animal studies were conducted with this material it was found that only small amounts of enzyme were taken up by the cells of the reticuloendothelial system, with almost all of the protein being taken up by hepatocytes [47]. During this period, other groups conducted clinical studies using purified β-glucocerebrosidase, but with mixed results. Beutler, et al. [48] and Ihler, et al. [50] attempted to improve efficacy by stabilizing β-glucocerebrosidase in erythrocyte ghosts while Gregoriadis, et al. [51] and Braidman and Gregoriadis [52] utilized liposomal encapsulation.

A major turning point in the development of an effective therapy occurred in 1978 when Stahl, et al. [53] identified the mannose receptor on alveolar macrophages that bound mannose-terminated glycoproteins. Brady and his colleagues reasoned that utilization of the mannose receptor should increase the delivery of β-glucocerebrosidase to macrophages. Initial studies involving targeting of this receptor to increase delivery to macrophages focused on covalent attachment of sugar chains to the enzyme. Addition of pentamannose was unsuccessful in increasing the amount of enzyme delivered to macrophages, whereas branched trimannosyl-dilysyl residues produced a modest increase in uptake into macrophages [54,55]. Subsequent studies utilized enzymatic modification of the carbohydrate chains and produced more impressive results. Sequential deglycosylation of β-glucocerebrosidase was carried out to remove the sialic acid, galactose, and N-acetylglucosamine from the complex oligosaccharides. Removal of the sialic acid alone increased clearance from the circulation owing to increased the uptake by the asialoglycoprotein receptor. Removal of the galactose residues increased uptake of β-glucocerebrosidase into the nonparenchymal cells of the liver 3.5-fold compared to nonremodeled β-glucocerebrosidase (Table 6.2). Removal of the N-acetylglucosamine residues resulted in a further 1.4-fold increase in uptake into the nonparenchymal

TABLE 6.2

Effect of Carbohydrate Remodeling on Liver Cell Uptake

Treatment	Cellular Distribution (U/10^6 Cells)	
	Nonparenchymal	Hepatocytes
Control (no enzyme)	6.6	104
None	48	256
Neuraminidase	16	337
Neuraminidase and galactosidase	170	380
Neuraminidase, galactosidase, and hexoseaminidase	245	290

cells [56]. These studies established the need for optimum carbohydrate remodeling for β-glucocerebrosidase enzyme replacement to be an effective therapy for treatment of Gaucher Disease.

6.5   Development of Ceredase

With the proof of concept demonstrated, significant effort was required to scale up the extraction and purification of placental glucocerebrosidase to make it clinically and commercially viable. The magnitude of this challenge can be appreciated by the fact that it took ~20,000 placentas to extract enough β-glucocerebrosidase to treat 1 patient for 1 year. Genzyme Corporation adapted the purification and carbohydrate remodeling schemes developed by Brady, et al., to improve both the purification efficiency and purity of the final product. Since the source material for the enzyme was human placentas, a great deal of care was taken to ensure that the final production process had sufficient viral reduction steps to eliminate any risk of viral contamination. In addition to scaling up the β-glucocerebrosidase purification, it was also essential to scale up the production of the three carbohydrate-remodeling enzymes and implement additional chromatographic steps for their removal. The resulting highly purified carbohydrate-remodeled β-glucocerebrosidase was formulated with 1% human serum albumin and sold commercially as Ceredase (Alglucerase).

The clinical trial that led to the approval of Ceredase was conducted on 12 patients, 4 adults and 8 children who were classified with Type I Gaucher Disease. Patients were given 60 IU of Ceredase/kg of body weight by intravenous infusion once every 2 weeks for between 9 and 12 months. Part way through the trial, the dose of two severely affected children was increased to 60 IU/kg every week. All patients in the trial showed a clinical response with a reduction in spleen volume and an increase in hemoglobin. Other clinical improvements observed in several patients included a reduction in liver size, reduction in plasma glucocerebroside and serum levels of tartrate-resistant acid phosphatase (a lysosomal enzyme that is elevated in some lysosomal storage diseases), and an increase in platelet count. Some evidence of an improvement in the bone disease was observed in three of the patients [57].

Since Ceredase was a natural product of human origin, a higher level of host protein impurities was allowed than would be typical of a recombinant product today. Detection of impurities was also challenging since the protein was formulated with a significant molar excess of human serum albumin. Following product approval and during the development of reversed-phase high-performance liquid chromatography (HPLC) methods to determine protein purity, two prominent (relative to other impurity peaks) protein impurity peaks were detected in the Ceredase preparations. Isolation and N-terminal sequence analysis identified the two peaks as the α and β subunits of human chorionic gonadotropin (HCG). Although product containing HCG had been given to several patients for an extended period of time, no serious adverse events were reported [58,59]. The low level (~2%) of HCG contamination and the fact that it was subjected to the carbohydrate remodeling process most likely contributed to the lack of adverse events associated with the presence of HCG. The carbohydrate remodeling step also resulted in the oligosaccharides of HCG terminating in mannose residues, producing a very short half-life relative to native HCG. Once the HCG impurity was identified, the purification scheme was modified to eliminate this impurity from later preparations.

Although the presence of a low level of placental protein impurity was acceptable, as the impurities were also human proteins and would not be expected to be immunogenic, complete removal of the three nonhuman-derived enzymes required for carbohydrate remodeling was essential, and development of specific and sensitive assays for detecting residual enzymes was required. The efficiency of the purification scheme in removing these proteins is demonstrated by the low level of immune response in patients who received Ceredase at doses often exceeding 100 mg per infusion [60].

6.6   Development of Cerezyme

Even before Ceredase received approval as a therapy for Gaucher Disease, its safety and efficacy were readily apparent. But it was also apparent that the clinical supply of Ceredase would eventually be limited by the availability of human placentas. Another important consideration at the time was the potential risk of viral contamination in a product derived from human tissue. This risk was extremely low in the case of Ceredase as placentas were screened for viral contamination, and the harsh detergent-based extraction procedure as well as the purification steps were very effective viral reduction steps. Given these considerations, development of a recombinant product, Cerezyme (Imiglucerase), was initiated even before the approval of Ceredase.

Since β-glucocerebrosidase is a large glycoprotein and carbohydrates are essential for correct folding and activity, a mammalian expression system was chosen. The cDNA for β-glucocerebrosidase was cloned into CHO cells using a dihydrofolate reductase (DHFR) expression system. Following amplification, highest producing clones were adapted to an anchorage-dependent serum-free microcarrier spinner culture system for production evaluation [61]. The highest producing line was then progressively scaled up from spinner flasks to production bioreactors of increasing size up to 2000 L. The bioreactors were operated in a continuous perfusion mode to maximize production efficiency and reduce the potential for proteolytic degradation or other posttranslational modifications of the product due to cell lysis. The Cerezyme purification process was similar to that used for the production of Ceredase and was based on standard chromatographic procedures. Since the bioreactors were harvested in a serum-free mode during production, the initial impurity burden on the purification scheme was less than that for the Ceredase purification process. But because Cerezyme was produced using recombinant technology in a CHO cell line, a significantly higher level of purity was required, necessitating modifications of the purification scheme. These increased purity requirements also necessitated the development of additional analytical tools such as an enzyme linked immunosorbent assay (ELISA) to detect host cell proteins, reversed-phase HPLC, and peptide-mapping methods.

In developing the recombinant product, it was also desirable to eliminate the human serum albumin that was used as a stabilizer in Ceredase to reduce further the risk of viral contamination. In the absence of a protein stabilizer, β-glucocerebrosidase is prone to aggregate at the concentrations required for a commercial product. This required a change from the liquid formulation used in Ceredase to the lyophilized formulation used today for Cerezyme.

One of the challenges of developing recombinant protein products is the potential for differences between the recombinant product and the naturally occurring protein. These differences can result in increased immunogenicity, altered biodistribution, efficacy, and safety. In many cases, direct comparison of the recombinant protein with the natural protein is not feasible owing to a lack of sufficient natural protein or processing of the enzyme during extraction or isolation, as may occur in plasma proteins isolated from urine. The availability of highly purified human placental β-glucocerebrosidase (Ceredase) allowed a detailed comparison of the recombinant product with to the placental protein. This comparison was subsequently used as the basis of comprehensive analyses for demonstrating product comparability during manufacturing scale-up and other process changes.

6.7 Biochemical Comparison of Cerezyme and Ceredase

The biochemical comparison of the two proteins was based on detailed structural protein analysis, enzymatic properties, and *in vitro* binding and uptake studies. One of the key methods incorporated in this analysis was peptide mapping. When the Cerezyme peptide-mapping procedure was developed, electrospray mass spectrometry was in its infancy and was just being developed for protein applications. Peptide mapping is a powerful tool for studying posttranslational modifications as well as differences in amino acid sequence and proteolytic processing. Without mass spectrometry, the power of the peptide map hinges on the resolution and reproducibility of enzymatic digestion, chromatographic separation, and identification of peptides by N-terminal sequencing.

For Cerezyme and Ceredase, trypsin was chosen for peptide mapping because it resulted in peptides of suitable length for both recovery from the HPLC column and N-terminal sequence analysis. Digestion of Cerezyme with trypsin produces 44 theoretical tryptic peptides (Table 6.3); however, the actual number of peptides observed differed from the theoretical value due to partial and nonspecific cleavages. When the peptide maps of Cerezyme and Ceredase were compared (Figure 6.2), the tryptic maps obtained were very similar even at the level of minor peaks, with the exception of four peaks (labeled A to D). Interestingly, the four differences observed between the Cerezyme and Ceredase tryptic maps all arise from a single amino acid substitution at position 495. The cDNA sequence published by Sorge [37] was used for the development of the Cerezyme-producing cell line. This sequence was subsequently found to contain a sequence error arising from a cloning artifact that resulted in the encoding of a histidine residue instead of an arginine residue [39]. The protein sequence of Cerezyme therefore differs from that of Ceredase at residue 495. In Ceredase, the C-terminal sequence is WRRQ and in Cerezyme the corresponding sequence is WHRQ. This results in tryptic cleavage at residue 495 in Ceredase compared with cleavage at residue 496 in Cerezyme. In the case of both Ceredase and Cerezyme, incomplete cleavage of the C-terminal peptide is observed to give rise to peak C in the Cerezyme map and peak D in the Ceredase map. The complete cleavage product, peak B in the Cerezyme map, is not present in the Ceredase map, presumably due to the presence of double arginines that apparently affect the tryptic cleavage. Peak A in the Cerezyme map arose from a chymotryptic-like cleavage at Y487, while a corresponding cleavage was not observed in the Ceredase map.

This single amino acid difference between the natural (Ceredase) and the recombinant protein (Cerezyme) does not have any significant effect on the enzymatic activity of the proteins since the two are enzymatically indistinguishable (Table 6.4).

The oligosaccharide structures present on placental β-glucocerebrosidase had previously been shown to be a combination of complex and oligomannose oligosaccharides, but the site-specific distribution of these structures had not been determined [43]. The carbohydrate remodeling process (Figure 6.3) used in the production of Ceredase remodels the complex structures down to the $GlcNAc_2 Man_3$ core structure but does not affect the oligomannose oligosaccharides, resulting in a combination of mannose-terminated core structures and oligomannose chains.

TABLE 6.3

Recombinant β-Glucocerebrosidase Tryptic Peptides

Peptide	Amino Acid Number	Sequence
T1	1–2	AR
T2	3–7	PCIPK
T3	8–39	SFGYS SVVCV CNATY CDSFD PPTFP ALGTF SR
T4	40–44	YESTR
T5	45–47	SGR
T6	48	R
T7	49–74	MELSM GPIQA NHTGT GLLLT LQPEQ K
T8	75–77	FQK
T9	78–79	VK
T10	80–106	GFGGA MTDAA ALNIL ALSPP AQNLL LK
T11	107–120	SYFSE EGIGY NIIR
T12	121–131	VPMAS CDFSI R
T13	132–155	TYTYA DTPDD FQLHN FSLPE EDTK
T14	156–157	LK
T15	158–163	IPLIH R
T16	164–170	ALQLA QR
T17	171–186	PVSLL ASPWT SPTWL K
T18	187–194	TNGAV NGK
T19	195–198	GSLK
T20	199–211	GQPGD IYHQT WAR
T21	212–215	YFVK
T22	216–224	FLDAY AEHK
T23	225–257	LQFWA VTAEN EPSAG LLSGY PFQCL GFTPE HQR
T24	258–262	DFIAR
T25	263–277	DLGPT LANST HHNVR
T26	278–285	LLMLD DQR
T27	286–293	LLLPH WAK
T28	294–303	VVLTD PEAAK
T29	304–321	YVHGI AVHWY LDFLA PAK
T30	322–329	ATLGE THR
T31	330–346	LFPNT MLFAS EACVG SK
T32	347–353	FWEQS VR
T33	354–359	LGSWD R
T34	360–395	GMQYS HSIIT NLLYH VVGWT DWNLA LNPEG GPNWV R
T35	396–408	NFVDS PIIVD ITK
T36	409–413	DTFYK
T37	414–425	QPMFY HLGHF SK
T38	426–433	FIPEG SQR
T39	434–441	VGLVA SQK
T40	442–463	NDLDA VALMH PDGSA VVVVL NR
T41	464–466	SSK
T42	467–473	DVPLT IK
T43	474–496	DPAVG FLETI SPGYS IHTYL W<u>H</u>R
T44	497	Q

Potential N-linked glycosylation sites are indicated by bold type. The Ceredase sequence differs from that given above by the substitution of H495 (underlined) by arginine.

Differences in glycosylation can have a significant impact on the half-life, bioavailability, and biodistribution of proteins. Since both the placental and recombinant β-glucocerebrosidase undergo the same carbohydrate-remodeling steps to produce mannose-terminated oligosaccharides, it was not expected that any major differences would arise in biological properties due to glycosylation differences. Nevertheless, a detailed comparison of the

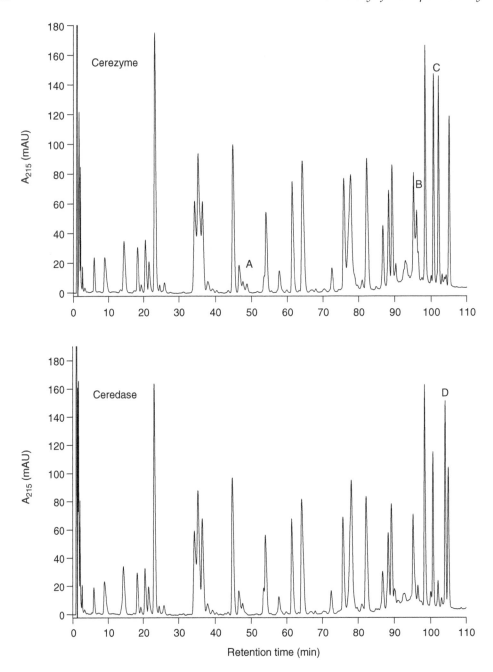

FIGURE 6.2
Tryptic peptide maps of reduced and pyridylethylated Cerezyme and Ceredase. The four peptides that differ between the two proteins are labeled A to D.

glycosylation was carried out in light of the importance of the carbohydrate remodeling process to the efficacy of Ceredase.

Monosaccharide compositional analysis is a convenient way to determine the efficiency of the oligosaccharide remodeling process since complete oligosaccharide remodeling should remove all of the galactose residues. Monosaccharide compositional analysis

TABLE 6.4

Kinetic Parameters for Ceredase and Cerezyme for the Hydrolysis of
p-Nitrophenyl β-D-Glucopyranoside

Sample	K_m^* (mM)	V_{max}^*(μmol/min/mg)
Ceredase	1.00 (0.04)	48.1 (2.0)
Cerezyme	1.01 (0.09)	48.4 (3.9)

*Mean (Standard Deviation)

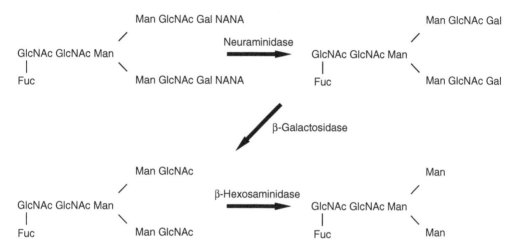

FIGURE 6.3   β-Glucocerebrosidase oligosaccharide-remodeling process.

performed before and after the oligosaccharide remodeling process (Table 6.5) indicated that the remodeling step was highly efficient for both Ceredase and Cerezyme, with only 4.5% of the galactose remaining in Ceredase and 10.5% remaining in Cerezyme. A difference in the level of fucosylation between the two proteins was also evident in this analysis, as was a slightly higher level of mannose residues in Ceredase.

A more detailed analysis of the glycosylation was performed by fluorophore-assisted carbohydrate analysis (FACE®). FACE is used to monitor the carbohydrate remodeling process as well as determine the structures at each of the four occupied glycosylation sites. In FACE analysis, released oligosaccharides are labeled with a charged fluorescent dye and separated on highly cross-linked, high-percentage acrylamide gels based on mass and charge. FACE analysis before and after oligosaccharide remodeling clearly showed the reduction of the complex oligosaccharides to $Man_3GlcNAc_2 \pm Fuc$ (Figure 6.4) and the presence of oligomannose structures on Ceredase that were not modified by the remodeling process. Interestingly, no oligomannose carbohydrate chains were detected in Cerezyme.

The location of the oligomannose and fucosylated structures and the efficiency of remodeling at each N-linked glycosylation site were determined by FACE analysis of the oligosaccharides isolated from individual glycopeptides (Figure 6.5). The main difference in fucosylation between the two proteins was observed at N146, which was more heavily fucosylated in Cerezyme. The oligomannose structures present on Ceredase are located at N19, and based upon the fluorescence intensity of the oligosaccharide bands, the predominant oligomannose structure is Man_6, with Man_5, Man_7, and Man_8 structures also present. Although the remodeled oligosaccharide structures differed between Cerezyme

TABLE 6.5

Monosaccharide Compositions of Placental and Recombinant Glucocerebrosidase Before and After Oligosaccharide Remodeling

Sample	Protein (mol/mol)			
	Fuc	GlcNAc	Gal	Man
Placental β-glucocerebrosidase	1.6	14.8	8.9	15.2
Ceredase	1.4	7.4	0.4	15.2
Recombinant human β-glucocerebrosidase	2.1	15	8.6	12
Cerezyme	2.1	7.9	0.9	12.3

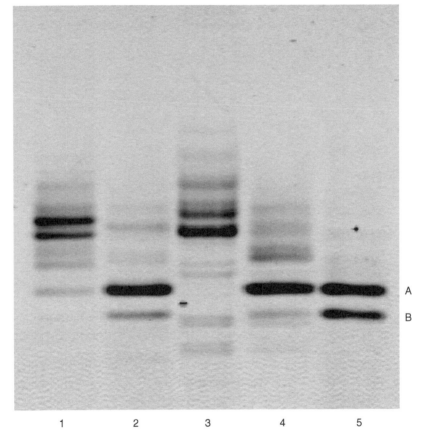

FIGURE 6.4

Fluorophore-assisted carbohydrate electrophoresis of β-glucocerebrosidase before and after carbohydrate modification. Lane 1 — Recombinant Human β-glucocerebrosidase; 2 — Cerezyme; 3 — Placental β-glucocerebrosidase; 4 — Ceredase; 5 — Labeled oligosaccharide standards: A = Man$_3$GlcNAc$_2$ Fuc, B = Man$_3$GlcNAc$_2$.

and Ceredase, due to the presence of oligomannose structures on Ceredase and fucose on N146 of Cerezyme, the oligosaccharide-remodeling process resulted in the generation of mannose-terminated structures in each case.

From the biochemical comparison of the two products, the most significant difference was observed in the type of N-linked oligosaccharides present at the N19 site. While

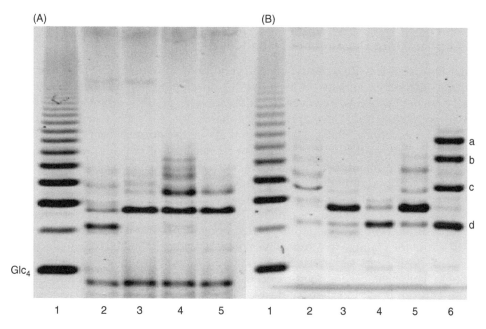

FIGURE 6.5
Fluorophore-assisted carbohydrate electrophoresis of oligosaccharides released from individual glycosylation sites of Cerezyme (A) and Ceredase (B). Lane 1 — dextran ladder standard with Glucose 4 band indicated. 2 — N19 oligosaccharides 3 — N59 oligosaccharides 4 — N146 oligosaccharides 5 — N270 oligosaccharides 6 — Oligomannose standards: (a) Man_9 (b) Man_7 (c) Man_5 (d) Man_3.

differences in glycosylation were observed in the unmodified proteins at the other three glycosylation sites, these differences were largely eliminated during the process of oligo-saccharide remodeling. Since the goal of the oligosaccharide remodeling process is to produce mannose-terminated residues, the difference between an oligomannose structure and the $Man_3GlcNAc_2 \pm Fuc$ found on Cerezyme at N19 was not expected to be significant with respect to the mannose-binding properties of the two proteins. To confirm this, cell uptake assays and biodistribution studies were performed [62]. The results from these studies indicated that, the recombinant enzyme had a slightly higher uptake into Kupffer cells than the placental enzyme.

6.8 Clinical Comparisons of Cerezyme and Ceredase

A goal often sought in the development of therapeutic proteins is to make the protein as similar to the normal human protein as possible. Cerezyme development was initi-ated based on extensive knowledge from the development of the placental product and comes very close to achieving this goal. The efficacy of Cerezyme was demonstrated in a clinical trial and has been confirmed by many subsequent studies [63,64]. The biochemical differences between the products that we can detect analytically are not apparent clinically. In a double-blind randomized parallel trial of 30 Type I patients, the efficacy and incidence of adverse events in the two products were comparable even though the incidence of IgG antibody formation was higher (40 vs. 20%) for Ceredase [63].

6.9 Orphan Drug Development Challenges

Gaucher Disease is classified as an "orphan condition" in the United States and Europe. This makes market exclusivity an incentive for developing therapeutics for such a rare disease. Gaucher Disease is, however, better described as an ultra-orphan condition, given the small population size. Development of a therapeutic for such a small population of patients raises additional challenges over and above the normal risks of drug development. Although the patient population is small, the cost of development of an orphan drug is no different than for a normal therapeutic protein. This cost is therefore divided among a few thousand rather than tens or hundreds of thousands of patients, resulting in high cost per patient. Although the clinical trials leading to approval may be small in size (tens vs. hundreds or thousands of patients), the costs per patient can be very high owing to the sophisticated clinical evaluation needed per patient as well as the need to transport patients across the country to a few clinical sites. Owing to the heterogeneous nature of the disease, dosing studies are difficult to conduct, and surrogate endpoints are often essential in lieu of clinical endpoints, since some pathological aspects can take decades to develop. This can result in extensive post marketing (phase IV) clinical requirements and the need for long-term monitoring of patients immune response to the drug. The cost of regulatory filings, sales and marketing, as well as distribution are significant on a per patient basis when there are only a few patients in a country. There are also significant ancillary costs associated with working with insurance companies, health organizations, and individual countries to obtain reimbursement for an expensive therapy for a disease that most people have never heard of.

Sensitivities to drug pricing have led to concerns over the cost of Cerezyme and Ceredase, which were among the most expensive (at the time) therapeutic products. With the success of Cerezyme, and the publicity surrounding the price of the product, there has been much interest in developing alternative expression systems [65] on the assumption that increased expression will significantly lower the price of the product. While it is certainly possible to develop expression systems with a higher productivity, such as insect cell, transgenic animal, and transgenic plant systems, the potential effect on the final price of the product is not as significant as many believe. Protein expression levels are only a minor portion of the final cost of this type of therapeutic protein. Purification, quality-control testing, fill-finish steps, distribution, sales and marketing, regulatory clinical support, and compassionate use programs are unaffected by expression levels and overall contribute significantly more to the final price of a product. A tenfold increase in expression level does not necessarily imply a significant reduction in the price of a therapeutic protein.

Ceredase and Cerezyme are two of the most, if not the most, effective and safe drugs ever developed. Clinical response is observed in all patients, and the treatment allows them (Type I patients) to live a normal life. Given the analytical tools available at the time and the limited experience in the production of recombinant proteins in mammalian expression systems, this success was a combination of hard work, skill, and some good fortune.

Acknowledgements

The successful development of two therapeutic proteins takes enormous dedication and effort from hundreds of people. I thank all of those involved in the development of Ceredase and Cerezyme as well as the courageous patients who took part in the initial clinical trials. I also thank Debra Barngrover, Edward Cole, Mark Hayes, Mike Hayes, Edward Kaye, and Willem Weperen for their helpful discussions and for reviewing this chapter.

References

1. Neufeld, E.F., Lysosomal storage diseases, *Annu. Rev. Biochem.*, 60, 257–280, 1991.
2. Glew, R.H., et al., Mammalian glucocerebrosidase: Implications for Gaucher Disease, *Lab. Invest.*, 58, 5–25, 1988.
3. Grabowski, G.A., Gaucher disease. Enzymology, genetics, and treatment, *Adv. Hum. Genet.*, 21, 377–441, 1993.
4. Beutler, E., Gaucher disease, *Blood Rev.*, 2, 59–70, 1988.
5. Pastores, G.M., Gaucher Disease. Pathological features, *Baillieres Clin. Haematol.*, 10, 739–749, 1997.
6. Parkin, J.L. and Brunning, R.D., Pathology of the Gaucher cell, *Prog. Clin. Biol. Res.*, 95, 151–175 1982.
7. Beutler, E. and Grabowski, G.A., Gaucher disease, in *The Metabolic and Molecular Bases of Inherited Disease*, Scriver, C.R., et al., Eds., McGraw-Hill, New York, 2001, pp. 3635–3668.
8. Vellodi, A., et al., Management of neuronopathic Gaucher disease: A European consensus, *J. Inherit. Metab. Dis.*, 24, 319–327, 2001.
9. Zhao, H. and Grabowski, G.A., Gaucher disease: Perspectives on a prototype lysosomal disease, *Cell Mol. Life Sci.*, 59, 694–707, 2002.
10. Brady, R.O., Kanfer, J., and Shapiro, D., The metabolism of glucocerebrosides. I. Purification and properties of a glucocerebroside-cleaving enzyme from spleen tissue, *J. Biol. Chem.*, 240, 39–43, 1965.
11. Brady, R.O., et al., Demonstration of a deficiency of glucocerebroside-cleaving enzyme in Gaucher Disease, *J. Clin. Invest.*, 45, 1112–1115, 1966.
12. Patrick, A.,D., A deficiency of glucocerebrosidase in Gaucher Disease, *Biochem. J.*, 97, 17–18, 1965.
13. Brady, R.O., The sphingolipidoses, *New Engl. J. Med.*, 275, 312–318, 1966.
14. Dale, G.L., Villacorte, D.G., and Beutler, E., Solubilization of glucocerebrosidase from human placenta and demonstration of a phospholipid requirement for its catalytic activity, *Biochem. Biophys. Res. Commun.*, 71, 1048–1053, 1976.
15. Blonder, E., Klibansky, C., and de Vries, A., Effects of detergents and choline-containing phospholipids on human spleen glucocerebrosidase, *Biochim. Biophys. Acta*, 431, 45–53, 1976.
16. Basu, A. and Glew, R.H., Characterization of the phospholipid requirement of a rat liver beta-glucosidase, *Biochem. J.*, 224, 515–524, 1984.
17. Pentchev, P.G., et al., Isolation and characterization of glucocerebrosidase from human placental tissue, *J. Biol. Chem.*, 248, 5256–5261, 1973.
18. Dale, G.L. and Beutler, E., Enzyme replacement therapy in Gaucher Disease: A rapid, high-yield method for purification of glucocerebrosidase, *Proc. Natl. Acad. Sci., USA*, 73, 4672–4674, 1976.
19 Furbish, F.S., et al., Enzyme replacement therapy in Gaucher Disease: Large-scale purification of glucocerebrosidase suitable for human administration, *Proc. Natl. Acad. Sci., USA*, 74, 3560–3563, 1977.
20. Dale, G.L., et al., Large scale purification of glucocerebrosidase from human placentas, *Birth Defects Orig. Artic. Ser.*, 16, 33–41, 1980.
21. Grabowski, G.A. and Dagan, A., Human lysosomal beta-glucosidase: Purification by affinity chromatography, *Anal. Biochem.*, 141, 267–279, 1984.
22. Murray, G.J., et al., Purification of beta-glucocerebrosidase by preparative-scale high-performance liquid chromatography: The use of ethylene glycol-containing buffers for chromatography of hydrophobic glycoprotein enzymes, *Anal. Biochem.*, 147, 301–310, 1985.

23. Osiecki-Newman, K.M., et al., Human acid beta-glucosidase: Affinity purification of the normal placental and Gaucher disease splenic enzymes on N-alkyl-deoxynojirimycin-sepharose, *Enzyme*, 35, 147–153, 1986.

24. Ho, M.W. and O'Brien, J.S., Gaucher Disease: Deficiency of 'acid' -glucosidase and reconstitution of enzyme activity *in vitro*, *Proc. Natl. Acad. Sci., USA*, 68, 2810–2813, 1971.

25. Ho, M.W. and Rigby, M., Glucocerebrosidase: Stoichiometry of association between effector and catalytic proteins, *Biochim. Biophys. Acta*, 397, 267–273, 1975.

26. Mraz, W., Fischer, G., and Jatzkewitz, H., Low molecular weight proteins in secondary lysosomes as activators of different sphingolipid hydrolases, *FEBS Lett.*, 67, 104–109, 1976.

27. Peters, S.P., et al., Isolation of heat-stable glucocerebrosidase activators from the spleens of three variants of Gaucher Disease, *Arch. Biochem. Biophys.*, 183, 290–297, 1977.

28. Peters, S.P., et al., Purification and properties of a heat-stable glucocerebrosidase activating factor from control and Gaucher spleen. *J. Biol. Chem.*, 252, 563–573, 1977.

29. Berent, S.L. and Radin, N.S., Mechanism of activation of glucocerebrosidase by co-beta-glucosidase (glucosidase activator protein), *Biochim. Biophys. Acta*, 664, 572–582, 1981.

30. Iyer, S.S., Berent, S.L., and Radin, N.S., The cohydrolases in human spleen that stimulate glucosyl ceramide beta-glucosidase, *Biochim. Biophys. Acta*, 748, 1–7, 1983.

31. Vaccaro, A.M., et al., An endogenous activator protein in human placenta for enzymatic degradation of glucosylceramide, *Biochim. Biophys. Acta*, 836, 157–166, 1985.

32. Morimoto, S., et al., Distribution of saposin proteins (sphingolipid activator proteins) in lysosomal storage and other diseases, *Proc. Natl. Acad. Sci., USA*, 87, 3493–3497, 1990.

33. Vaccaro, A.M., et al., Structural analysis of saposin C and B. Complete localization of disulfide bridges, *J. Biol. Chem.*, 270, 9953–9960, 1995.

34. Weiler, S., et al., Synthesis and characterization of a bioactive 82-residue sphingolipid activator protein, saposin C, *J. Mol. Neurosci.*, 4, 161–172, 1993.

35. Christomanou, H., Kleinschmidt, T., and Braunitzer, G., N-terminal amino-acid sequence of a sphingolipid activator protein missing in a new human Gaucher disease variant, *Biol. Chem. Hoppe Seyler*, 368, 1193–1196, 1987.

36. Qi, X., Leonova, T., and Grabowski, G.A., Functional human saposins expressed in *Escherichia coli*. Evidence for binding and activation properties of saposins C with acid beta-glucosidase, *J. Biol. Chem.*, 269, 16746–16753, 1994.

37. Sorge, J., et al., Molecular cloning and nucleotide sequence of human glucocerebrosidase cDNA, *Proc. Natl. Acad. Sci., USA*, 82, 7289–7293, 1985.

38. Tsuji, S., et al., Nucleotide sequence of cDNA containing the complete coding sequence for human lysosomal glucocerebrosidase, *J. Biol. Chem.*, 261, 50–53, 1986.

39. Sorge, J., et al., Correction: Molecular cloning and nucleotide sequence of human glucocerebrosidase cDNA, *Proc. Natl. Acad. Sci., USA*, 83, 3567, 1986.

40. Dvir, H., et al., X-ray structure of human acid-beta-glucosidase, the defective enzyme in Gaucher disease, *EMBO Rep.*, 4, 704–709, 2003.

41. Erickson, A.H., Ginns, E.I., and Barranger, J.A., Biosynthesis of the lysosomal enzyme glucocerebrosidase, *J. Biol. Chem.*, 260, 14319–14324, 1985.

42. Edmunds, T., Cerezyme: A case study, *Dev. Biol. Stand.*, 96, 131–140, 1998.

43. Takasaki, S., et al., Structure of the N-asparagine-linked oligosaccharide units of human placental beta-glucocerebrosidase, *J. Biol. Chem.*, 259, 10112–10117, 1984.

44. Aerts, J.M., et al., Glucocerebrosidase, a lysosomal enzyme that does not undergo oligosaccharide phosphorylation, *Biochim. Biophys. Acta*, 964, 303–308, 1988.

45. Brady, R.O., et al., Replacement therapy for inherited enzyme deficiency. Use of purified glucocerebrosidase in Gaucher Disease, *New Engl. J. Med.*, 291, 989–993, 1974.

46. Brady, R.O., Murray G.J., and Barton N.W., Modifying exogenous glucocerebrosidase for effective replacement therapy in Gaucher disease, *J. Inherit. Metab. Dis.*, 17, 510–519, 1994.

47. Furbish, F.S., et al., The uptake of native and desialylated glucocerebrosidase by rat hepatocytes and Kupffer cells, *Biochem. Biophys. Res. Commun.*, 81, 1047–1053, 1978.

48. Beutler, E., et al., Enzyme replacement therapy in Gaucher Disease: Preliminary clinical trial of a new enzyme preparation, *Proc. Natl. Acad. Sci., USA*, 74, 4620–4623, 1977.

49. Ihler, G.M., Erythrocytes as carriers for glucocerebrosidase, *Prog. Clin.Biol. Res.*, 95, 655–667, 1982.

50. Ihler, G.M., Glew, R.H., and Schnure, F.W., Enzyme loading of erythrocytes, *Proc. Natl. Acad. Sci., USA*, 70, 2663–2666, 1973.
51. Gregoriadis, G., et al., Experiences after long-term treatment of a type I Gaucher disease patient with liposome-entrapped glucocerebroside: Beta-glucosidase, *Birth Defects Orig. Artic. Ser.*, 16, 383–392, 1980.
52. Braidman, I. and Gregoriadis, G., Preparation of glucocerebroside beta-glucosidase for entrapment in liposomes and treatment of patients with adult Gaucher Disease, *Biochem. Soc. Trans.*, 4, 259–261, 1976.
53. Stahl, P.D., et al., Evidence for receptor-mediated binding of glycoproteins, glycoconjugates, and lysosomal glycosidases by alveolar macrophages, *Proc. Natl. Acad. Sci., USA*, 75, 1399–1403, 1978.
54. Doebber, T.W., et al., Enhanced macrophage uptake of synthetically glycosylated human placental beta-glucocerebrosidase, *J. Biol. Chem.*, 257, 2193–2199, 1982.
55. Murray, G.J., et al., Targeting of synthetically glycosylated human placental glucocerebrosidase, *Biochem. Med.*, 34, 241–246, 1985.
56. Furbish, F.S., et al., Uptake and distribution of placental glucocerebrosidase in rat hepatic cells and effects of sequential deglycosylation, *Biochim. Biophys. Acta*, 673, 425–434, 1981.
57. Barton, N.W., et al., Replacement therapy for inherited enzyme deficiency-macrophage-targeted glucocerebrosidase for Gaucher Disease, *New Engl. J. Med.*, 324, 1464–1470, 1991.
58. Whittington, R. and Goa, K.L., Alglucerase. A review of its therapeutic use in Gaucher Disease. *Drugs*, 44, 72–93, 1992.
59. Grabowski, G.A., Leslie, N., and Wenstrup, R., Enzyme therapy for Gaucher disease: The first 5 years, *Blood Rev.*, 12, 115–1133, 1998.
60. Richards, S.M., Olson, T.A., and McPherson, J.M., Antibody response in patients with Gaucher disease after repeated infusion with macrophage-targeted glucocerebrosidase, *Blood*, 82, 1402–1409, 1993.
61. Hoppe, H., Cerezyme-recombinant protein treatment for Gaucher Disease, *J. Biotechnol.*, 76, 259–261, 2000.
62. Friedman, B., et al., A comparison of the pharmacological properties of carbohydrate remodeled recombinant and placental-derived beta-glucocerebrosidase: Implications for clinical efficacy in treatment of Gaucher disease, *Blood*, 93, 2807–2816, 1999.
63. Grabowski, G.A., et al., Enzyme therapy in type 1 Gaucher disease: Comparative efficacy of mannose-terminated glucocerebrosidase from natural and recombinant sources, *Ann. Intern. Med.*, 122, 33–39, 1995.
64. Weinreb, N.J., et al., Effectiveness of enzyme replacement therapy in 1028 patients with type 1 Gaucher disease after 2 to 5 years of treatment: A report from the Gaucher Registry, *Am. J. Med.*, 113, 112–119, 2002.
65. Cramer, C.L., et al., Bioproduction of human enzymes in transgenic tobacco, *Ann. N. Y. Acad. Sci.*, 792, 62–71, 1996.

7

α-Galactosidase

Debra Barngrover

CONTENTS

7.1   Introduction

α-Galactosidase (EC 3.1.2.22), a lysosomal enzyme, is a part of the degradation pathway for glycolipids that is involved in the sequential removal of the glycans, leaving behind the core lipid, ceramide (Figure 7.1). An abnormal gene causes a deficiency in the activity of this enzyme, which leads to Fabry's Disease (Anderson–Fabry's Disease in the United Kingdom). This deficiency results in the steady accumulation of several glycolipids, mainly globotriaosylceramide (GL-3), in multiple cell types. This progressive glycosphingolipid accumulation leads to life-threatening clinical sequelae in renal, cardiac, and cerebrovascular systems [1]. Without renal dialysis or kidney transplantation, the mean age at death for

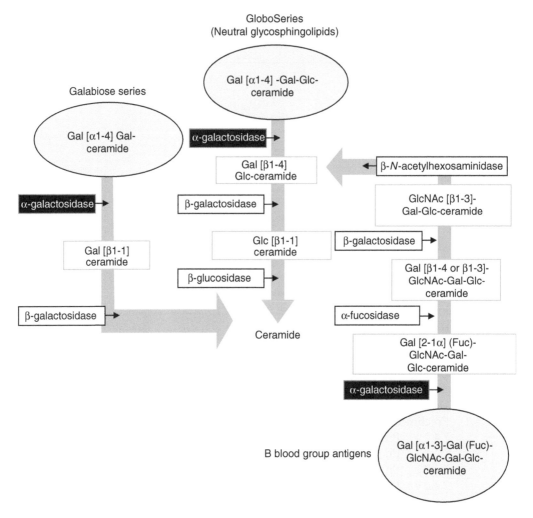

FIGURE 7.1
Pathways of glycolipid catabolism in the lysosome, showing sequential removal of the glycans. Circled species accumulate in Fabry's disease.

patients with classical Fabry's disease was 41 years [2], although even after the advent of dialysis and transplantation, the mean age at death has still only increased to 50 years [3].

Fabrazyme® (agalsidase beta, Genzyme Corporation, Cambridge, MA), the recombinant form of human α-galactosidase, replaces the missing enzyme activity in affected patients. Infused once every 2 weeks at a recommended dose of 1 mg/kg [4], the enzyme has demonstrated significant reduction in GL-3 deposits in the microvasculature of the kidney. Studies are being conducted to assess its clinical benefits in patients [5–8].

7.2   Detailed Biochemical Characteristics of the Enzyme

Human α-galactosidase is a noncovalently-linked homodimeric glycoprotein with molecular mass of approximately 100 kDa. On the basis of matrix-assisted laser desorption ionization time-of-flight mass spectrometry, the subunit in Fabrazyme® is calculated to have a monomeric molecular mass of 51.2 kDa [9]. A minor component with a molecular weight of 47.5 kDa is also visible on sodium dodecyl sulfate–polyacrylamide gels (SDS–PAGE) run under reducing conditions. Although attempts have been made to map the disulfide bonds internal to the enzyme's subunits, these have been unsuccessful owing to disulfide scrambling with sample reduction.

The complementary deoxyribonucleic acid (cDNA) for the mature enzyme was first cloned in 1985 [10], with the complete cDNA sequence [11] and genomic sequence [12] following soon after in 1987. The complete cDNA encodes a protein of 429 amino acids (aa), including a 31-aa signal peptide and a 398-aa mature peptide [12]. The potential for mRNA editing, which results in a single-nucleotide conversion near the 3' end of the coding region (resulting in a F296Y substitution), has been reported for this enzyme [13]. Examination of the recombinant protein by peptide mass fingerprinting has found no evidence for the appearance of this variant protein in Fabrazyme®, and extensive analysis of amplified mRNAs from ten normal donors found no edited sequences [14].

Although the amino acid sequence contains four consensus sites for N-terminal glycosylation, only three, namely, N108, N161, and N184, are found to be occupied. Expression of an N377E mutant in COS-1 cells gave a protein with the same molecular mass as the wild type [15]. The potential glycosylation site at N377 is very close to the C terminus of the protein. Additionally, the sequence Asn-X-Pro is often not glycosylated owing to the presence of proline. These two factors are consistent with the lack of glycosylation at this site. Expression of mutant glycoforms with 1, 2, or 3 of the occupied sites obliterated indicate that occupancy of N184 is essential for enzyme solubility and stability. Similarly, treatment of the recombinant enzyme with endoglycosidase-H, which removes most of the high mannose chains on N161 and N184, also results in protein aggregation and precipitation. The oligosaccharides present in a sample of Fabrazyme® have been mapped [9], with N108 typically containing a complex structure and N161 and N184 typically containing high mannose and hybrid structures (Table 7.1). Since the enzyme is a homodimer, the active molecule actually contains six oligosaccharide chains, as depicted in Figure 7.2, thus resulting in nearly 250,000 potential glycoforms.

The optimum pH of the enzyme is typical for a lysosomal enzyme and ranges from 3.8 to 4.6, depending on the substrate used [16]. The *in vitro* hydrolysis of the natural substrate, GL-3, requires the presence of a detergent such as sodium taurocholate to hold the substrate in micelles. Evidence from *in vitro* studies with recombinant α-galactosidase indicates that an activator protein, termed sphingolipid activator protein B (SAP-B or saposin B), is probably required for *in vivo* enzyme activity [17]. SAP-B is an ~8.5 kDa peptide that is derived by posttranslational cleavage from a precursor protein, termed prosaposin, that encodes four similar peptides in tandem, SAP A, B, C, and D [18,19]. Since the natural glycolipid substrates are poorly soluble in water and difficult to obtain in a pure state, several artificial substrates have been developed to facilitate diagnosis of Fabry's disease and enzyme analysis. The most commonly used substrates include 4-methylumbelliferyl-α-D-galactoside, which yields a fluorescent compound upon hydrolysis, and *p*-nitrophenyl-α-D-galactoside, which yields a colored compound. The published assay methods with each of these substrates need to be carefully evaluated (see, for example, [9]), because even these substrates have a low aqueous solubility. The preparation of the substrate may need to be adjusted, for example, by the addition of a small amount of an organic solvent, such as ethanol or dimethyl sulfoxide (DMSO), to ensure that the assay is performed with sufficient substrate, preferably double the K_M concentration. The K_M and V_{max} were determined for Fabrazyme® with each of these substrates (Table 7.2).

Reversed phase-high performance liquid chromatography (RP-HPLC) analysis performed using a YMC 2.1 mm × 100 mm octyl column eluted with a linear trifluoracetic acid–acetonitrile gradient gives a profile with three distinct protein peaks [9]. Liquid chromatographic mass spectrometric analysis (LC/MS) of tryptic peptides from the protein demonstrates

TABLE 7.1

Site-Specific Glycosylation in Fabrazyme

Structure	Percentage of Total Glycoforms
Asn108	
Tetraantennary fucosylated tetrasialylated	13
Tetraantennary fucosylated trisialylated	1
Tetraantennary fucosylated disialylated	1
Triantennary fucosylated trisialylated	**44**
Triantennary fucosylated disialylated	5
Biantennary fucosylated disialylated	31
Biantennary fucosylated monosialylated	5
Asn161	
Biphosphorylated oligomannose 8	4
Biphosphorylated oligomannose 7	2
Phosphorylated oligomannose 7	**39**
Phosphorylated oligomannose 6	15
Oligomannose 6	1
Oligomannose 5	2
Phosphorylated hybrid	12
Biantennary fucosylated disialylated	1
Biantennary disialylated	19
Biantennary monosialylated	3
Asn184	
Biphosphorylated oligomannose 7	**36**
Phosphorylated oligomannose 6	**35**
Phosphorylated oligomannose 5	7
Oligomannose 5	5
Phosphorylated hybrid	13
Triantennary fucosylated trisialylated	2
Triantennary fucosylated disialylated	2

The major oligosaccharide species at each site is indicated in bold.

that the enzyme has the predicted amino acid sequence from the cDNA, except for C-terminal heterogeneity. The predominant peak seen in the RP-HPLC analysis of Fabrazyme® is the full-length enzyme, with smaller amounts of two C-terminally truncated species (either lacking the terminal leucine or the two terminal leucine residues, respectively). It is worth noting that during the initial development of the Fabrazyme® production process, the predominant species seen was C-terminally truncated, missing two leucine residues. During scale-up and improvement of the production process, additional controls were implemented, resulting in a substantial reduction in the degree of C-terminal truncation. This suggests that the appearance of the C-terminally truncated species is due to proteolytic processing of the mature full-length protein. Interestingly, there is a report of a sixfold increase in specific activity in enzyme expressed from truncated cDNAs, resulting in the removal of between 2 and 10 C-terminal amino acids [20]. However, activity measurements of a large number of lots with variable levels of C-terminally truncated species have revealed no such difference in specific activity of Fabrazyme®.

Through a series of studies with somatic cell hybrids and finally *in situ* hybridization using radiolabeled cDNA as a probe, the α-galactosidase gene was localized to the Xq22 region of the long arm of the X chromosome [16]. The α-GAL cDNA isolated from most libraries contains either no 3' untranslated region or, at most, a short region of 6 to 7

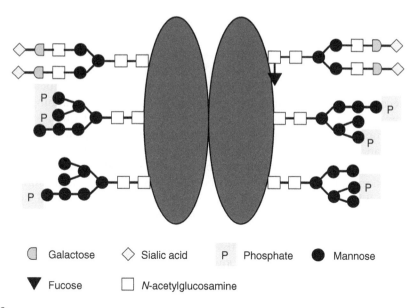

FIGURE 7.2

Model of α-galactosidase molecule, showing dimeric protein chains in the center and possible oligosaccharide chains on N108, N161, and N184, (top to bottom).

TABLE 7.2

Enzyme Kinetic Values for Fabrazyme® with 33 mM p-nitrophenyl-α-D-Galactoside (pNP-Gal) and 10 mM 4-methylumbelliferyl-α-D-Galactoside (4MU-Gal)

Specific Activity (μmol/min/mg)		V_{max} (μmol/min/mg)		K_M (mM)	
pNP-Gal	4MU-Gal	pNP-Gal	4MU-Gal	pNP-Gal	4MU-Gal
65.0 ± 0.3	64.0 ± 3.0	83.2 ± 4.8	79.5 ± 2.2	7.0 ± 0.6	2.0 ± 0.2

nucleotides [21]. The complete genomic clone is 12 kB and contains seven exons [22]. No pseudogenes have been found and only one other human gene bears some similarity, namely, α-N-acetylgalactosaminidase [16]. This enzyme can also cleave α-galactosides and was originally named α-galactosidase B. It was differentiated from the A form by different thermal stability (A was thermolabile, and B was thermostable) and inhibition by myoinositol. The presence of this activity confounded early studies of Fabry patients, because it appeared that they had 10 to 25% normal levels of α-galactosidase activity. Initial studies seemed to indicate that the two enzymes were isozymes, with perhaps different glycosylation patterns accounting for their different biochemical properties. Eventually, the lack of cross-reaction by polyclonal antibodies and the mapping of the two enzymes to different chromosomes confirmed that they were related but different enzymes [16]. A deficiency in the enzyme α-N-acetylgalactosaminidase has been linked to Schindler disease, an even rarer, highly heterogeneous lysosomal storage disease [23]. Enzyme assays of patient samples (leukocytes, serum, tears) for the diagnosis of Fabry's disease must include an inhibitor of α-N-acetylgalactosaminidase, such as N-acetylgalactosamine, to avoid a misdiagnosis [24]. Several inhibitors of α-galactosidase A, most notably, imino sugars such as 1-deoxy-galactonojirimycin, α-galacto-homonojirimycin, α-allo-homonojirimycin, and β-1-C-butyl-deoxygalactonojirimycin [25], have been described.

α-Galactosides are a major constituent of plant seed walls and must often be degraded during seed germination. Thus, there are a variety of plant-derived α-galactosidases, mostly with neutral pH optima, that have been used or proposed for a variety of human, veterinary, and botanical applications. Beano® (GlaxoSmithKline, London) or Bean-zyme™ (Mikeska Products, Santa Barbara, CA) are commercially available products in the United States, derived from fungal extracts that are mixed with legume-containing food prior to consumption. These products are said to reduce the discomfort often associated with legume consumption by reducing the amount of undigested α-galactosides that reach the large intestine and are degraded by the microflora present there (http://www.bean-zyme.com). α-Galactosidases derived from coffee bean [26] or soybean [27] have been proposed for the conversion of B-blood group erythrocytes (by removal of the terminal α-galactosides from the B-blood group antigen, see Figure 7.1) into the universal donor type O erythrocytes. Similarly, removal of the xenoantigens, notably, α-galactoside-containing epitopes, from pig erythrocytes or pig organs has been proposed to allow the use of these components in humans [28]. The nutritive value of soybean meal can be improved by treatment with an α-galactosidase [29]. Downregulating the expression of α-galactosidase, on the other hand, has been demonstrated to enhance the freeze tolerance of petunia plants [30]. These are just a few of the many roles and proposed uses of α-galactosidases.

7.3   Fabry's Disease and the Role of Fabrazyme® Enzyme Replacement Therapy

7.3.1   Introduction to Fabry's Disease

Fabrazyme® is approved for long-term enzyme replacement therapy (ERT) in patients with a confirmed diagnosis of Fabry's disease (α-galactosidase A deficiency). Fabry's disease is a rare, inherited, X-linked lysosomal storage disorder with multisystemic effects. The disease, also known as Anderson–Fabry's disease, Morbus Fabry, and angiokeratoma corporis diffusum universale, was first described just over a century ago by two dermatologists working independently—Johannes Fabry, in Dortmund, Germany, and William Anderson, in London, England [31,32]. The cause of the disease was identified to be fatty deposits in blood vessels throughout the body in an autopsy report in 1947, by Pompen, et al. [33], who recognized the disease as a generalized storage disorder [33]. The structures of the primary lipids were identified as GL-3 and galabiosylceramide in 1963 and thus the disease was classified as a sphingolipidosis [34]. Brady, et al. [35] identified the deficient enzyme as a galactosyl hydrolase in 1967, while Kint further identified the enzyme as an α-galactosyl hydrolase (α-GAL) in 1970 [36]. With the defect identified, research in the early 1970s turned to attempting to replace the missing activity, first by infusing normal human plasma [37], and then with a single dose of partially purified enzyme from human placenta [38]. Sufficient enzyme was purified from human plasma and spleen by Desnick, et al. [39] in 1979 to allow for six doses to two brothers. This pioneering work not only demonstrated the potential for ERT to clear GL-3 from the plasma, but also demonstrated the importance of the oligosaccharides on the enzyme. A similar dose of the plasma-derived enzyme cleared 25 times more substrate than the splenic form, with a prolonged depletion of the substrate. This difference was correlated with a longer plasma half-life for the plasma-derived enzyme, attributed to a higher level of sialylation of the enzyme. This therapy was not initially pursued because of the difficulty in purifying sufficient amounts of α-GAL from human tissue. Effective ERT had to wait until the enzyme could be expressed by recombinant means and produced using large-scale cell culture.

In patients with Fabry's disease, the absence of sufficient α-GAL causes lipids, particularly GL-3 (also known as Gb3 and ceramide trihexoside, CTH), to accumulate progressively in the lysosomes of many cell types throughout the body [16,40]. GL-3 accumulation in the vascular endothelium is a major cause of renal, cardiac, and cerebrovascular complications in Fabry's disease. Progressive pathological changes in the kidney result in renal failure by midlife in most classical Fabry cases. Before the availability of dialysis or transplantation, the average age of death for patients with classical Fabry's disease was 41 years [2]; today, average life expectancy is still only 50 years [3]. Until the advent of ERT, Fabry's disease could only be managed by palliative and nonspecific measures, such as analgesia, stroke prophylaxis, cardiac interventions, dialysis, and kidney transplantation. These measures have limited effectiveness because they do not address the lack of α-GAL and the resultant intracellular GL-3 accumulation. The availability of Fabrazyme®, recombinant human α-GAL, provides an important, disease-specific treatment for patients with Fabry's disease. Fabrazyme® has been evaluated in several clinical trials (see Section 7.4). These studies demonstrate that Fabrazyme® treatment results in significant GL-3 reduction from the vascular endothelium of the kidney, heart, skin, and from certain other cell types. The reduction of GL-3 inclusions suggests that Fabrazyme® may ameliorate disease expression; however, the relationship of GL-3 inclusion reduction to specific clinical manifestations has not been established.

7.3.2 Inheritance of Fabry's Disease

Estimates of the incidence of Fabry's disease range from 1 in 40,000 in males [16] to 1 in 117,000 in the general population [41], and the disease is found to be panethnic. Since Fabry's disease is X-linked, it predominantly affects males, but females may have manifestations of this disease to a greater extent than previously thought [42]. This is probably because of the random inactivation of one of the two X chromosomes (Lyonization), which occurs in every somatic cell of females. A skewed inactivation of the chromosome containing the normal allele of the gene could potentially lead to different clinical outcomes in heterozygotes [43]. A recent survey of 42 Fabry patients identified on dialysis in the United States found that 12% of them were females, demonstrating the possibility for severe outcomes in this population [44]. Males with Fabry's disease (hemizygotes) pass the defective gene to all of their daughters and none of their sons. Females (heterozygotes) have a 50% chance of passing on the defective gene to both their sons and daughters (Figure 7.3). The defects in the α-GAL gene are heterogeneous, and most families have private mutations [45]. To date, over 300 mutations of the α-GAL gene (locus Xq22.1) have been recorded in the Human Mutation Database [46]. The wide range of mutations may explain variations in clinical presentation; however, efforts to establish phenotype–genotype correlations have been limited [16].

7.3.3 Diagnosis and Disease Manifestations

Fabry's disease has been classified into two types, classical and atypical, which roughly correlate with the amount of residual activity of α-GAL present. Although classical Fabry's disease usually presents in childhood with pain, fever, hypohidrosis, fatigue, and/or exercise intolerance (Table 7.3), the disease often goes unrecognized by physicians until adulthood, when the underlying pathology is advanced [47,48]. In a study of 30 large pedigrees, the mean age of diagnosis of index cases was 29 years [49]. A second, more recent study of the prevalence of lysosomal storage disorders in Australia from 1980 through 1996, found the median age of diagnosis of Fabry's disease to be 28.6 years [41]. Delayed diagnosis may be due to under-recognition of the disease. In addition, Fabry's disease symptoms are mistaken for those of other disorders, such as rheumatoid or juvenile arthritis, rheumatic fever, erythromelalgia, neurosis, Raynaud's syndrome, multiple sclerosis, lupus, acute

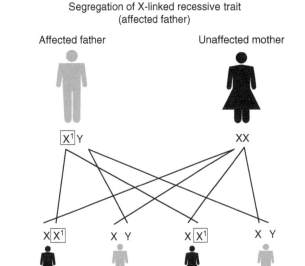

Segregation of X-linked recessive trait
(affected father)

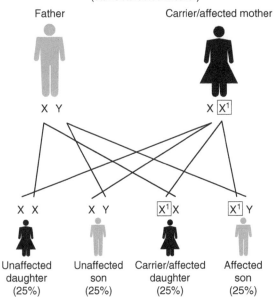

Segregation of X-linked recessive trait
(carrier/affected mother)

FIGURE 7.3
Inheritance patterns for Fabry's disease.

appendicitis, "growing pains" or malingering, petechiae, or collagen vascular disease [16,49]. Clinical diagnosis of classical Fabry's disease is based upon some (or all) of the following: family history, history of childhood fevers in association with pain in the extremities, characteristic skin lesions (angiokeratomas), characteristic "whorled" corneal opacity, and the presence of lipid-laden cells in urinary sediment or biopsied tissues. Diagnosis is confirmed biochemically by demonstration of very low or undetectable α-GAL activities in plasma, serum, leukocytes, tears, or biopsied tissue, using an assay

TABLE 7.3

Symptoms of Fabry's Disease

Early Manifestations (Childhood to Adolescence)

Intermittent paresthesia and acroparesthesia — chronic, burning, tingling pain, usually in the extremities, and beginning in early childhood, can occur daily

Episodic "Fabry crises" of agonizing, incapacitating pain — lasting for minutes to days, can disappear or worsen with adulthood, experienced by 80–90% of patients

Recurrent fever — accompanying pain and associated with an elevated erythrocyte sedimentation rate

Angiokeratomas — appear in adolescence and worsen with adulthood

Corneal and lenticular opacities

Hypohidrosis or anhidrosis

Heat or cold intolerance

Exercise intolerance

Mild proteinuria and urinary sediment containing globotriaosylceramide (GL-3)

Gastrointestinal problems — abdominal pain, diarrhea, vomiting, nausea

Psychological problems — depression, denial of symptoms

Later Manifestations (Adolescence to Adulthood)

Renal dysfunction leading to uremia and hypertension and progressing to end-stage renal disease

Cardiovascular dysfunction — myocardial infarction, left venticular hypertrophy, valvular abnormalities, arrhythmias

Cerebrovascular complications — risk of early stroke, hemiplegia, hemianesthesia, transient ischemic attacks

Pulmonary complications — airflow obstruction, dyspnea

Neurological complications — vertigo, tinnitus, hearing loss, hyperacusis, nystagmus, diplopia

---

with a synthetic substrate of α-GAL and with N-acetylgalactosamine in the reaction mixture to inhibit α-N-acetylgalactosaminidase (galactosidase B) activity [24].

Atypical variants can be identified by low α-GAL activity. These patients are usually diagnosed after the onset of cardiac manifestations or serendipitously during evaluation of other medical problems.

In classical Fabry's disease, multiple organs are typically affected clinically. In the kidney, progressive endothelial GL-3 accumulation is thought to promote inflammation, which reduces blood flow to tubules and glomeruli, leading eventually to irreparable nephron damage. Because of compensatory mechanisms and the vast reserve in normal kidney function, patients can remain relatively asymptomatic despite significant loss of function [50]. However, after a critical number of nephrons are damaged, adequate glomerular filtration cannot be maintained and there is rapid onset of kidney failure.

Common cardiac manifestations of Fabry's disease include left ventricular hypertrophy, valvular disease (especially mitral valve prolapse and regurgitation), and conduction abnormalities leading to congestive heart failure, arrhythmias, and myocardial infarction [16].

Many cerebrovascular abnormalities have been documented in Fabry's disease, including early stroke, thromboses, transient ischemic attacks, hemiparesis, vertigo/dizziness, diplopia, dysarthria, nystagmus, nausea and vomiting, headache, hemiataxia, and ataxia of gait [51,52]. Both cardiac and cerebrovascular involvement are progressive and become more severe with age.

In atypical Fabry's disease, clinical manifestation may be limited to only one organ. Both cardiac and renal variants have been described. A recent study of one 75-year-old cardiac variant patient found significant GL-3 deposits in the podocytes, which may have been associated with the mild proteinuria seen in this patient. These deposits were absent in mesangial, interstitial, and vascular endothelial and smooth-muscle cells, which probably accounted for the long-term preservation of renal function in this patient compared with the classically affected Fabry patient [53].

7.3.4   Active Site and Possible Mechanism

Although human α-galactosidase has been crystallized, only a preliminary X-ray analysis has been made and no structure has been published yet [54]. Garman and Garboczi [55] and Garman, et al. [56] have constructed a model based on their determination of the structure of chicken α-*N*-acetylgalactosaminidase to 1.9Å resolution

The two proteins share 54% amino acid sequence. In their model, there are 13 amino acids involved in the active site, which are widely spaced across the molecule (W47, D92, D93, Y134, C142, K168, D170, C172, E203, L206, Y207, R227, and D231). Eleven of these residues are conserved between the chicken and human enzymes, while the two nonconserved amino acids (E203 and L206) are larger in the human α-galactosidase, making the active site smaller. This is consistent with the restricted substrate specificity of the human α-GAL enzyme. The authors mapped 245 of the now more than 300 identified mutations causing Fabry's disease and as expected, confirmed that most of the mutations were either in the active site or reduced the stability of the enzyme.

7.3.5   Targeting of the Enzyme

Enzymes used to treat lysosomal storage diseases are unique in that they are not active in circulation or at the cell membrane, as they tend to show little activity at the neutral pH of plasma. Thus, the traditional measures of drug efficacy, which test for dosing regimens that give a consistent or therapeutically sufficient plasma level, are not relevant to the measurement of lysosomal enzymes. For these enzymes to be active, they must not only be precisely targeted to the correct organ and cell types within these organs, but even to the correct organelle within the cell, namely the lysosome. The stability of the enzyme activity within the lysosome is a key attribute of drug efficacy, but this measurement is difficult to obtain.

There are three known receptors that may be involved in the binding and transport of Fabrazyme® to cellular lysosomes. All three of these receptors bind specific carbohydrates found in the oligosaccharide chains and are thus relatively insensitive to the protein backbone. The first is the mannose-6-phosphate (M6P) receptor, which plays a role in the targeting of newly produced lysosomal enzymes to the lysosome as well as reuptake of enzymes that were secreted. This role of M6P in the targeting of lysosomal hydrolases was first hypothesized by Sando and Neufeld [57] in 1972 while studying I-cell disease, which is a lysosomal storage disorder characterized by the deficiency of multiple enzymes. The underlying defect was determined to be in the production of the M6P targeting signal, which requires the activity of the two enzymes in the Golgi apparatus [58]. The potential for this receptor to play a role in the uptake of exogenously supplied enzyme was demonstrated by Sando and Neufeld [57] in uptake studies with another lysosomal hydrolase, α-L-iduronidase, and by Kaplan, et al. [59] in studies using β-glucuronidase. Later Mayes, et al. [60] confirmed that the M6P receptor was responsible for the uptake of α-galactosidase by fibroblasts derived from Fabry patients. This trafficking is depicted in Figure 7.4, which shows that the most newly synthesized lysosomal enzymes are recognized by the M6P receptor at the Golgi, which translocates them to the lysosomes, their final intracellular location. A proportion of the enzymes are also secreted into circulation and can be recaptured through a variety of receptors and delivered to lysosomes. This receptor pathway makes it possible for the intravenously delivered enzyme to reach its target, i.e., — the lysosome, where substrate storage occurs. Fabrazyme® was confirmed to contain approximately 3 mol of M6P/mol protein (Table 7.4). Biphosphorylated oligosaccharide chains, which are known to bind well to the M6P receptor, are found in the site-specific analysis (Table 7.1). The role of the M6P receptor in the uptake of Fabrazyme® by fibroblast cell lines

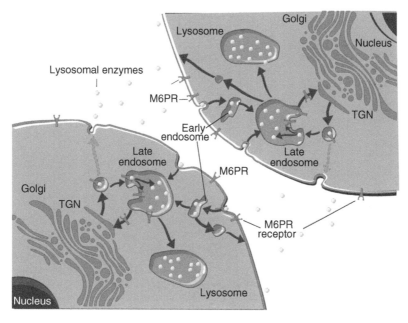

FIGURE 7.4

Trafficking of lysosomal enzymes, demonstrating intracellular transport to the lysosome and uptake of exogenous enzyme. TGN = transGolgi network; M6PR = mannose-6-phosphate receptor.

TABLE 7.4

Monosaccharide Composition of a Typical Lot of Fabrazyme®

Monosaccharide	mol/mol Protein
Fucose	1.8 ± 0.1
Galactose	8.0 ± 0.4
N-acetylglucosamine	18.4 ± 0.8
Mannose	25.7 ± 1.8
Mannose-6-phosphate	3.1 ± 0.1
N-acetylneuraminic acid (sialic acid)	7.0 ± 1.0
Sialic acid/galactose ratio	0.88

is demonstrated by a significant decrease in the uptake by the addition of M6P, but not mannose-1-phosphate (M1P) in an *in vitro* cell-uptake experiment (Figure 7.5).

A second carbohydrate receptor that could be involved in the uptake of Fabrazyme® is the asialoglycoprotein receptor. This receptor recognizes the penultimate galactose on complex chains, which is exposed when the terminal sialic acid is removed [61]. This receptor is predominantly found in the reticuloendothelial cells of the liver and spleen. Since these organs are not severely affected in Fabry's disease, it is desirable to minimize the amount of enzyme taken up by these organs. Coverage of nearly 90% of the galactose in the complex chains of Fabrazyme® (see Table 7.4) would minimize binding to this receptor.

The third known mechanism of uptake is through mannose receptors. This is a family of receptors with varying specificities and locations, found predominantly on macrophages and endothelial cells [62]. Achord, et al. [63] demonstrated the role of these receptors in the uptake of the "low uptake" (missing phosphate) form of β-glucuronidase in reticuloendothelial cells in the liver.

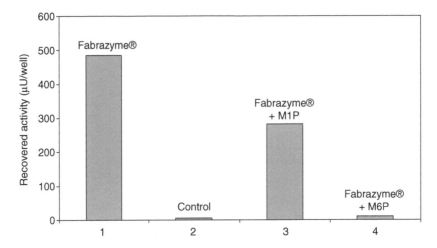

FIGURE 7.5
Uptake of Fabrazyme® by Fabry fibroblasts in culture. Cells were incubated with (1) 1330 µU/well Fabrazyme®, (2) 0 µU/well Fabrazyme®, (3) 5 mM mannose-1-phosphate, 1330 µU/well Fabrazyme®, and (4) 5 mM mannose-6-phosphate, 1330 µU/well Fabrazyme® at 37°C/5% CO_2 for 24 h. Activity of the cell lysate was assayed for each condition to determine the uptake.

7.3.6   Detailed Information on the Cell Line

The cell line that produces Fabrazyme® begins with the genetic modification of a host cell (Chinese hamster ovary [CHO] cell line) to produce human α-GAL. Genzyme chose the CHO cell line for the following reasons:

1. The demonstrated safety profile of multiple products produced using this cell line
2. The species barrier to infection with human viruses
3. Experience with successfully using material from this system to replace the native human enzyme for another inherited disorder (Gaucher disease)
4. The known ability of CHO cells to glycosylate recombinant proteins (mannose-6-phosphate and sialylation)
5. Experience with large-scale production of enzymes using this system

The human α-GAL gene was isolated, spliced into a bacterial plasmid, and then inserted into the CHO cell. The α-GAL gene was attached to a gene for dihydrofolate reductase (DHFR), which allows for amplification of both genes (copy number increase) by stepwise increases in the concentration of methotrexate (which inhibits DHFR). As a lysosomal enzyme, most of the enzyme produced would be retained intracellularly in the lysosome and not secreted. The recovery of this intracellular enzyme would therefore require the production of large quantities of very expensive cells, lysing these cells and then recovering the desired product from a highly heterogeneous mix of intracellular proteins and cellular DNA. A key finding by Desnick, et al. [64] was that stable overexpression of the enzyme results in secretion of the enzyme into the extracellular medium. This greatly simplified the recovery and purification process, since the level of protein impurities and host cell DNA would be significantly lower. The final cell line was cloned in the absence of DHFR and the most stable, high-producing clone was picked for further production. Multiple vials of this clone have been frozen in a master cell bank (MCB). Periodically, one vial of the MCB is thawed and expanded to produce multiple vials of a working cell bank. For each bioreactor run, one vial of the working cell bank is thawed and expanded. In this manner, consistency of the cell bank is assured over the life of the product (Figure 7.6). The

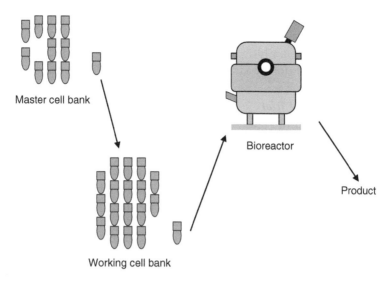

FIGURE 7.6   Cell banking scheme for the production of Fabrazyme®.

cell banks have been thoroughly tested to confirm their genetic stability and the absence of viruses, mycoplasma, and bacteria. The banks are split and stored in several locations.

7.4   Development History of the Product

7.4.1   Development Strategy

Since Fabry's disease is a serious, life-threatening disease with a slow progression to organ failure, Fabrazyme® was filed with the Food & Drug Administration (FDA) under an accelerated approval mechanism. Under the FDA's Accelerated Approval regulations, marketing approval may be granted on the basis of adequate and well-controlled clinical trials. These trials are designed to establish that the product has an effect on a surrogate endpoint that is reasonably likely to predict clinical benefit. Approval under these regulations requires that the applicant study the product further to verify the clinical benefit. Genzyme chose GL-3 reduction in renal interstitial capillary endothelial cells as the surrogate marker, since it is believed that reduction of this lipid will likely predict benefit to the patient. Postmarketing studies are being conducted to verify the degree of clinical benefit to patients.

7.4.2   Preclinical and Clinical Studies

7.4.2.1   *Preclinical Studies*

Preclinical studies of the active ingredient in Fabrazyme® (agalsidase *beta*, recombinant human α-GAL) were performed in several animal models, including the α-GAL knock-out mouse (Fabry mouse). These studies assessed the safety and pharmacodynamics of agalsidase *beta* as well as the pattern of GL-3 removal. A dose-finding study in the Fabry mouse demonstrated GL-3 depletion in a dose-dependent manner in the plasma, liver, heart, and kidneys of enzyme-treated animals. The half-life of the enzyme was estimated to be 48 h in the liver and 36 h in the spleen, indicating that enzymatic activity was stable after uptake into organs [65]. *In vitro* studies using indium-111-DTPA labeled α-GAL demonstrated that the enzyme was relatively stable to proteolysis in the lysosomal environment, in contrast to a nonlysosomal protein such as albumin [66]. These results provided the rationale and dosing strategy for a phase 1/2 trial in humans.

7.4.2.2   Phase 1/2 Clinical Trial

The phase 1/2 clinical trial of Fabrazyme® was a single-center, open-label, dose-ranging study that involved 15 male patients with classical Fabry's disease (plasma α-GAL activity <1.5 nmol/h/mL). Five dosing regimens, 0.3, 1.0, or 3.0 mg/kg every 2 weeks and 1.0 or 3.0 mg/kg every 48 h, were employed for a total of five infusions. The study was conducted to evaluate the safety and pharmacokinetics of Fabrazyme® infusions in patients with Fabry's disease and to provide preliminary efficacy data for ERT in Fabry's disease. Efficacy assessments were based on change from baseline to end of study in plasma GL-3 concentration, urine sediment, and GL-3 concentration in tissue biopsies as evaluated by light and electron microscopy. The results of this small study provided preliminary data on the safety, pharmacokinetics, and *in vivo* activity of Fabrazyme® in patients with Fabry's disease and provided the basis for the phase 3 placebo-controlled study [67].

7.4.2.3   Phase 3 Clinical Trial

A double-blind, randomized, placebo-controlled phase 3 clinical study was conducted in eight centers in the United States and Europe [68]. The 58 participants (56 men and 2 women) had Fabry's disease with below normal α-GAL activity (<1.5 nmol/h/mL in plasma, and <4 nmol/h/mg in leukocytes), and ranged in age from 16 to 61 years, with an average age of approximately 30 years. Patients were randomized to receive an infusion of Fabrazyme® ($n=29$) or placebo ($n=29$) every 2 weeks for 20 weeks (11 doses). There were no statistically significant differences in baseline characteristics (including age, height, weight, gender, and race) between the placebo and Fabrazyme® groups. Patients who were dependent on prophylactic drugs or analgesics for pain relief were allowed to continue on these medications for the duration of the trial. All patients were pretreated with acetaminophen and an antihistamine.

Since renal failure is a common devastating feature of Fabry's disease, and accumulation of GL-3 in renal endothelial cells may play a role in renal failure, reduction in GL-3 inclusions in renal interstitial capillary endothelial cells was chosen prospectively as the primary efficacy endpoint of this study. The endpoint was assessed by light examination of tissue biopsy samples obtained before and after 20 weeks of treatment. Three independent expert pathologists, who were blinded to treatment assignment and time of biopsy, examined an average of 195 capillaries in each specimen and assigned each biopsy a composite score of 0 (normal or near normal) to 3 (severe vessel inclusions). On the basis of pathophysiological considerations, treatment success was defined as a score of 0 at week 20.

Other endpoints evaluated included GL-3 reduction in the vascular endothelium of the heart and skin; reduction of GL-3 in plasma; maintenance of mean serum creatinine levels; and pain reduction as determined by the McGill Pain Questionnaire (Short Form).

Fabrazyme® infusions resulted in statistically significant ($p < 0.001$) reduction to normal or near-normal levels of GL-3 from the renal capillary endothelium. Twenty of the twenty-nine Fabrazyme®-treated patients (69%) achieved a score of 0 (no or trace vessel inclusions) at 20 weeks. Of the remaining 9 Fabrazyme®-treated patients, 8 achieved scores of 1 (including 5 who improved and 3 who had a score of 1 at baseline); the remaining patient had a missing biopsy and was assigned a score of 3. In contrast, none of the 29 patients treated with placebo had a 0 score ($p < 0.001$). Figure 7.7 shows the difference between the appearance of the kidney vasculature at baseline and after 20 weeks of treatment in one representative patient.

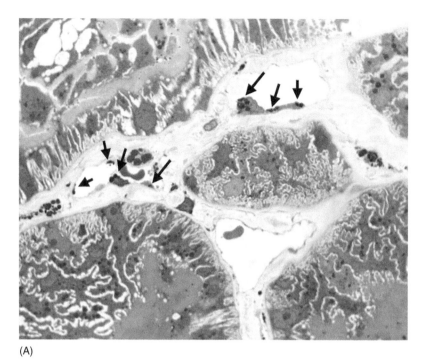

(A)

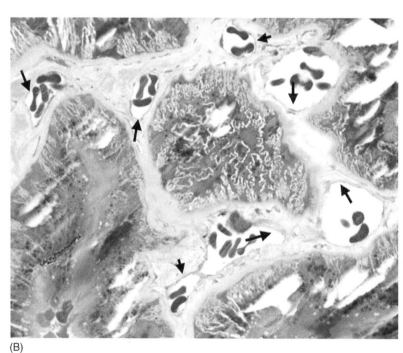

(B)

FIGURE 7.7

Renal capillary endothelium before and after Fabrazyme®. These photomicrographs of the kidney (methylene blue/azure II stain) are from a patient in the phase 3 placebo-controlled study who received 11 treatments with Fabrazyme®. Before treatment (A), the capillary endothelium is heavily laden with glycosphingolipid inclusions (histology score of 3). After treatment (B), glycosphingolipid inclusions have been reduced in the capillary endothelium (histology score of 0).

The percentage of patients after 20 weeks of treatment with mean capillary endothelium scores of 0 were 69% in the kidney, 100% in the skin, and 72% in the heart. Plasma GL-3 levels decreased to below the limit of detection in the treated patients, which correlated with histological findings in the kidney vasculature. The reduction in GL-3 inclusions suggests that Fabrazyme® may ameliorate disease expression; however, the relationship between GL-3 reduction and specific clinical manifestations of Fabry's disease has not been established.

Mean serum creatinine values were normal at baseline and remained normal to week 20 in both treatment groups. No differences between groups in symptoms or renal function were observed during this 5 month study. Pain scores improved significantly from baseline to week 20 in both treatment groups, but since there was no statistically significant difference between the groups, an actual effect could not be told apart from a placebo effect.

In the phase 3 placebo-controlled study, a statistically significant difference was observed for three adverse events that were reported more frequently in patients treated with Fabrazyme® compared with placebo. These adverse experiences were rigors (15/29 [52%] vs. 4/29 [14%], $p=0.004$), fever (14/29 [48%] vs. 5/29 [17%], $p=0.024$), and skeletal pain (6/29 [21%] vs. 0/29 [0%], $p=0.023$). Skeletal pain reported during this study represents isolated musculoskeletal events and is probably not due to the infusion of Fabrazyme®. Rigors and fever represent primarily infusion-associated reactions. The initial presentation of these symptoms most often coincided with IgG seroconversion, which occurred in 83% of patients treated with Fabrazyme®. When rigors and fever occurred, they were generally mild to moderate in nature and were successfully managed by a temporary reduction in infusion rate and treatment with acetaminophen and diphenhydramine.

7.4.2.4   *Phase 3 Extension Study*

All 58 patients from the phase 3 placebo-controlled study chose to enroll in an open-label extension study. After 6 months, all 22 former placebo patients with available biopsies attained a score of 0 for renal vasculature. Overall (after 6 or 12 months of Fabrazyme®), 47/49 (96%) biopsied patients had a histologic score of 0 for vascular endothelium in kidney; 32/40 (80%) had a score of 0 in the heart vasculature; and 51/53 (96%) had a score of 0 in the skin vasculature. Reduction in GL-3 levels was maintained in the superficial and deep vessel skin capillary endothelium for up to 36 months of treatment. After 12 or 18 months of Fabrazyme® therapy, plasma GL-3 levels remained below the limit of detection in all patients. Mean serum creatinine values continued to remain normal from baseline with treatment for up to 30 months.

In addition to reversing GL-3 accumulation in endothelial cells in the kidney vasculature, Fabrazyme® reduced GL-3 to normal or near-normal levels in other renal cell types, such as interstitial capillary endothelium, glomerular capillary endothelium, mesangial cells, interstitial cells, and noncapillary endothelium. But GL-3 was still present in vascular smooth-muscle cells, tubular epithelium, and podocytes, at variably reduced levels.

After 24 to 30 months of Fabrazyme® treatment in the phase 3 extension study, the most common adverse events were rigors, somnolence, temperature-change sensitivity, fever, rhinitis, nausea, and headache. The adverse events associated with Fabrazyme® infusions were successfully managed using standard medical practices. All patients were pretreated with antipyretics with or without an antihistamine. Infusion reactions occurred in some patients after receiving antipyretics, antihistamines, and oral steroids. Infusion reactions declined in frequency with continued use of Fabrazyme®; however, serious infusion reactions occurred after extended durations of Fabrazyme® treatment. Ninety-one percent of patients completed one or more full infusions in ≤2.5 h, and 76% completed one or more full infusions in ≤2.0 h.

Since male Fabry patients do not produce a normal α-galactosidase enzyme protein, most might be expected to recognize the infused enzyme as "foreign" and develop antibodies to this protein. Fifty-two out of 58 (89%) patients developed anti- Fabrazyme® IgG antibodies; however, after 24 to 30 months of treatment, antibody titers decreased in approximately half of all seroconverted patients. The clinical relevance of a decrease in antibody titers is unknown. Seven patients stopped producing IgG antibodies but continued to be monitored long-term. Only a small number of patients experienced reactions suggestive of immediate (Type 1) hypersensitivity. Some patients were successfully reinfused with Fabrazyme® after developing these reactions.

7.4.2.5 Additional Studies

The safety and efficacy of Fabrazyme® was also assessed in a phase 2 open-label study of 13 Japanese patients who were treated with 1.0 mg/kg of Fabrazyme® every 2 weeks for 20 weeks. The phase 2 Japanese study results were consistent with the results of the phase 3 placebo-controlled study.

A double-blind, placebo-controlled phase 4 study of Fabrazyme® in over 80 patients with Fabry's disease and impaired renal function is currently in progress. The endpoint of this multicenter, multinational study is the length of time to occurrence of clinically significant progression of renal disease, cardiac disease, cerebrovascular disease, or death. The phase 4 study ended in January 2004 and patients were enrolled into an open-label extension study. These patients will be followed for an additional 18 months to evaluate the mean change in serum creatinine levels.

Genzyme has also sponsored a prospectively defined, epidemiological study of the natural history of Fabry's disease. The natural decline in renal function has not been well documented, and there is a need for a rigorously compiled, broader historical database that can be used to model and predict the course of Fabry's disease. The data from this study consist of medical records from 447 patients at 27 sites in 5 countries. Genzyme is conducting a phase 2 open-label pediatric study to assess the safety and pharmacokinetics of Fabrazyme® in children. Anticipated trial duration is 60 weeks.

7.5 Details of Enzyme Product Manufacture

To start a production run, a vial of the working cell bank is thawed and expanded over several generations. Once a sufficient cell density is achieved, the cells are seeded into a bioreactor and cell expansion is continued. After the target cell density is achieved, the culture is perfused over several days with a maintenance medium to slow cell growth and maintain a stable metabolic environment. During the harvest phase of several days, medium is continuously added to the culture and the enzyme is drawn off and collected for purification. The enzyme goes through a multistep purification process, including four chromatography steps and nanofiltration, capable of removing potential virus particles and other impurities. To help ensure that the product meets worldwide regulatory authority standards and specifications, testing takes place during every stage of the manufacturing process. The purified α-GAL is stabilized with excipients (mannitol and phosphate buffer) and undergoes double-sterile filtration before it is distributed into vials under aseptic conditions. The vials are lyophilized in either 20 cc (35 mg) or 5 cc (5 mg) configurations to enhance stability and storage. Both vials contain the same concentration of active ingredient

(5 mg/mL) and can be used interchangeably to generate a patient dose. After lyophilization, vials are ready for final quality-control testing.

For clinical trials and early commercial production, the production process was carried out in a pilot facility (Figure 7.8). As product demand increased, the process was scaled-up more than sixfold to a commercial facility (Figure 7.9). This scale-up was carefully planned to allow a smooth transition from material produced at one scale to material produced at the second scale. The planning process included evaluation of the following:

1. The scope of the proposed change — which steps had to be scaled-up, which parameters (e.g., column loads and flow rates, column bed heights, so on) were to be held constant.
2. The probable impact of the proposed changes such as any potential change in levels of impurities.
3. The possibility of unintended consequences such as changes in column operation that may affect resin lifetime, intermediate stability, or cleaning effectiveness.
4. The scope of the necessary validation — whether to revalidate the entire process or only the affected steps.
5. The analyses and product characterization needed to demonstrate comparability.
6. The stability data needed to demonstrate comparability, including any information available from accelerated or forced degradation studies.
7. The impact on in-process controls, which may need to be modified to maintain acceptable product quality.
8. A plan to collect data not only on parameters which changed during the scale-up, but also to confirm what parameters have not changed (e.g., impurity load in the initial harvest pool).
9. The inventory of material from the small-scale process necessary to ensure adequate supply during the validation and regulatory approval from all markets, as well as a transition plan for each market.

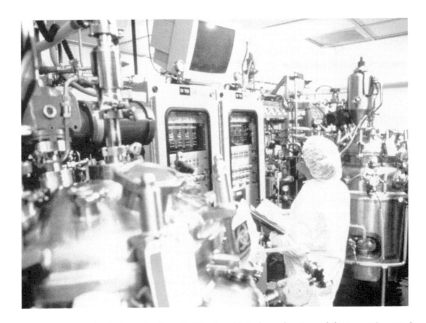

FIGURE 7.8 Fully automated pilot production facility for clinical production of therapeutic proteins.

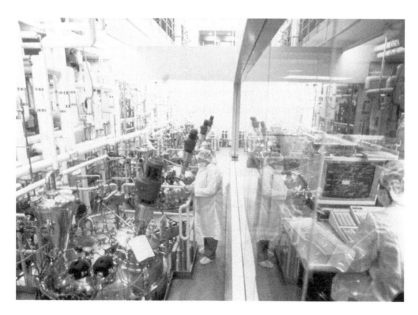

FIGURE 7.9 Bioreactor hall of a commercial production facility.

The package of comparability data, which was prepared to support this change, was multilayered and involved intimate knowledge of the smaller scale process. The data package included information on:

1. Characterization of the product from the large-scale process in comparison to a reference standard from the smaller scale process, using a number of assays beyond those used for normal product release — this is what is typically considered a "comparability data package."
2. Evaluation of the range of results on the release assays from a number of large-scale lots in comparison to the range of results seen with the lots produced at the smaller scale to determine whether the large-scale lots were within the approved specifications for this product, and also whether the range of results seen had shifted with the new process.
3. Comparison of the in-process data collected at each step during the validation runs (e.g., impurities seen at each column step, yields at each step) to determine if each step was functioning as intended at the two scales.
4. Comparison of stability data on the final product, as well as process intermediates to determine if there were any differences between the two scales.
5. A detailed listing of each process change between the two scales, the potential impact of each change on the product, and the data collected to evaluate this impact.

The depth and breadth of information used to complete a thorough evaluation of manufacturing process changes requires a detailed knowledge of the process, which is gained through experience during process development by the innovator manufacturer. It is important to note that such a comparability exercise must take into account all the steps identified above to ensure that the product subject to change will maintain the same efficacy and safety profile demonstrated in clinical trials.

7.6   Conclusion

Fabrazyme® has been approved in over 30 countries worldwide (as of February 2004). Due to the limited patient population (approximately 5000 worldwide and 2000 in the United States), the drug was designated an orphan drug by the FDA, and thus has a 7-year market exclusivity in the United States. Recently, an expert panel was convened to consider the diagnosis and management of Fabry patients. After reviewing the available therapies and clinical data available for ERT, the panel concluded that recombinant α-galactosidase was safe and effective in reducing substrate burden in the patients. They further stated that "Enzyme replacement therapy in all males with Fabry's disease (including those with end-stage renal disease) and female carriers with substantial disease manifestations should be initiated as early as possible" [1, p. 338].

Acknowledgements

The author thanks Rebecca Sendak, Karen Lee, Kate Zhang, Jennifer Baker-Malcolm, and Denise Honey for sharing their data and Tim Edmunds, Adam Sherman, and Mark Hayes for their help in editing and reviewing this chapter.

References

1. Desnick, R.J., et al., Fabry's disease, an under-recognized multisystemic disorder: Expert recommendations for diagnosis, management and enzyme replacement therapy, *Ann. Intern. Med.*, 138, 338–346, 2003.
2. Colombi, A., et al., Angiokeratoma corporis diffusum — Fabry's disease, *Helv. Medica Acta*, 34, 67–83, 1967.
3. Branton, M.H., et al., Natural history of Fabry renal disease — Influence of a-galactosidase A activity and genetic mutations on clinical course, *Medicine*, 81, 122–138, 2002.
4. Fabrazyme. Summary of product characteristics. http://www.emea.eu.int/humandocs/humans/epar/fabrazyme/fabrazyme.htm.
5. Banikazemi, M. and Desnick, R., Fabry's disease: Enzyme replacement therapy (ERT) improves gastrointestinal symptoms, presented at *Annual Meeting of the European Society of Human Genetics*, Birmingham, England, 2003, p. 536.
6. DeSchoenmakere, G., Chauveau, D., and Grunfeld, J., Enzyme replacement therapy in Anderson–Fabry's disease: Beneficial clinical effect on vital organ function, *Nephrol. Dialysis Transplant.*, 18, 33–35, 2003.
7. Weidemann, F., et al., Improvement of cardiac function during enzyme replacement therapy in patients with Fabry's disease — A prospective strain rate imaging study, *Circulation*, 1299–1301, 2003.
8. Germain, D., et al., Effects of enzyme replacement therapy on renal function in Fabry's disease, presented at *Annual Meeting of the European Society of Human Genetics*, Birmingham, England, 2003, p. 533.
9. Lee, K., et al., A biochemical and pharmacological comparison of enzyme replacement therapies for the glycolipid storage disorder Fabry's disease, *Glycobiology*, 13, 305–313, 2003.
10. Calhoun, D.H., et al., Fabry's disease: Isolation of a cDNA clone encoding human alpha-galactosidase a, *Proc. Natl. Acad. Sci., USA*, 82, 7364–7368, 1985.

11. Tsuji, S., et al., Signal sequence and DNA-mediated expression of human lysosomal alpha-galactosidase A, *Eur. J. Biochem.*, 165, 275–280, 1987.

12. Quinn, M., et al., A genomic clone containing the promoter for the gene encoding the human lysosomal enzyme, alpha-galactosidase A, *Gene*, 58, 177–188, 1987.

13. Novo, F.J., et al., Editing of human alpha-galactosidase RNA resulting in a pyrimidine to purine conversion, *Nucleic Acids Res.*, 23, 2636–2640, 1995.

14. Blom, D., et al., Recombinant enzyme therapy for Fabry's disease: Absence of editing of human alpha-galactosidase A mRNA, *Am. J. Hum. Genet.*, 72, 23–31, 2003.

15. Ioannou, Y.A., et al., Human α-galactosidase A: Glycosylation site 3 is essential for enzyme solubility, *Biochem. J.*, 332, 1–9, 1998.

16. Desnick, R.J., Ioannou, Y.A., and Eng, C.M., A-galactosidase a deficiency: Fabry's disease, in *Metabolic and Molecular Bases of Inherited Disease*, 8th ed., Scriver, C.R., Beaudet, A.L., Sly, W.S., and Valle, D., Eds., McGraw-Hill, New York, 2001, pp. 3733–3774.

17. Kase, R., et al., Only sphingolipid activator protein b (sap-b or saposin b) stimulates the degradation of globotriaosylceramide by recombinant human lysosomal alpha-galactosidase in a detergent-free liposomal system, *FEBS Lett.*, 393, 74–76, 1996.

18. O'Brien, J.S. and Kishimoto, Y., Saposin proteins: Structure, function and role in human lysosomal storage disorders, *FASEB J.*, 5, 301–308, 1991.

19. Rorman, E.G., Scheinker, V., and Grabowski, G.A., Structure and evolution of the human prosaposin chromosomal gene, *Genomics*, 13, 312–318, 1992.

20. Miyamura, N., et al., A carboxy-terminal truncation of human alpha-galactosidase A in a heterozygous female with Fabry's disease and modification of the enzymatic activity by the carboxy-terminal domain — increased, reduced, or absent enzyme activity depending on number of amino acid residues deleted, *J. Clin. Invest.*, 98, 1809–1817, 1996.

21. Bishop, D.F., Kornreich, R., and Desnick, R.J., Structural organization of the human alpha-galactosidase A gene: Further evidence for the absence of a 3′ untranslated region, *Proc. Natl. Acad. Sci., USA*, 85, 3903–3907, 1988.

22. Kornreich, R., Desnick, R.J., and Bishop, D.F., Nucleotide sequence of the human alpha-galactosidase A gene, *Nucleic Acids Res.*, 17, 3301–3302, 1989.

23. Desnick, R.J. and Bishop, D.F., Fabry's disease: Alpha-galactosidase deficiency; Schindler disease: Alpha-*N*-acetylgalactosaminidase deficiency, in *Metabolic Basis of Inherited Disease*, 6th ed., Scriver, C.R., Beaudet, A.L., Sly, W.S., and Valle, D., Eds., McGraw-Hill, New York, 1989, pp. 1751–1796.

24. Mayes, J.S., et al., Differential assay for lysosomal alpha-galactosidases in human tissues and its application to Fabry's disease, *Clin. Chim. Acta*, 112, 247–251, 1981.

25. Asano, N., et al., *In vitro* inhibition and intracellular enhancement of lysosomal alpha-galactosidase A activity in Fabry lymphoblasts by 1-deoxygalactonojirimycin and its derivatives, *Eur. J. Biochem.*, 267, 4179–4186, 2000.

26. Goldstein, J. and Zhu, A., 1995, New recombinant coffee bean alpha-galactosidase — Used for cleaving alpha 1, 3-linked galactose residues on the surface of cells for production of blood products, WO 9507088, 16 Mar 1995.

27. Davis, M.O., et al., Cloning, expression and characterization of a blood group B active recombinant alpha-D-galactosidase from soybean (*Glycine max*), *Biochem. Mol. Biol. Int.*, 39, 471–485, 1996.

28. Doucet, J., et al., Modification of xenoantigens on porcine erythrocytes for xenotransfusion, *Surgery*, 135, 178–186, 2004.

29. Ghazi, S., Rooke, J., and Galbraith, H., Improvement of the nutritive value of soybean meal by protease and alpha-galactosidase treatment in broiler cockerels and broiler chicks, *Br. Poultry Sci.*, 44, 410–418, 2003.

30. Pennycooke, J., Jones, J., and Stushnoff, C., Down-regulating alpha-galactosidase enhances freezing tolerance in transgenic petunia, *Plant Physiol.*, 133, 901–909, 2003.

31. Fabry, J., Ein beitrag zur kenntnis der purpura haemorrhagica nodularis (purpura papulosa hemorrhagica hebrae), *Arch. Dermatol. Syphilis*, 43, 187–200, 1898.

32. Anderson, W., A case of "angeio-keratoma", *Br. J. Dermatol.*, 10, 113–117, 1898.

33. Pompen, A.W.M., Ruiter, M., and Wyers, H.J.G., Angiokeratoma corporis diffusum (universale) Fabry, as a sign of an unknown internal disease: Two autopsy reports, *Acta Med. Scand.*, 128, 234–255, 1947.

34. Sweeley, C.C. and Klionsky, B., Fabry's disease: Classification as a sphingolipidosis and partial characterization of a novel glycolipid, *J. Biol. Chem.*, 238, PC3148–PC3150, 1963.

35. Brady, R.O., et al., Enzymatic defect in Fabry's disease: Ceramidetrihexosidase deficiency, *New Engl. J. Med.*, 276, 1163–1167, 1967.

36. Kint, J.A., Fabry's disease: Alpha-galactosidase deficiency, *Science*, 167, 1268–1269, 1970.

37. Mapes, C.A., et al., Enzyme replacement in Fabry's disease, an inborn error of metabolism, *Science*, 169, 987–989, 1970.

38. Brady, R.O., et al., Replacement therapy for inherited enzyme deficiency. Use of purified ceramidetrihexosidase in Fabry's disease, *New Engl. J. Med.*, 289, 9–14, 1973.

39. Desnick, R.J., et al., Enzyme therapy in Fabry's disease: Differential *in vivo* plasma clearance and metabolic effectiveness of plasma and splenic alpha-galactosidase A isozymes, *Proc. Natl. Acad. Sci., USA*, 76, 5326–5330, 1979.

40. Peters, F.P.J., Vermeulen, A., and Kho, T.L., Anderson–Fabry's disease: α-Galactosidase deficiency, *Lancet*, 357, 138–140, 2001.

41. Meikle, P.J., et al., Prevalence of lysosomal storage disorders, *JAMA*, 281, 249–254, 1999.

42. MacDermot, K.D., Holmes, A., and Miners, A.H., Natural history of Fabry's disease in affected males and obligate carrier females, *J. Inherited Metab. Dis.*, 24 (Suppl. 2), 13–14, 2001.

43. Ropers, H.-H., et al., Evidence for preferential X-chromosome inactivation in a family with Fabry's disease, *Am. J. Hum. Genet.*, 29, 361–370, 1977.

44. Thadhani, R., et al., Patients with Fabry's disease on dialysis in the United States, *Kidney Int.*, 61, 249–255, 2002.

45. Ashton-Prolla, P., et al., Fabry's disease: Comparison of enzymatic, linkage and mutation analysis for carrier detection in family with novel mutation, *Am. J. Med.*, 84, 420–424, 1999.

46. See http:archive.uwcm.ac.uk/uwcm/mg/search/119272.html.

47. Shelley, E.D., Shelley, W.B., and Kurczynski, T.W., Painful fingers, heat intolerance, and telangiectases of the ear: Easily ignored childhood signs of Fabry's disease, *Pediat. Dermatol.*, 12, 215–219, 1995.

48. Menkes, D.L., O'Neil, T.J., and Saenz, K.K.P., Fabry's disease presenting as syncope, angiokeratomas, and spike-like cataracts in a young man: Discussion of the differential diagnosis, *Military Med.*, 162, 773–776, 1997.

49. Morgan, S. and d'A Crawfurd, M., Anderson–Fabry's disease, *Br. Med. J.*, 297, 872–873, 1988.

50. Obrador, G.T. and Pereira, B.J.G., Systemic complications of chronic kidney disease — pinpointing clinical manifestations and best management, *Post Grad. Med. J.*, 111, 115–122, 2002.

51. Grewal, R.P., Stroke in Fabry's disease, *J. Neurol.*, 241, 153–156, 1994.

52. Mitsias, P. and Levine, S.R., Cerebrovascular complications of Fabry's disease, *Ann. Neurol.*, 40, 8–17, 1996.

53. Meehan, S., et al., Fabry's disease: Renal involvement limited to podocyte pathology and proteinuria in a septuagenarian cardiac variant. Pathologic and therapeutic implications, *Am. J. Kidney Dis.*, 43, 164–171, 2004.

54. Murali, R., et al., Crystallization and preliminary x-ray analysis of human alpha-galactosidase A complex, *J. Mol. Biol.*, 239, 578–580, 1994.

55. Garman, S.C. and Garboczi, D.N., Structural basis of Fabry's disease, *Mol. Genet. Metab.*, 77, 3–11, 2002.

56. Garman, S.C., et al., The 1.9 angstrom structure of alpha-*N*-acetylgalactosaminidase: Molecular basis of glycosidase deficiency diseases, *Structure*, 10, 425–434, 2002.

57. Sando, G.N. and Neufeld, E.F., Recognition and receptor-mediated uptake of a lysosomal enzyme alpha-l-iduronidase, by cultured fibroblasts, *Cell*, 12, 619–627, 1977.

58. Kornfeld, S., Trafficking of lysosomal enzymes, *FASEB J.*, 1, 462–468, 1987.

59. Kaplan, A., Achord, D.T., and Sly, W., Phosphohexosyl components of a lysosomal enzyme are recognized by pinocytosis receptors on human fibroblasts, *Proc. Natl. Acad. Sci., USA*, 74, 2026–2030, 1977.

60. Mayes, J.S., et al., Endocytosis of lysosomal alpha-galactosidase A by cultured fibroblasts from patients with Fabry's disease, *Am. J. Hum. Genet.*, 34, 602, 1982.

61. Ashwell, G. and Harford, J., Carbohydrate-specific receptors of the liver, *Annu. Rev. Biochem.*, 51, 531–554, 1982.

62. McKenzie, E.J., Su, Y.P., and Martinez-Pomares, L., The mannose receptor, a bi-functional lectin with roles in homeostasis and immunity, *Glycosci. Glycotechnol.*, 14, 273–283, 2002.

63. Achord, D.T., et al., Human beta-glucuronidase: *In vivo* clearance and *in vitro* uptake by a glyco-protein recognition system on reticuloendothelial cells, *Cell*, 15, 269–278, 1978.

64. Desnick, R.J., Bishop, D.F., and Ioannou, Y.A., Cloning and expression of biologically active human alpha-galactosidase A, U.S. Patent 5,356,804, Oct 18, 1994.

65. Ioannou, Y.A., et al., Fabry's disease: Preclinical studies demonstrate the effectiveness of alpha-galactosidase A replacement in enzyme-deficient mice, *Am. J. Hum. Genet.*, 68, 14–25, 2001.

66. Duncan, J.R. and Welch, M.J., Intracellular metabolism of indium-111-DTPA-labeled receptor targeted proteins, *J. Nucl. Med.*, 34, 1728–1738, 1993.

67. Eng, C.M., et al., A phase 1/2 clinical trial of enzyme replacement in Fabry's disease: Pharmacokinetic, substrate clearance, and safety studies, *Am. J. Hum. Genet.*, 68, 711–722, 2001.

68. Eng, C.M., et al., Safety and efficacy of recombinant human alpha-galactosidase A replacement therapy in Fabry's disease, *New Engl. J. Med.*, 345, 9–16, 2001.

8

Urate Oxidase

Alain Bayol, Françoise Lascombes, Denis Loyaux, Jean-Marc Bras, Gérard Loison, René Couderc, and Pascual Ferrara

CONTENTS

8.1   Introduction

Urate oxidase (EC 1.7.3.3), also called uricase or urate oxygen oxidoreductase, is an enzyme of the purine breakdown pathway, that catalyzes the oxidation of uric acid in the presence of oxygen to allantoin and hydrogen peroxide through a complex reaction mechanism [1,2]. Urate oxidase, derived from *Aspergillus flavus*, has been used therapeutically under the name Uricozyme® for the last 20 years in patients with primary or secondary hyperuricemia, including those treated with cytoreductive drugs for a malignant hemopathy [3]. The complementary deoxyribonucleic acid (cDNA) coding this enzyme has been cloned and expressed in several microorganisms [4,5]. *Saccharomyces cerevisiae* was finally chosen for production scale because of the higher yield obtained. The recombinant enzyme accumulates intracellularly in an active and soluble form. The resulting purified enzyme, rasburicase (international nonproprietary name of the drug), is now available and has recently been approved in Europe and the United States under the trade names Fasturtec® and Elitek®, respectively.

8.2   Biochemical Characteristics of the Enzyme

8.2.1   Structure

Rasburicase and native urate oxidase from *A. flavus* have the same structure: a tetramer with identical subunits of 34 kDa [6], which are not linked by disulfide bridges. The N-terminal amino acid of the monomer is an N-α-acetylated serine [4]. The enzyme does not contain metal ions [6]. Isoelectricfocusing shows a main band at pI 7.6 in agreement with the calculated pI, and three minor bands (pI = 7.7, 7.3, and 7.2), which are also catalytically active [7]. A pH of 8.0 was found to be optimal for the enzyme's stability [8].

   X-ray analysis shows that the tetramer is composed of two dimers superimposed face-to-face to form a tunnel-shaped protein [9]. The four active sites (one per monomer) are located in a pocket opening toward the exterior of the protein.

   In the presence of oxygen, urate oxidase degrades uric acid into 5-hydroxyisourate and hydrogen peroxide. This unstable intermediate is then degraded to allantoin and CO_2 [1,2] (Figure 8.1). Improvement of crystallization conditions [10,11] by addition of polyethylene glycol allowed the study of the enzyme crystallized with several inhibitors: 8-Azaxanthin, 9-methyl uric acid, and oxonic acid [12]. The inhibitor is maintained in the active site by hydrogen bonds with Q228 and R176, and by stacking with F159. N-interaction with T57 (of a second monomer) and water-mediated interactions are present; K10 was also found to be essential for activity. A reaction mechanism was proposed where uric acid is bound to urate oxidase as a dianion, allowing the radical abstraction of the uric acid hydrogen N_9 and leading, in a subsequent reaction step with a water molecule, to 5-hydroxyisourate.

   A comparative study showed that rasburicase has a higher purity and specific activity than Uricozyme [7]. The differences observed for Uricozyme in the study are probably a result of the purification process, which modifies the enzyme. Uricozyme contains a mixture of urate oxidase molecules, one of which is a cysteine adduct on C103 (rasburicase-S-S-Cys). Rasburicase did not reveal any cysteine adduct, but it was possible to obtain the same modification by simple incubation of the enzyme with cysteine. The purification process of rasburicase maintains the structure of the molecule. Its specific enzyme activity is about 50% higher than that of Uricozyme. A higher degree of purity of the recombinant product and a better control of the production process should guarantee better safety.

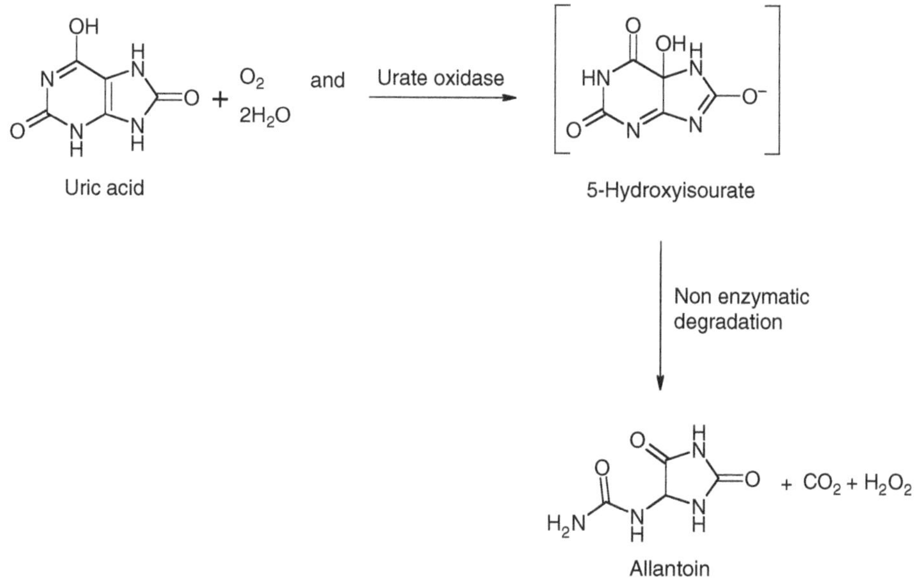

FIGURE 8.1 Metabolic conversion of uric acid into allantoin by urate oxidase.

8.2.2 Kinetic Parameters

Two different approaches have been used for measuring urate oxidase activity. The first one is based on monitoring substrate decrease (uric acid or oxygen), and the second is based on monitoring product increase.

Uric acid consumption is classically observed by spectrophotometry at 290 nm [13]. Nevertheless, the strong absorbance of uric acid at 292 nm limits the usable concentrations and may not permit a good estimation of urate oxidase kinetic parameters. Moreover, some reaction intermediates produced during the urate oxidation reaction absorb in the region from 270 to 330 nm [14] and thus interfere with uric acid quantification, particularly in the estimation of urate oxidase initial velocities. Dioxygen consumption can be monitored with a Clark-type electrode [15]; however, this method is not easily transposable for routine determination.

A 96-well plate assay of urate oxidase activity based on peroxidase quantitation of hydrogen peroxide was developed. The method has been applied to the determination of the kinetic parameters of rasburicase and a K_M value of 47.3 μM was found [16] at 30°C and pH 8.9.

8.2.3 Related Proteins

After treatment with hydrogen peroxide, the characterization of rasburicase revealed that C103 is modified into cysteic acid and cysteine sulfinic acid significantly whereas C35 and C90 are not affected. The kinetics of this reaction (Figure 8.2) show the formation of cysteic acid and sulfinic acid corresponding to the two known oxidation stages of cysteine.

Methionine sulfoxide was characterized in the same way. It was detected only after 5 h for M234 post incubation with hydrogen peroxide, and after 16 h for M231 and M109. No change was detected for M32. These modified products do not exceed 3% of the total methionine content. No methionine sulfone was detected.

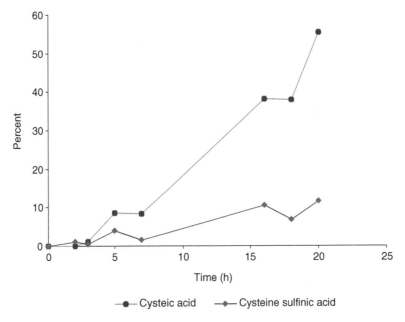

FIGURE 8.2
Kinetics of cysteine oxidation oxidized with hydrogen peroxide at a concentration of 3.1 mM in a 25 mM tris (aminomethane) buffer (pH 8.0) as revealed by mass spectrometry (ESI/MS) after alkylation and trypsin digestion.

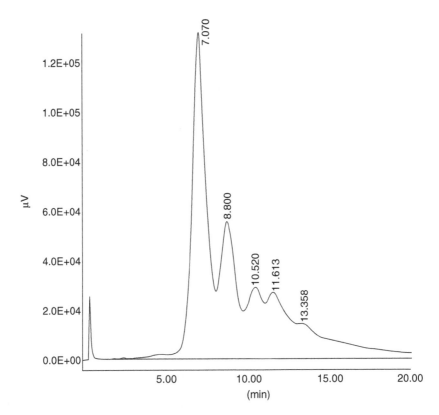

FIGURE 8.3 Ion-exchange chromatography profile after oxidation.

The microheterogeneity of rasburicase revealed by anion-exchange chromatography after oxidation (Figure 8.3) can be explained by the structural complexity of the protein, a tetramer composed of four identical monomers. From a theoretical point of view, a single change in one amino acid could result in up to five forms (one native tetramer and different combinations, i.e., 1:4, 2:4, 3:4, and 4:4, of native and oxidized monomer). Two changes on separate monomers could result in 15 forms, three changes in 35 forms, and so on, according to the mathematical law of nonordered arrangements. This complexity has been recognized for multimeric proteins [17].

8.3 Indications for which the Enzyme is Approved

8.3.1 Hyperuricemia

8.3.1.1 Mechanism of Uric Acid Production

Evolutionary genetic mutations have resulted in the loss of gene expression for urate oxidase in humans (and some higher primates), with the result that uric acid is the end product of the catabolism of purines. Purines can be derived from several major sources: (1) the breakdown of nucleic acids as a result of cellular turnover; (2) dietary ingestion of nucleic acids; (3) nucleic acid degradation following major cellular trauma, e.g., burns and crushing injuries; and (4) following cytotoxic chemotherapy as a result of rapid cell death.

Excess purine nucleotides and deoxynucleotides undergo a series of catabolic reactions to ultimately form uric acid. Several of the intermediates in the formation of uric acid may also be salvaged by pathways in nucleic acid synthesis. Given that human beings lack urate oxidase, uric acid is the final common product from several purine catabolic pathways (Figure 8.4).

Increase in uric acid production may be detected in any patient afflicted with a rapidly proliferating malignancy. Nucleic acid contained in the cytoplasm and nuclei is catabolized as a result of increased cell turnover. This increase in purine metabolism leads to hyperuricemia.

Further, aggressive cancer chemotherapy regimens also cause an important increase in cell lysis, releasing purine metabolites (the lysis driving tumor lysis syndrome [TLS]) and intracellular substances into the bloodstream. Hyperuricemia, hyperphosphatemia, hypocalcemia, hyperkaliemia, and azotemia constitute TLS. These substances are eliminated by renal excretion. Following treatment of some lymphomas and leukemias, plasma uric acid concentrations increase severalfold, generally ranging from 15 to $\geq$40 mg/dL, while normal ranges are 2 to 4 mg/dL in children and 2.5 to 7.5 mg/dL in adults. Urinary excretion of uric acid also increases severalfold, ranging from 2 to 3 g every 24 h [18–21].

8.3.1.2 Consequences of Hyperuricemia

A moderate and chronic increase of plasma uric acid level is responsible for gout, which is manifested by recurrent attacks of acute arthritis; in which crystals of monosodium urate monohydrate are demonstrable by tophi, which are aggregated deposits of urate, uric acid nephropathy and uric acid urolithiasis.

In contrast, an acute increase in plasma levels of uric acid seen in rapidly proliferating malignancy and during aggressive chemotherapy may lead to acute renal failure (ARF) caused by the precipitation of crystals of uric acid in renal tubules. The precipitation of uric acid is higher in acidic urine. Renal function can be further compromised by calcium

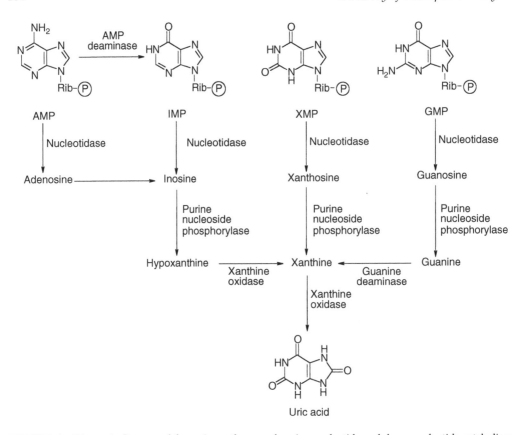

FIGURE 8.4 Schematic diagram of the major pathways of purine nucleotide and deoxynucleotide catabolism.

phosphate precipitation. ARF is the most feared immediate complication of hematological malignancies, as it requires dialysis and has a negative impact on the outcomes of patients with malignancies [22–31].

8.3.2 Medical Conditions Requiring Uricolytic Therapy

Gout, a chronic disease, is controlled by uricosuric agents which enhance the renal excretion of uric acid, or by xanthine oxidase inhibitors such as allopurinol. Uricolytic therapy is not the treatment of choice for gout, as it requires continuous treatment rather than a decrease in plasma uric acid concentration within a few hours. In contrast, since ARF, a consequence of acute hyperuricemia, is a life-threatening condition, any acute increase in uric acid plasma concentration has to be urgently treated or, ideally, prevented. Uricolytic therapy, through its fast-acting and highly effective action, fully meets these requirements.

8.3.2.1 Physiopathology

Malignant cells contain more nucleic acid than normal cells, and have a much higher cellular turnover. Although malignancies with high tumor burden and high proliferative rate may lead to spontaneous hyperuricemia, chemotherapy more readily induces TLS, since malignant cells are sensitive to treatment. These patients, even those who present with normal plasma uric acid concentrations, are metabolically unstable and at risk of metabolic perturbations triggered by dehydration and chemotherapy-induced tumor lysis. Thus, chemotherapy can be initiated only in metabolically stable patients with controlled plasma uric acid concentrations, and uricolytic therapy must be initiated prior to starting cytoreductive therapy in patients with or at risk of TLS.

8.3.2.2   Diseases and Causes of Acute Hyperuricemia

Diseases with high tumor burden or high tumor cell proliferation rate and tumors with high sensitivity to cytotoxic drugs present the highest risk of TLS and, therefore, hyperuricemia. These diseases are myeloproliferative diseases and hemopoietic tumors occurring in children and adults. Among myeloproliferative diseases and hemopoietic tumors, acute lymphoblastic leukemia, acute myeloid leukemia, acute undifferentiated leukemia, chronic lymphocytic leukemia, blastic crises of chronic myeloid leukemia, and non-Hodgkin's lymphoma are the most frequently associated with TLS. Plasma cell disorders, such as multiple myeloma and myelodysplastic syndrome, may be responsible for TLS as well. Among lymphomas and leukemias, advanced-stage Burkitt's lymphoma and B-cell acute lymphoblastic leukemia, high-proliferative-rate diseases, are at the highest risk for severe TLS and subsequent renal failure [32]. Solid tumors have been reported to induce TLS, among which are germ cell tumors and small-cell lung cancer. White blood cell count and lactate dehydrogenase are parameters of tumor load. Elevated plasma levels are good indicators of high risk of TLS [29,31].

Treatment must be started prior to initiation of cytotoxic therapy, to control plasma uric acid concentration and avoid renal complications. This treatment must be fast-acting to avoid any delay in chemotherapy initiation in potentially curable patients at risk of threatening symptoms associated with a high tumor burden and high proliferation rate, such as hyperleukocytosis and hyperviscosity syndrome.

Gout is a disease characterised by chronic hyperuricemia and a mild plasma uric acid concentration increase, and therefore does not represent an indication to be treated by rasburicase. Nevertheless, a few patients with allopurinolallergy, and allograft transplant recipients were successfully treated by rasburicase [33,34].

8.4   Developmental History of the Enzyme

8.4.1   Rasburicase

Urate oxidase is present in most mammals, but primates and humans have lost this enzyme owing to genetic mutations that took place during the evolutionary process. The pharmacokinetics of rasburicase following a 30 min intravenous (IV) infusion is linear over the dose range of 0.05 to 0.20 mg/kg. Rasburicase is a protein enzyme with a low clearance rate (2.3 to 3.8 mL/h/kg) and has a mean volume of distribution similar to the vascular space. The mean elimination half-life is approximately 18 h and is independent of the dose administered. There is no significant correlation between hepatic function and uricolytic activity, and the renal elimination of rasburicase is a minor pathway for rasburicase clearance. There is no need for dose adjustments with respect to the regarding gender and age of the patients, provided that rasburicase is dosed in a mg/kg manner. Like other proteins, rasburicase is expected to be hydrolyzed with reincorporation of amino acids into new cellular proteins. No drug–drug interactions were observed from preclinical studies or reported from clinical use.

Rasburicase is active at the end of the purine catabolic pathway. The recommended dose of rasburicase is 0.15 or 0.20 mg/kg/d, administered once daily. The median treatment duration is 3 to 5 d [21,29,39].

8.4.1.1   Mechanism of Action

Rasburicase is a recombinant urate oxidase enzyme that catalyzes the enzymatic oxidation of uric acid into allantoin, as shown in Figure 8.1. In contrast to uric acid, allantoin is readily water-soluble, facilitating its elimination by urinary excretion. The reactive by-product of this reaction, hydrogen peroxide, is then neutralized by catalase to form oxygen and water.

8.4.2   Safety of Rasburicase

Rasburicase is well tolerated. The most important safety concern is allergic reactions, such as anaphylaxis, which may occur because rasburicase is an heterologous protein. Allergic reactions tend to occur within 10 min after beginning infusion of the first dose. The incidence of hypersensitivity reactions is 1% [29,35,40], while the incidence of severe allergic reactions is 0.5% [29] or less [31,36,37].

Rasburicase may induce hemolysis in patients with glucose-6-phosphate dehydrogenase (G6PD) deficiency because hydrogen peroxide, an oxidizing agent, is one of the major by-products of the conversion of uric acid into allantoin. Hemolysis and methemoglobinemia have been reported in patients with an incidence of 0.5% [38] or less [36]. It is not known whether patients with deficiency of methemoglobine reductase are at increased risk for methemoglobinemia or hemolytic anemia.

Other adverse events have been recorded during treatment with rasburicase but the relationship to rasburicase was not known as the adverse events might also have been related to the underlying disease state and its treatment with cytotoxic chemotherapy. The most frequent adverse events reported were headache, nausea, fever, and vomiting, with an incidence of about 5%.

Rasburicase should not be administered to patients with a known history of anaphylactic reactions or known history of hypersensitivity reactions to rasburicase or any of the excipients. Rasburicase is contraindicated in patients with known G6PD deficiency.

8.4.3   Results of Rasburicase Treatment

Rasburicase has been successfully used in patients with myeloproliferative diseases and hemopoietic tumors, leading to hyperuricemia or at risk of TLS.

Rasburicase efficacy is assessed by plasma uric acid concentration measurements. Caution has to be taken to ensure accurate uric acid measurements. Rasburicase will cause enzymatic degradation of the uric acid within blood samples left at room temperature, resulting in spuriously low uric acid levels. Blood must be collected in prechilled tubes containing heparin anticoagulant and immediately immersed and maintained in an ice water bath. Plasma samples must be assayed within 4 h of sample collection.

Rasburicase produces rapid and pronounced reduction in plasma uric acid concentrations in patients, regardless of whether they are hyperuricemic at baseline [21,29,31,36,39,41,42–44]. Mean plasma uric acid concentration is reduced by more than 80% 4 h after the first dose of rasburicase in patients. Rasburicase effectively prevents secondary increases of uric acid concentration ≥8 mg/dL in most of the patients, and plasma uric acid remains controlled 24 h after the last dose of rasburicase, as shown in Figure 8.5.

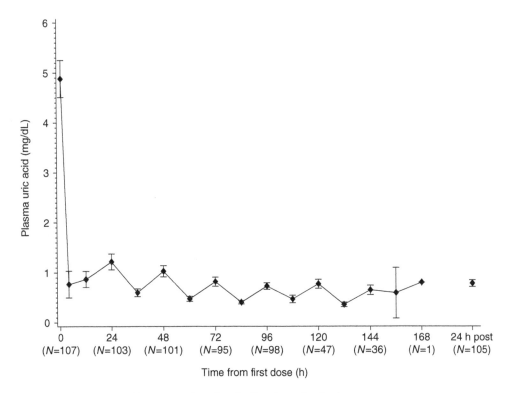

FIGURE 8.5 Plasma uric acid concentration after the first dose of rasburicase.

Through its rapid onset of action, rasburicase enables the initiation of chemotherapy treatment in a timely manner and without delay, which constitutes a critical issue in the treatment of proliferative diseases [40,45,46].

An improvement in renal function has been observed in patients with baseline-elevated serum creatinine. In these patients, serum creatinine levels dropped within a few days (Figure 8.6).

The frequency of ARF was significantly decreased when rasburicase was used in the management of TLS [21,29,31,36,39–43,47]. It has been clearly established that maintenance of renal function is a factor of great importance in the management of these patients who receive chemotherapy and who therefore require dose adjustments to minimize toxicity. Furthermore, these patients are candidates for potentially curative chemotherapy and at risk for late complications from the treatment of their original malignancy. In this context, early preservation of renal function appears highly desirable.

Rasburicase has been commercially available since 2002. Rasburicase is indicated for:

1. The treatment of hyperuricemia due to rapid tumor lysis in pediatric and adult patients
2. The prevention of chemotherapy-induced hyperuricemia in pediatric and adult patients who have malignancies associated with rapid tumor lysis

Compared with previous treatments of TLS, i.e., hydration alkalinization and allopurinol therapy, rasburicase reduces uric acid levels more rapidly and more effectively, and improves renal function with a good safety profile. Rasburicase used to prevent and treat

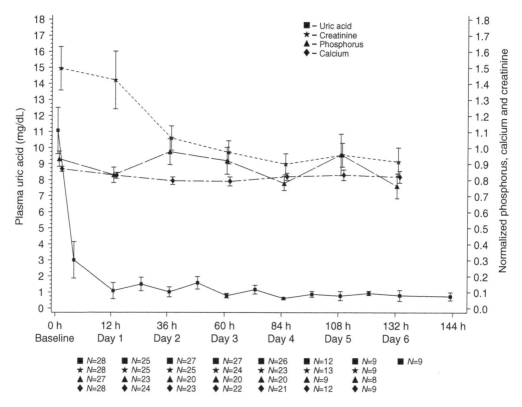

FIGURE 8.6   Creatinine, calcium, phosphorus, and uric acid concentration after rasburicase treatment.

hyperuricemia avoids strong alkalinization. A high urine pH is associated with decreased phosphate excretion, which can favor the precipitation of calcium-phosphate salts in the renal tubules, a cause of renal failure [46]. By reintroducing an enzyme present in most of the mammals but lost in humans following genetic mutations, this enzymatic therapy provides an important therapeutic breakthrough.

8.5   Characteristics of the Producing Strain

A laboratory strain of baker's yeast (*S. cerevisiae*) has been chosen as a host system for rasburicase production. Yeast presents several advantages over *A. flavus*. First, *S. cerevisiae* is a urate oxidase-lacking microorganism that is generally recognized as safe. This is not the case with *A. flavus* which, under certain conditions, can produce highly carcinogenic toxins known as aflatoxins. Second, *S. cerevisiae* can be grown at a relatively high cell density. In addition, there is a strong industrial know-how with yeast cultures, based on industrial practices for more than a century. Finally, the genetics of *S. cerevisiae* allow the use of a number of powerful and versatile techniques that greatly facilitate the tasks of strain construction and improvement.

8.5.1 The Expression Vector (pEMR547)

The urate oxidase expression plasmid, pEMR547, is an *Escherichia coli–S. cerevisiae* shuttle vector composed of the following elements:

1. The *Pvu*II–*Eco*RI fragment (2.3 kb) of the bacterial vector pBR322 [49,50], which contains the origin of replication and the ampicillin resistance gene, enabling DNA plasmid propagation and amplification in *E. coli*.
2. A *Pst*I–*Xba*I fragment (1.3 kb) derived from the B form of the yeast endogenous 2 μm plasmid [51]. This segment encompasses the replication origin (also known as autonomous replication sequence, ARS) and the stabilization (STB) locus [52]. The ARS sequence is required to allow the maintenance of the vector in an extrachromosomal state. The STB is involved in the 2 μm partition process during mitosis. STB requires a set of three proteins encoded by 2 μm plasmid genes [53]. As these genes are not present in the expression vector itself, correct partition of the expression vector is dependent on the presence of the endogenous 2 μm plasmid in the production cells. As already mentioned, the expression vector and the yeast endogenous plasmid share DNA sequences present on both plasmids. These sequences have been shortened to a minimum so as to prevent intermolecular recombination events that could occur between both plasmid species, while still retaining the desired characteristics. As a result, the expression plasmid is stable, both with respect to structure and to mitotic segregation, even in cells growing in the absence of any selection pressure.
3. The vector also carries a defective selectable marker, *LEU2*-d, which lacks promoter sequences essential for normal level expression. This selectable marker, which encodes β-isopropylmamate dehydrogenase, was originally constructed by Beggs [54]. However, whereas in the original construction, pJDB207, the *LEU2*-d gene was inserted in an otherwise contiguous 2 μm region, this is not the case with pEMR547. In the latter plasmid, the *LEU2*-d marker flanks, but is not inside, the 2 μm fragment. This modification improves stability by preventing gene conversion back to the wild-type situation, which would result in the loss of the *LEU2*-d sequence at a high frequency. Since the *LEU2* gene is defective, it is very poorly expressed. This weak level of expression has to be compensated by a very high number of plasmid copies, ~100 copies per haploid genome. This considerably high number is obtained through a cell transformation procedure especially designed for that purpose [5].

8.5.1.1 The Urate Oxidase-Encoding Sequence

The urate oxidase-encoding sequence used for urate oxidase production in yeast was isolated from an *A. flavus* cDNA library, using synthetic oligonucleotides as probes. As a control, the *A. flavus* urate oxidase-encoding gene, *uaZ*, was also cloned. The gene and cDNA sequences were compared by alignment to ensure the absence of mutation in the urate oxidase-encoding cDNA. Both sequences were indeed found to be identical, except for the addition of two introns in the genomic sequence. The cDNA sequence was used for expression in yeast. Some codons in the urate oxidase open reading frame were changed with the aim of improving expression, but these changes did not alter the sequence of the resulting translation product. A galactose-regulated artificial promoter was designed to drive the transcription of the urate oxidase-encoding sequence at a very high level and in a strictly controlled fashion [5]. This promoter combined sequences obtained from two yeast gene promoters, the upstream sequence of the *gal7* gene promoter and the downstream sequence of the *adh2* promoter. The construction was found to be more powerful than each of the natural promoters it derives from, and one of the most efficient promoters for the expression of foreign proteins. Urate oxidase biosynthesis is maximally induced in the presence of galactose when glucose is absent. Expression is repressed in the presence of glucose.

8.5.2 The Host Strain

The host strain has been chosen from several laboratory yeast strains on the basis of the following criteria: adequate growth characteristics, very high level of urate oxidase production with minimal amounts of degradation products under appropriate induction conditions, and stable maintenance of the plasmid at a high copy number, whether cells are grown under selective pressure conditions or not. Under optimal expression conditions, urate oxidase accumulates at a level exceeding 20% of cell proteins. This high level of expression, combined with an optimized fermentation process, results in improved biomass and high productivity. This accounts for a 100- to 1000-fold increase in urate oxidase production level per unit fermentation volume, as compared to the mold fermentation process. The host strain lacks β-isopropylmamate dehydrogenase as a result of several mutations in the *LEU2* locus. It is also deficient in various vacuolar protease activities.

8.5.3 The Cell Bank System

A cell bank system has been established to guarantee batch-to-batch consistency of the product during successive production runs. A single master cell bank (MCB) has been constituted. It is composed of cryotubes containing samples of a culture of the urate oxidase production strain grown in rich medium under nonselective conditions. The cryotubes are stored in liquid nitrogen, which ensures strain viability and stability on a long-term basis.

Each working cell bank (WCB) is prepared from one cryotube of the MCB by the inoculation of a synthetic minimal medium, adequately supplemented to fulfil the strain requirement. The culture for the preparation of each WCB is performed in a leucine-free medium that is selective for plasmid-containing cells. Later culture stages are no longer performed under conditions selective for plasmid-containing cells; however, plasmid-free cells represent a very low percentage of the total cells in the culture (<1%). The generation number for the WCB is ~10.

8.5.4 Genetic Stability

The genetic stability of the urate oxidase production strain was investigated during storage of the cell banks and during production by routine testing and by specific studies. An unlimited lifespan has been attributed to the MCB stored in liquid nitrogen. The stability of the production strain was investigated with samples of two WCBs stored in liquid nitrogen for 3 and 2 years, respectively. No change in colony appearance, cell viability, and plasmid structure was detected at any time during the storage period.

Genetic stability was evaluated in experiments designed to reproduce the production process in the preculture, and cultures in the bioreactor were kept identical with the real production situation. However, to increase the total number of generations, two subsequent preculture steps were added between the regular preculture and the final culture in the bioreactor; each represented nine generations, bringing the final number of generations to 42 or 43, i.e., 18 more than those that reacted during the production process. No genetic drift of the production strain was detected in this experiment, as shown by characterization of the production strain, the production plasmid, and the urate oxidase production pattern. Although all these steps were performed under growth medium conditions that were not selective for plasmid-containing cells, plasmid-free cells were not found to accumulate in the culture, and still represented a small percentage of total cells (<1%). Thus, the stability of the production strain was considered to be satisfactory.

8.6   Enzyme Manufacture Process

8.6.1   Production Process

The production process of urate oxidase involves three steps:

1. Fermentation, during which a high but consistent quantity of enzyme is produced corresponding to a high cell density at the end of the culture
2. Extraction of intracellular enzyme: the cells are first collected, washed, and disrupted in order to obtain a cell crude extract from which urate oxidase will be isolated
3. Purification, during which the host cell proteins and the other contaminating molecules are removed by several steps of ultrafiltration or chromatography

8.6.1.1   *Fermentation*

8.6.1.1.1   *Preparation of Inoculum*

The producing strain is stored in liquid nitrogen under the seed lot system: a single MCB from which are prepared the successive WCBs. WCBs are controlled and released by Quality Control in accordance with the existing monographs.

One cryotube of the current WCB is thawed and the content is aseptically transferred under laminar flow into a flask containing the sterile preculture medium.

This flask is then incubated at 30°C in a rotary shaker. Samples are taken before inoculation and at the end of the preculture in order to check the sterility of the medium and the purity of the culture at the end of incubation, respectively, prior to inoculation of the fermenter.

8.6.1.1.2   *Culture into Fermenter*

The fermentation process was developed to produce a consistently high level of urate oxidase, and to ensure strain stability and culture purity.

The culture in the production fermenter consists of two successive phases that differ in the carbon source used:

1. Glucose during the first half of the culture phase, during which the synthesis of urate oxidase does not occur, as it is repressed by small amounts of glucose
2. Alcohol and galactose during the second half of the culture phase, during which enzyme biosynthesis is induced by the galactose of the culture medium. During this phase, ethanol is the main carbon source

We have determined that at ethanol concentrations >7.5 g/L, the growth rate decreases proportionally to the ethanol concentration. Therefore, during fermentation, alcohol concentration is kept lower than this inhibiting value.

During the glucose phase, a part of the carbon source is converted into ethanol (Crabtree effect); thus, the initial glucose concentration has been set in order to keep the maximum ethanol concentration consistently lower than 7.5 g/L (Figure 8.7). Of course, the specific growth rate is lower with restricted than with higher glucose concentration, but the yield of the fermentation (weight of biomass produced by weight of glucose metabolized) is higher.

The 450 L bioreactor (Figure 8.8) is inoculated with the preculture prepared in a shaken flask. When glucose is exhausted, the ethanol produced previously is consumed and at the same time, more glucose is gradually added with a feeding pump in order to increase the biomass content of the broth.

After 26 h of culture, glucose feeding is stopped and the alcohol-fed batch medium containing the inducer of the biosynthesis of urate oxidase is added by another feeding pump. The liquid alcohol concentration is calculated using an algorithm from ethanol concentrations obtained by gas chromatography on-line analysis. Typical growth curves, showing the consistency of successive fermentations, are given in Figure 8.9 and Figure 8.10.

The culture is stopped when the biomass content in the broth is higher than the specification set in the dossier. The sterility of the media before inoculation and the purity of the culture at the end of the fermentation are tested.

8.6.1.2 *Extraction*

The yeast cells containing the enzyme are collected by tangential flow microfiltration (porosity of membranes: 0.14 μm), washed with purified water filtered on-line (diafiltration), and then placed in a buffer. After this, the cells are disrupted by a high pressure homogenizer; the cell debris is removed by another loop of tangential flow microfiltration (same porosity as previously), washed with the same buffer, and the permeate is filtered through a 0.22-μm membrane filter.

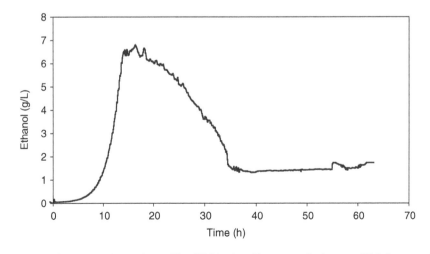

FIGURE 8.7 Ethanol concentration, estimated by GPC in the effluent gas, during one 450 L fermentation.

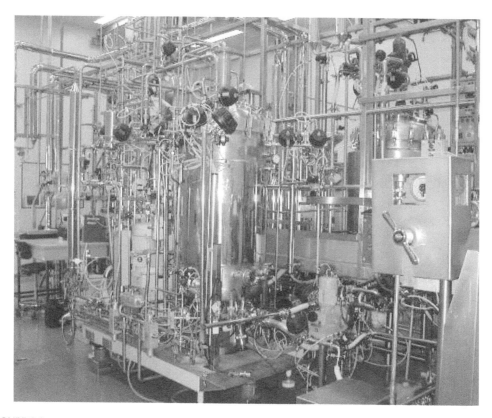

FIGURE 8.8
View of the 450 L fermenter (center) and high-pressure homogenizer (right). The process is fully automated, particularly for sterilization, culture parameters control, and cleaning in place to enhance process reliability.

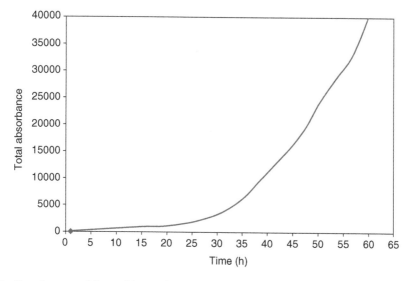

FIGURE 8.9 Growth curve of *S. cerevisiae* producing strain in 450 L fermenter.

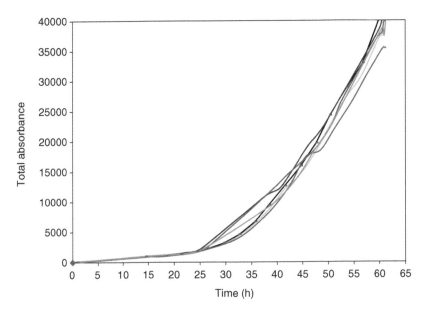

FIGURE 8.10   Reproducibility of cultures in 450 L fermenter.

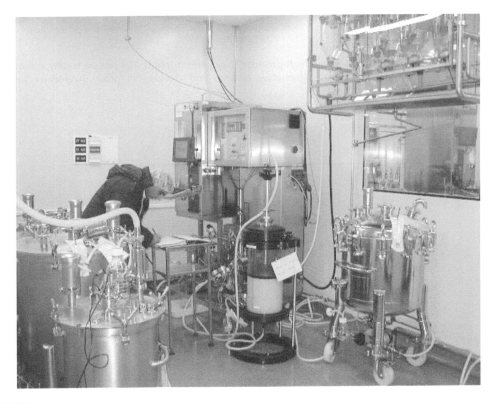

FIGURE 8.11
View of a room for purification of urate oxidase by chromatography. All purification steps are automated (center); stainless-steel vessels for buffers prepared with WFI, and intermediates (left and right); fraction collector (top).

8.6.1.3 Purification

The purification process consists of several ultrafiltration and chromatography steps (Figure 8.11). It has been validated for the elimination of DNA and host cell proteins of the producing strain. To prevent contamination:

1. Water for injection (WFI) is used throughout the entire purification process
2. All buffers used are previously filtered through a 0.22-μm filtration membrane
3. Purification intermediates are collected in stainless-steel vessels that have been cleaned, rinsed with WFI, and autoclaved for 30 min at 121°C
4. All purification intermediates are stored at 4°C. Furthermore, they are previously filtered through a 0.22-μm filter prior to storage if they must be stored for more than 24 h at 4°C
5. Columns and ultrafiltration membranes are cleaned immediately after each run and stored under conditions that prevent microbial growth

For all the purification steps, samples are collected from stainless-steel tanks for physicochemical and microbiological controls by using a syringe through a septum membrane.

All intermediates must comply with the physicochemical and microbiological acceptance criteria set. If not, the batch is rejected.

A closed system, first autoclaved for 30 min at 121°C, is used for the final filtration and filling of the bulk drug substance vessels.

8.7 Main Quality Control Evaluations Undertaken during Production

In-process controls are performed throughout the production process. The media used for preculture and culture steps are controlled to verify the absence of viable contaminating microorganisms. At the preculture step, the inoculum is controlled to verify normal cell growth (absorbance at 600 nm), morphology, and the microbial purity. At the culture step, the final fermentation broth is subjected to the same controls as well as tests for production strain stability: uracil auxotrophy and plasmid segregation. In the cell disruption step, the cell homogenate is controlled to determine the level of enzyme activity and specific activity of the disrupted biomass. Finally, after cell filtration, the crude extract is controlled for the amount of rasburicase prior to purification.

For purification, in-process control tests are performed to ensure process consistency. They were developed considering the need to obtain rapidly the results necessary for determining whether to proceed to the next step and to keep the fractions. Thus, these methods differ slightly from those used to control the drug substance and the drug product. Microbiological controls at each step confirm that the process is conducted in a proper manner.

The drug substance is controlled by a comprehensive set of release tests that ensure its adequate characterization. The drug substance is adequately identified by peptide mapping that is related to the primary structure, size-exclusion chromatography (SEC); and ion-exchange chromatography (IEC), that is related to the tetramer (size and microheterogeneity) and enzyme activity.

DNA testing is no longer routinely performed because its elimination has been demonstrated by spiking experiments.

Three chromatography complementary methods (IEC, SEC, and reverse phase chromatography [RPC]), separating the different molecules on the basis of charge, polarity, and size, respectively, are performed. Electrophoresis (SDS–PAGE) is also performed to detect related proteins separated by size under denaturing conditions. As explained above, IEC reveals the tetrameric heterogeneity of the drug substance and RPC gives a limit for the modified monomers. The IEC method is preferred to isoelectricfocusing because it is more quantitative. An immunoassay has been developed to assess the absence of *S. cerevisiae* proteins at a level less than 50 ppm.

Two assays are performed. The enzyme activity assay is easy to perform *in vitro* and is representative of the enzyme's biological activity *in vivo*. Rasburicase content is determined by SEC. The principal peak consists of all the active tetrameric forms. The drug substance specifications are based on a selection of tests for identity, purity and impurities, and biological activity. They have been established on the basis of the data for batches of drug substance used for toxicology, clinical, and stability studies.

8.8 Final Enzyme Product Formulation

To ensure a long storage period, a freeze-dried formulation has been developed to guarantee molecular integrity and enzyme activity. The formula with a mannitol/alanine ratio of 0.7 is found to be the best composition [48].

The first marketing authorization was granted in February 2001 for Fasturtec 1.5 mg. Fasturtec/Elitek is administered as a once-daily IV infusion, and the recommended dose is 0.2 mg/kg/d. A new presentation, Fasturtec 7.5 mg, has been developed, as its need was obvious: as an example, only two vials will be necessary (instead of ten vials) for a patient weighing 75 kg. The drug is stored at 5°C with a shelf life of 36 months, but it remains within the acceptance limits up to 5 months at 25°C.

References

1. Kahn, K., Serfozo, P., and Tipton, P.A., Identification of the true product of the urate oxidase reaction, *J. Am. Chem. Soc.*, 119, 5435–5442, 1997.
2. Kahn, K., Theoretical study of intermediates in the urate oxidase reaction, *Bioorg. Chem.*, 27, 351–362, 1999.
3. Kissel, P., et al., Treatment of malignant haemopathies and urate oxidase, *Lancet*, 25, 229, 1975.
4. Legoux, R., et al., Cloning and expression in *Escherichia coli* of the gene encoding *Aspergillus flavus* urate oxidase, *J. Biol. Chem.*, 267, 8565–8570, 1992.
5. Leplatois, P., Le Douarin., and Loison, G., High-level of a peroxisomal enzyme: *Aspergillus flavus* uricase accumulates intracellularly and is active in *Saccharomyces cerevisiae*, *Gene*, 122, 139–145, 1992.
6. Conley, T.G. and Priest, D.G., Thermodynamics and stoichiometry of the binding of substrate analogues to uricase, *Biochem. J.*, 187, 727–732, 1980.
7. Bayol, A., et al., Modification of a reactive cysteine explains differences between rasburicase and Uricozyme®, a natural *Aspergillus flavus* uricase, *Biotechnol. Appl. Biochem.*, 36, 21–31, 2002.
8. Bayol, A., et al., Study of pH and temperature-induced transitions in urate oxidase (Uox-EC 1.7.3.3.) by microcalorimetry (DSC), size exclusion chromatography (SEC) and enzymatic activity experiments, *Biophys. Chem.*, 54, 229–235, 1995.
9. Colloc'h, N., et al., Crystal structure of the protein drug urate oxidase–inhibitor complex at a 2.05 Å resolution, *Nat. Struct. Biol.*, 4, 947–952, 1997.

10. Bonneté, F., et al., Interactions in solution and crystallization of *Aspergillus flavus* urate oxidase, *J. Crystal Growth*, 232, 330–339, 2001.
11. Vivarès, D. and Bonneté, F., X-ray scattering studies of *Aspergillus flavus* urate oxidase: Towards a better understanding of PEG effects on the crystallization of large proteins, *Acta Crystallogra.*, D 58, 472–479, 2002.
12. Retailleau, P., et al., Complexed and ligan-free high-resolution structures of urate oxidase (Uox) from *Aspergillus flavus*: A reassignment of the active-site binding mode, *Acta Crystallogra.*, D 60, 453–462, 2004.
13. Kalckar, H.M., Differential spectrophotometry of purine compounds by means of specific enzymes, *J. Biol. Chem.*, 167, 429, 1947.
14. Priest, D.G. and Pitts, O.M., Reaction intermediate effects on the spectrophotometric uricase assay, *Anal. Biochem.*, 50, 195–205, 1972.
15. Pitts, O.M. and Priest, D.G., A steady-state kinetic investigation of the uricase reaction mechanism, *Arch. Biochem. Biophys.*, 163, 359–366, 1974.
16. Fraisse, L., et al., A colorimetric 96-well microtiter plate assay for the determination of urate oxidase activity and its kinetic parameters, *Anal. Biochem.*, 309, 173–179, 2002.
17. Herman, A., FDA Characterization of Biotech Pharmaceutical Products Workshop, Washington, December 11, 13, 1993.
18 Hande, K.R., Hyperuricemia, uric acid nephropathy, and the tumor lysis syndrome, in *Renal Complications of Neoplasia*, McKinney, TD, Ed., Praeger, New York, 1986, pp. 134–156.
19. Rieselbach, R.E., et al., Uric acid excretion and renal function in the acute hyperuricemia of leukemia. Pathogenesis and therapy of uric acid nephropathy, *Am. J. Med.*, 37, 872–884, 1964.
20. Primikirios, N., Stutzman, L., and Sandberg, A.A., Uric acid excretion in patients with malignant lymphomas, *Blood*, 17, 701–718, 1961.
21. Pui, C.-H., Rasburicase: A potent uricolytic agent, *Expert Opin. Pharmacother.*, 3, 1–10, 2002.
22. Cohen, L.F., et al., Acute tumor lysis syndrome. A review of 37 patients with Burkitt's lymphoma, *Am. J. Med.*, 68, 486–491, 1980.
23. Arrambide, K. and Toto, R.D., Tumor lysis syndrome, *Semin. Nephrol.*, 13, 273–280, 1993.
24. Wibe, E., et al., Tumor lysis syndrome: A life-threatening complication during cytostatic treatment of chemosensitive types of cancer, *Tidsskr. Nor. Laegeforen*, 111, 2435–2437, 1991.
25. Jones, P.D., et al., Renal dysfunction and hyperuricemia at presentation and relapse of acute lymphoblastic leukemia, *Med. Pediatr. Oncol.*, 18, 283–286, 1990.
26. Stokes, D.N., The tumour lysis syndrome: Intensive care aspects of paediatric oncology, *Anaesthesia*, 44, 133–136, 1989.
27. Andreoli, S.P., et al., Purine excretion during tumor lysis in children with acute lymphocytic leukemia receiving allopurinol: Relationship to acute renal failure, *J. Pediatr.*, 109, 292–298, 1986.
28. Pochedly, C., Hyperuricemia in leukemia and lymphoma, *Postgrad. Med.*, 55, 93–98, 1974.
29. Navolanic, P.M., et al., Elitek™-rasburicase: An effective means to prevent and treat hyperuricemia associated with tumor lysis syndrome, A Meeting Report, Dallas, Texas, January 2002; *Leukemia*, 17, 499–514, 2003.
30. Conger, J.D. and Falk, S.A., Intrarenal dynamics in the pathogenesis and prevention of acute urate nephropathy, *J. Clin. Invest.*, 59, 86, 1977.
31. Bosly, A., et al., Rasburicase (Recombinant Urate Oxidase) for the management of hyperuricemia in patients with cancer, *Cancer*, 98, 1048–1054, 2003.
32. Ablin, A., et al., Nephropathy, xanthinuria, and orotic aciduria complicating Burkitt's lymphoma treated with chemotherapy and allopurinol, *Metabolism*, 21, 771–778, 1972.
33. Fam, A.G., Difficult gout and new approaches for control of hyperuricemia in the allopurinol-allergic patient, *Curr. Rheumatol. Reports (US)*, 3, 29–35, 2001.
34. Rozenberg, S., Koeger, A.C., and Bourgeois, P., Urate oxidase for gouty arthritis in cardiac transplant recipients, *J. Rheumatol.*, 20, 2171, 1993.
35. Jeha, S., et al., Recombinant urate oxidase (Elitek) is safe and effective in prevention and treatment of malignancy-associated hyperuricemia in adult patients, *Blood*, 100, 556a, 2002.
36. Patte, C., et al., Urate-oxidase in the prevention and treatment of metabolic complications in patients with B-cell lymphoma and leukemia, treated in the Société Française d'Oncologie Pédiatrique LMB89 protocol, *Ann. Oncol.*, 13, 789–795, 2002.

37. Pui, C.-H., et al., Recombinant urate oxidase (rasburicase) in the prevention and treatment of malignancy-associated hyperuricemia in pediatric and adult patients: Results of a compassionate-use trial, *Leukemia*, 15, 1505–1509, 2001.
38. Pui, C.-H., et al., Recombinant urate oxidase (Rasburicase, Elitek) for prevention and treatment of malignancy-associated hyperuricemia: Updated results of a compassionate use trial, *Blood*, 100, 555a, 2002.
39. Coiffier, B., et al., Efficacy and safety of Rasburicase (recombinant urate oxidase) for the prevention and treatment of hyperuricemia during induction chemotherapy of aggressive non-Hodgkin's lymphoma: Results of the Graal1 (Groupe d'Etude des Lymphomes de l'Adulte Trial on Rasburicase Activity in Adult Lymphoma) Study, *J. Clin. Oncol.*, 21, 4402–4406, 2003.
40. Ribeiro, R.C. and Pui, C.-H., Recombinant urate oxidase for prevention of hyperuricemia and tumor lysis syndrome in lymphoid malignancies, *Clin. Lymphoma*, 3, 225–232, 2003.
41. Pui, C.-H., et al., Recombinant urate oxidase for the prophylaxis or treatment of hyperuricemia in patients with leukaemia or lymphoma, *J. Clin. Oncol.*, 19, 697–704, 2001.
42. Goldman, S.C., et al., A randomized comparison between rasburicase and allopurinol in children with lymphoma or leukaemia at high risk for tumor lysis, *Blood*, 97, 2998–3003, 2001.
43. Pui, C.-H., Rasburicase: A viewpoint, *Paediatric Drugs*, 3, 438, 2001.
44. Pui, C.-H., et al., Urate oxidase in prevention and treatment of hyperuricemia associated with lymphoid malignancies, *Leukemia*, 11, 1813–1816, 1997.
45. Yim, B.T., Sims-McCallum, R.P., and Chong P.H., Rasburicase for the treatment and prevention of hyperuricemia, *Ann. Pharmacother.*, 37, 1047–1054, 2003.
46. Ribeiro, R.C. and Pui, C.-H., Hyperuricemia in patients with cancer, *Am. J. Cancer*, 1, 409–422, 2002.
47. Goldman, S., Rasburicase: A viewpoint, *Paediatric Drugs*, 3, 438–439, 2001.
48. Bayol, A., et al., Stable Freeze-Dried Formulation Comprising a Protein Assay Kit, EP0682944B1 (1999)/U.S. Patent 5,763,409, 1998.
49. Bolivar F., et al., Construction and characterization of new cloning vehicles. II. A multipurpose cloning system, *Gene*, 2, 95–113, 1977.
50. Sutcliffe, J.G., Complete nucleotide sequence of the *Escherichia coli* plasmid pBR322, *Cold Spring Harb. Symp. Quant. Biol.*, 43, 77–90, 1979.
51. Hartley, J.L. and Donelson, J.E., Nucleotide sequence of the yeast plasmid, *Nature*, 286, 860–865, 1980.
52. Kikuchi, Y., Yeast plasmid requires a *cis*-acting locus and two plasmid proteins for its stable maintenance, *Cell*, 35, 487–493, 1983.
53. Broach, J.R. and Volkert, F.C., Circular DNA plasmids of yeasts, in *Molecular and Cellular Biology of the Yeast Saccharomyces*, Vol. 1, J.R. Broach, E.W. Jones, and J.R. Pringle, Eds., CSH Press, Cold Spring Harbor, 1991, pp. 297–331.
54. Beggs J.D., Transformation of yeast by a replicating hybrid plasmid, *Nature*, 275, 104–108, 1978.

9

L-*Asparaginase Review of Pharmacology, Drug Resistance, and Clinical Applications*

Christine Mauz-Körholz, Volker Wahn, and Dieter Körholz

CONTENTS

9.1 Historical Background

In 1953, Kidd [1,2] demonstrated that the growth of mouse lymphoma cells was inhibited by guinea pig serum but not by rabbit or horse serum. During the following years, Broome [3] established that the content of L-asparaginase (L-Asp) in guinea pig serum was responsible for the serum's antineoplastic effects. The high concentration of L-Asp in guinea pig serum was first described by Clementi [4] in 1922. Purification to chemical homogeneity was achieved by Yellin and Wriston [5], which facilitated the large-scale production of the enzyme. The first clinical trial was undertaken by Dolowy et al. [6] in 1966. Today, there are only three preparations with clinical significance: (1) *Escherichia coli*-derived L-Asp; (2) *Erwinia chrysanthemi*-derived L-Asp; and (3) polyethylene glycol (PEG)-modified L-Asp [7].

9.2 Pharmacology of L-Asp

9.2.1 Chemistry

Native asparaginase is purified from different *E. coli* strains [8]. Most isoenzymes have a molecular mass of about 120 kDa. Those with a mass in the region of 240 kDa exhibit a lower specific enzyme activity. L-Asp consists of four identical subunits with one active center. The specific activity ranges between 300 and 400 μM substrate consumption per min per mg of protein or enzyme. In addition to asparaginase activity, all enzyme preparations, even recombinant proteins, contain about 10% L-glutaminase activity [9,10].

Similar to *E. coli*-asparaginase *(E. coli*-Asp), *Erwinia*-asparaginase *(Erwinia*-Asp) has a molecular mass of 138 kDa and a similar specific activity [11]. However, both enzymes differ significantly in their isoelectric point (pH 5.0 for *E. coli*-Asp and pH 8.7 for *Erwinia*-Asp).

Besides unmodified L-Asp preparations, chemically modified forms were introduced in order to reduce the immunogenicity of this enzyme, as this is one of the limiting factors in clinical use. The enzyme has been coupled to PEG [12], dextran [13], or poly-DL-alanyl peptides [14]. However, only PEG-asparaginase (PEG-Asp), formed by the covalent binding of monomethoxypolyethylene glycol to *E. coli*-Asp, has gained clinical usage. Coupling of PEG to asparaginase preserves the active center of the enzyme and reduces the immunogenicity of the protein dramatically [15,16].

9.2.2 Pharmacokinetics

In one study using 2500 U/m^2 PEG-Asp as intramuscular (i.m.) injection, serum levels of PEG-Asp peaked on day 5 after injection with a plasma level of 1 U/mL. Clearance by noncompartment model was 0.169 L/m^2/d. In contrast, native *E. coli*-Asp peaked 4 h after i.m. injection of 6000 U/m^2 with plasma levels of 2 U/mL. The elimination half-life was 1.1 d [17]. Pretreatment asparagine concentrations ranged between 41 ± 4 and 55 ± 5 μM for patients treated with native or PEG-Asp in this cohort. At a plasma concentration of 0.1 U/mL asparagine, asparagine levels decreased below 3 μM. Other reports have suggested that a plasma concentration of 0.03 U/mL asparagine is sufficient to reduce asparagine to below 0.1 μM [18]. However, asparagine levels tend to be lower at the same asparaginase plasma activity when native L-Asp instead of PEG-Asp is used. In addition, colony-stimulating factor (CSF) asparagine levels decreased with increasing plasma concentrations of asparaginase. Earlier studies have shown that an L-Asp plasma activity above 100 U/mL is sufficient to reduce asparagine levels in CSF [19,20].

In contrast to E.coli asparaginase of PEG-asparaginase, the half-life of *Erwinia*-Asp seems to be much shorter. It was reported to be about 6 h [21]. Similar results were also obtained in other studies comparing the three different L-Asp preparations. Asslin [7] showed that half-lives significantly differed between *E. coli*-Asp, *Erwinia*-Asp, and PEG-Asp. In children with newly diagnosed acute lymphoblastic leukemia (ALL), the half-life ranged from 0.65 d (*Erwinia*-Asp) to 1.25 d (*E. coli*-Asp) and 5.73 d (PEG-Asp). Similarly, the number of days with significant asparagine depletion was quite different and was shortest for *Erwinia*-Asp (7 to 15 d), followed by *E. coli*-Asp (14 to 23 d), and PEG-Asp (26 to 34 d).

9.3   Mechanism of Action, Drug Resistance, and *In Vitro* Testing

The depletion of extracellular asparagine levels was first believed to be the major mechanism of cytotoxicity because leukemia cells, but not normal cells, have an asparagine synthetase deficiency. Thus, leukemia cells essentially depend on the supply of L-asparagine. Resistance to asparaginase was explained by two different mechanisms as given below.

9.3.1   Asparagine Synthetase Activity in Leukemic Cells

In patients with ALL clinically resistant to L-Asp, an increased asparagine synthetase activity was noticed [22]. This was also described in some murine lymphoma cell lines [23,24]. Thus, it was supposed that these leukemic cells became independent of asparagine supply and, therefore, resistant to L-Asp treatment.

9.3.2   Formation of Asparaginase-Specific Antibodies and Silent Inactivation

A second mechanism of resistance seemed to be the production of neutralizing antibodies. The clinical significance of the formation of antibodies against L-Asp is still unclear. Some studies have shown that the development of antibodies was associated with increased asparagine levels. However, there is no clear evidence that the development of specific antibodies is truly associated with a decreased event-free survival (EFS) rate. In a trial that included 154 children presenting with ALL, Woo et al. [25] found that in 54 patients, antibodies against asparaginase occurred and that 30 of the 154 patients developed a hypersensitivity reaction during L-Asp infusion. Of the remaining 100 patients with antibodies, 18 developed an allergic reaction. Of the 48 patients with allergic reactions, 36 were subsequently treated with *Erwinia*-Asp. In only 7 out of the 36, allergic reactions against this L-Asp preparation occurred. However, the EFS for patients with antibodies was $83 \pm 6\%$ vs. $76 \pm 5\%$ in patients without antibodies, and $82 \pm 6.5\%$ for patients with allergic reactions, and $78 \pm 5\%$ for patients without reactions against asparaginase. Similar results were also obtained in patients with antibodies against *Erwinia*-Asp. In a case-control study, formation of antibodies to *Erwinia*-Asp did not reveal a significantly worse outcome in those patients [26]. However, the missing effect of antibody-mediated inactivation of L-Asp on clinical outcome might be inferior to the power of the multidrug treatment schedules. A study by Albertsen et al. [21] clearly showed that the formation of high-titered antibodies against *E. coli*-Asp or *Erwinia*-Asp led to decreased serum L-Asp activity, which resulted in increased L-asparagine plasma levels, thereby indicating an inactivation of L-Asp activity.

In patients with hypersensitivity to *E. coli*-Asp, a switch to PEG-Asp has been proposed. However, a recent study by Müller et al. [27] showed that in two thirds of these patients, a prolonged L-Asp plasma activity of >100 U/mL could be obtained, whereas in one third of the patients, a rapid clearance of PEG-Asp activity was seen, although none of these patients developed a hypersensitivity reaction. This phenomenon is called "silent inactivation" of L-Asp. Thus, pharmacological monitoring seems to be advisable in patients who switch from *E. coli*-Asp to PEG-Asp due to a hypersensitivity reaction.

9.3.3   Induction of Apoptosis by L-Asp

During the past few years, induction of apoptosis as a major mechanism of drug-mediated toxicity has been described in several tumor models [28]. The drugs seem to interact with their specific cellular targets, which in the second phase leads to changes in the mitochondrial potential and subsequently to the release of cytochrome *c*. Cytochrome *c* then interacts with Apaf-1 and procaspase-9 to form the apoptosome complex [29–31]. Finally, caspase-9 is activated and initiates the cleavage of the effector caspases-3 and -7. These enzymes cleave a number of regulatory and structural proteins such as poly (ADP-ribose) polymerase (PARP), leading to the morphological feature of apoptosis.

Recently, it has been shown that incubation of leukemic cells obtained from ALL patients with L-Asp leads to caspase-3 activation and inactivation of PARP. Resistance to L-Asp was inversely correlated with caspase-3 activation and PARP inactivation, demonstrating that mutations of the apoptotic system or an imbalance of pro- and antiapopototic factors within the tumor cells might cause resistance to L-Asp [32]. However, it is still unclear how resistance to apoptosis induction is correlated with the intracellular levels of asparagine synthetase. Thus, to date, it is not yet clear if the aforementioned mechanisms of drug inactivation are correlated with the resistance to L-Asp-mediated apoptosis. However, *in vitro* resistance testing to L-Asp by the use of the dimethylthiazol-diphenyltetratzolium bromide (MTT) assay is clearly correlated with the outcome of the patients.

Recently, it has been demonstrated that *in vitro* sensitivity to L-Asp, prednisolone, and vincristine is strongly associated with the outcome of patients with ALL. EFS for patients with a high PVA (prednisone, vincristine, L-Asp) score (7 to 9; i.e., relatively resistant cells) is $69 \pm 7\%$, while it is 84% for patients with a score of 3 or 4 and $83 \pm 4.4\%$ for a score of 5 and 6 [33]. This test system is now being used by the German cooperative ALL (CoALL) study group to stratify high- and low-risk patients with ALL. It might also become suitable to extend the indications for clinical application of L-Asp. Recently, Okada et al. [34] reported on *in vitro* resistance testing of acute myeloblastic leukemia (AML) blasts by using the MTT assay. They could demonstrate that French–American–British (FAB)-type M1 blasts seem to be as sensitive to L-Asp as common-ALL (c-ALL) blasts, while M2, M3, and M7 type blasts were relatively insensitive to L-Asp.

9.4   Clinical Applications

After the large-scale production of L-Asp was established, Clavell et al. [35] published excellent results of patients with ALL who were treated with prednisone, vincristine, methotrexate, doxorubicin, as well as with L-Asp. Today, L-Asp is used in most of the leukemia treatment protocols.

In the 1990s, L-Asp derived from *E. coli* or *Erwinia chrysanthemi* was used in treatment protocols in equal doses and schedules, as if these substances were one and the same drug. Often, *Erwinia*-Asp was used as a substitute for *E. coli*-Asp in patients with hypersensitivity to *E. coli*-Asp. However, there are quite important differences in pharmacology between both preparations. The half-life of *E. coli*-Asp is longer that that of *Erwinia*-Asp, and so is the time of L-Asp depletion as mentioned above. Recently, Duval et al. [36] reported on a randomized trial including 700 children with ALL who received

10000 U/m^2 of *E. coli*- or *Erwinia*-Asp. While coagulation abnormalities were more frequent in patients treated with *E. coli*-Asp (30.2% vs. 11.9%) other toxicities were not significantly different. However, EFS and overall survival (OS) were significantly better in children treated with *E. coli*- than with *Erwinia*-Asp (EFS: 73.4% vs. 59.8%, OS: 83.9% vs. 75.1%), suggesting that preferentially, *E. coli*-Asp should be used in children with ALL.

E. coli-Asp and PEG-Asp have recently been used in a randomized trial including 118 children with standard risk ALL [17]. Patients received either 2 doses of 2500 U/m^2 PEG-Asp or 15 doses of 6000 U/m^2 native *E. coli*-Asp. Treatment with PEG-Asp led to a more rapid clearance of leukemic blasts from the bone marrow. Adverse effects, hospitalization days, and infections were similar in both groups. Although 26% of patients treated with native asparaginase but only 2% of patients treated with PEG-Asp had high-titered antibodies, the outcome of patients in both groups was similar, again demonstrating that antibody formation toward L-Asp probably does not affect the efficacy of leukemia treatment in a multidrug protocol. Pharmacoeconomic studies comparing the costs of native and PEG-Asp found no significant differences when societal costs (transportation, lodging, missed workdays, food, babysitter, etc.) and payer costs (frequency of encounters) were taken into account [37]. Thus, application of PEG-Asp instead of native *E. coli*-Asp in the frontline treatment of ALL has been suggested by these authors.

9.5   Adverse Effects

9.5.1   Hypersensitivity Reactions

Since bacteria-derived proteins appear foreign to the human immune system, it is not surprising that the parenteral administration of such proteins is followed by an immune response, although these patients concomitantly receive a strong immunosuppressive treatment that normally prevents successful immunization with, for example, tetanus antitoxin [38–41].

In our own studies, we could show that patients with a hypersensitivity reaction toward *E. coli*-Asp had significantly elevated IgG and IgM antibody levels toward *E. coli*-Asp. The mechanism of hypersensitivity was related to immune complex formation and subsequent complement activation [42,43].

Besides IgG and IgM, a few patients developed specific IgE antibodies, causing a typical type-I allergic reaction. This mechanism was experimentally confirmed by using the sera of these patients for passive sensitization of basophils of a healthy blood donor. The cells then released histamine upon incubation with L-Asp [44]. These different mechanisms of L-Asp hypersensitivity might explain why patients without detectable IgG and IgM antibodies could experience allergic reactions to asparaginase [45].

In a study by Wang et al. [46], antibody formation was investigated in patients receiving native *E. coli*-Asp, PEG-Asp, and *Erwinia*-Asp. This study showed that antibodies to *E. coli*-Asp exhibited high cross-reactivity to PEG-Asp but not to *Erwinia*-Asp, and vice versa. This might explain why all of the patients with a hypersensitivity reaction during *E. coli*-Asp treatment will not develop a hypersensitivity reaction during subsequent treatment with *Erwinia*-Asp. The role of L-Asp-specific antibody formation during chemotherapy is also described extensively by Wahn [47].

9.5.2   Effects on Blood Coagulation

Both thrombotic as well as hemorrhagic events have been described in patients with L-Asp treatment [47]. Thrombosis might eventually occur in the central venous sinus, but today, thromboses are most likely to be located in close connection with the central lines used in these patients.

L-Asp induces several changes in the coagulation system, including a decrease of anti-coagulatory proteins such as antithrombin III (ATIII) [48–51], plasminogen, or protein C [52–54]. An acquired protein S deficiency is rarely associated with L-Asp treatment [55].

Nowak-Göttl et al. [56] found that the risk of developing thrombosis during treatment with prednisone and L-Asp is significantly elevated in patients with genetic thrombophilic risk factors. However, in contrast to these results of patients treated according to the BFM protocol (where BFM = Berlin/Frankfurt/Münster), we found that thrombotic events are very rare in patients treated according to the CoALL study [57]. In this study, asparaginase is not combined with steroids at an early time of induction treatment. In a subsequent matched-pair analysis between patients of both study groups, we found that the combination of steroids and L-Asp early in the induction treatment might be a potent prothrombotic risk factor, especially in patients with genetic prothrombotic risk factors [58]. Therefore, a randomized trial was initiated to investigate the role of the corticosteroid source in thromboembolism. The results of this study show that the risk of thrombosis was significantly higher if L-Asp was combined with prednisone compared with a combination of L-Asp and dexamethasone [59].

9.5.3   Endocrine Abnormalities

When L-Asp is used in combination with either prednisone or dexamethasone, about 10% of the patients experience a transient inhibition of insulin secretion and subsequent development of a temporary diabetic metabolism requiring insulin supplementation [60]. While this event should not lead to a complete discontinuation of L-Asp treatment, L-Asp should not be further administered in patients presenting with acute pancreatitis during L-Asp treatment. This very rare event is characterized by abdominal pain, vomiting, and elevation of serum amylase and lipase. In some severe cases, pseudocyst development and death have been reported [61]. Interestingly, the incidence of pancreatitis seems to depend on the L-Asp preparation administered. Recently, it was shown that the incidence of pancreatitis is higher after application of PEG-Asp than after native *E. coli*-Asp (18% vs. 1.9%, respectively). Thus, clinicians should be aware of this complication associated with the administration of PEG-Asp [62].

In addition to these changes in pancreatic function, other endocrine organs might be affected by L-Asp. Thyroxine-binding globulin, the major thyroid transport protein, is transiently but markedly decreased during L-Asp treatment [63,64], resulting in decreased T3 and T4 levels [65].

9.5.4   Neurological Abnormalities

Neurological abnormalities such as headache, somnolence, coma, and lethargy are well described in adults being treated with asparaginase, but they are quite rare in children [62,65]. In some patients, these symptoms are related to increased levels of ammonia. However, there are also patients with elevated serum levels of ammonia who do not manifest any neurological symptoms [66].

9.6   Conclusions

Since its use as an antineoplastic agent was discovered, L-Asp plays a fundamental role in ALL treatment. However, asparaginase treatment might be associated with severe and sometimes life-threatening side effects. Owing to its particular pharmacokinetics and low immunogenicity, today, PEG-modified *E. coli* L-Asp has been proposed to be the drug of choice, while *Erwinia*-Asp should not be used routinely because of its documented low efficacy in ALL treatment.

References

1. Kidd, J.G., Regression of transplanted lymphomas induced *in vivo* by means of normal guinea pig serum. I. Course of transplanted cancers of various kinds in mice and rats given guinea pig serum, horse serum or rabbit serum, *J. Exp. Med.*, 97, 565, 1953.
2. Kidd, J.G., Regression of transplanted lymphomas induced *in vivo* by means of normal guinea pig serum. II. Studies on the nature of the active serum constituent: Histological mechanism of the regression: Tests for effects of guinea pig serum on lymphoma cells *in vitro*, *J. Exp. Med.*, 98, 583, 1953.
3. Broome, J.J.D., Evidence that the L-Asparaginase activity of guinea pig serum is responsible for its antilymphoma effects, *Nature*, 191, 1114, 1961.
4. Clementi, A., La désamidation enzymatique de L-asparagine chez les differentes espèces animales et la signification physiologique de sa présence dans l'organisme, *Arch. Int. Physiol.*, 19, 369, 1922.
5. Yellin, T.O. and Wriston, J.C., Jr., Purification and properties of guinea pig serum asparaginase, *Biochemistry*, 5, 1605–1612, 1966.
6. Dolowy, W.C., et al., Toxic and antineoplastic effects of L-asparaginase. Study of mice with lymphoma and normal monkeys and report on a child with leukemia, *Cancer*, 19, 1813–1819, 1966.
7. Asslin, B.L., The three asparaginases. Comparative pharmacology and optimal use in childhood leukemia, *Adv. Exp. Med. Biol.*, 457, 621, 1999.
8. Irion, E. and Arens, A., Biochemical characterization of L-asparaginase from *E. coli*, in *Experimental and Clinical Effects of L-Asparaginases*, Grundmann, E. and Oettgen, H.F., Eds., RRCR, Springer, Heidelberg, 1979, p. 39.
9. Campbell, H.A. and Mashburn, L.T., L-Asparaginase EC-2 from *Escherichia coli*. Some substrate specificity characteristics, *Biochemistry*, 8, 3766–3775, 1969.
10. Swain, A.L., et al., Crystal structure of *Escherichia coli* L-asparaginase, an enzyme used in cancer therapy, *Proc. Natl. Acad. Sci., USA*, 90, 1474–1478, 1993.
11. Müller, H.J. and Boos, J., Use of L-asparaginase in childhood ALL, *Crit. Rev. Oncol. Hematol.*, 28, 97–113, 1998.
12. Abuchowski, A., et al., Treatment of L5178Y tumor-bearing BDF1 mice with a nonimmunogenic L-glutaminase-L-asparaginase, *Cancer Treat. Rep.*, 63, 1127–1132, 1979.
13. Davis, F.F., et al., Reduction of immunogenicity and extension of circulating half-life of peptides and proteins, in *Peptide and Protein Drug Delivery*, Lee, V.H.L., Ed., Marcel Dekker, Inc., New York, 1991, p. 831.
14. Uren, J.R. and Ragin, R.C., Improvement in the therapeutic, immunological and clearance properties of *Escherichia coli* and *Erwinia carotovora* L-asparaginases by attachment of poly-DL-alanyl peptides, *Cancer Res.*, 39, 1927–1933, 1979.
15. Park, Y.K., et al., Pharmacology of *Escherichia coli*-L-asparaginase polyethylene glycol adduct, *Anticancer Res.*, 1, 373–376, 1981.

16. Abuchowski, A., et al., Cancer therapy with chemically modified enzymes. I. Antitumor properties of polyethylene glycol-asparaginase conjugates, *Cancer Biochem. Biophys.*, 7, 175–186, 1984.
17. Avramis, V.I., et al., A randomized comparison of native *Escherichia coli* asparaginase and polyethylene glycol conjugated asparaginase for treatment of children with newly diagnosed standard-risk acute lymphoblastic leukemia: A Children's Cancer Group study, *Blood*, 99, 1986–1994, 2002.
18. Holcenberg, J.S. and Roberts, J., Enzymes as drugs, *Ann. Rev. Pharmacol. Toxicol.*, 17, 97–116, 1977.
19. Riccardi, R., et al., L-asparaginase pharmacokinetics and asparagine levels in cerebrospinal fluid of rhesus monkeys and humans, *Cancer Res.*, 41, 4554–4558, 1981.
20. Boos, J., et al., Monitoring of asparaginase activity and asparagine levels in children on different asparaginase preparations, *Eur. J. Cancer*, 32A, 1544–1550, 1996.
21. Albersten, B.K., et al., Comparison of intramuscular therapy with *Erwinia* asparaginase and asparaginase Medac: Pharmacokinetics, pharmacodynamics, formation of antibodies and influence on the coagulation system, *Br. J. Haematol.*, 115, 983–990, 2001.
22. Haskell, C.M. and Canellos, G.P., L-asparaginase resistance in human leukemia — Asparagine synthetase, *Biochem. Pharmacol.*, 18, 2578–2580, 1969.
23. Kiriyama, Y., et al., Biochemical characterisation of U937 cells resistant to L-asparaginase: The role of asparagine synthetase, *Leukemia*, 3, 294–297, 1989.
24. Hutson, R.G., et al., Amino acid control of asparagine synthetase: Relation to asparaginase resistance in human leukemia cells, *Am. J. Physiol.*, 272, C1691–C1699, 1997.
25. Woo, M.H., et al., Hypersensitivity or development of antibodies to asparaginase does not impact treatment outcome of childhood acute lymphoblastic leukemia, *J. Clin. Oncol.*, 18, 1525–1532, 2000.
26. Klug-Albertsen, B., et al., Anti-*Erwinia* asparaginase antibodies during treatment of childhood acute lymphoblastic leukemia and their relationship to outcome: A case-control study, *Cancer Chemother. Pharmacol.*, 50, 117–120, 2002.
27. Müller, H.J., et al., Pharmacokinetics of native *Escherichia coli* asparginase and hypersensitivity reactions in ALL-BFM 95 reinduction treatment, *Br. J. Haematol.*, 114, 794–799, 2001.
28. Friesen, C., et al., Involvement of the CD95 (APO-1/FAS) receptor/ligand system in drug induced apoptosis in leukemia cells, *Nat. Med.*, 2, 574–577, 1996.
29. Green, D.R. and Reed, J.C., Mitochondria and apoptosis, *Science*, 281, 1309–1312, 1998.
30. Castedo, M., et al., Mitochondria perturbations define lymphocytes undergoing apoptotic depletion *in vivo*, *Eur. J. Immunol.*, 25, 3277–3284, 1995.
31. Li, P., et al., Cytochrome c and dATP-dependent formation of Apaf-1/caspase-9 complex initiates an apoptotic protease cascade, *Cell*, 91, 479–489, 1997.
32. Holleman, A., et al., Resistance to different classes of drugs is associated with impaired apoptosis in childhood acute lymphoblastic leukemia, *Blood*, 102, 4541–4546, 2003.
33. Den Boer, M.L., et al., Patient stratification based on prednisolone–vincristine–asparaginase resistance profiles in children with acute lymphoblastic leukemia, *J. Clin. Oncol.*, 21, 3262–3268, 2003.
34. Okada, S., et al., *In vitro* efficacy of L-asparaginase in childhood acute myeloid leukemia, *Br. J. Haematol.*, 123, 802–809, 2003.
35. Clavell, L.A., et al., Four-agent induction and intensive asparaginase therapy for treatment of childhood acute lymphoblastic leukaemia, *New Engl. J. Med.*, 315, 657–663, 1986.
36. Duval, M., et al., Comparison of *Escherichia coli* asparaginase with *Erwinia* asparaginase in the treatment of childhood lymphoid malignancies: Results of a randomized European Organisation for Research and Treatment of Cancer-Children's Leukemia Group phase 3 trial, *Blood*, 99, 2734–2739, 2002.
37. Kurre, H.A., et al., A pharmacoeconomic analysis of Pegaspargase versus native *Escherichia coli* L-asparaginase for the treatment of children with standard-risk, acute lymphoblastic leukemia: The Children Cancer Group study (CCG-1962), *J. Pediatr. Hematol. Oncol.*, 24, 175–181, 2002.
38. Khan, A. and Hill, J.M., Neutralizing precipitin in the serum of a patient treated with L-asparaginase, *J. Lab. Clin. Med.*, 73, 846–852, 1969.
39. Peterson, R.G., Handschumacher, R.E., and Mitchell, M.S., Immunological responses to L-asparaginase, *J. Clin. Invest.*, 50, 1080–1090, 1971.

40. Maral, R., et al., Studies on the immunosuppressive activity of L-asparaginase, in *Experimental and Clinical Effects of L-Asparaginase* Grundmann, E.E. and Oettgen, H.F., Eds., Springer, Berlin, 1970, p. 160.
41. Dellinger, C.T. and Miale T.D., Compariason of anaphylactic reaction to asparaginase derived from *Escherichia coli* and *Erwinia* cultures, *Cancer,* 38, 1843–1846, 1976.
42. Elhag, K.M., Bettelheim, K.A., and Huber, T.J., Antibodies to bacterial L-asparaginases, *New Zealand Med. J.,* 86, 280–281, 1977.
43. Fabry, U., et al., Anaphylaxis to L-asparaginase during treatment of acute lymphoblastic leukemia in children — Evidence of a complement-mediated mechanism, *Pediatr. Res.,* 19, 400–408, 1985.
44. Körholz, D., et al., Bildung spezifischer IgG-Antikörper unter L-Asparaginasebehandlung, *Mschr. Kinderheilkd.,* 135, 325–328, 1987.
45. Körholz, D., et al., Allergische Reaktionen unter der Behandlung mit L-Asparaginase — Bedeutung spezifischer IgE-Antikörper, *Mschr. Kinderheilkd.,* 138, 23–25, 1990.
46. Wang, B., et al., Evaluaton of immunologic cross-reaction of antiasparaginase antibodies in acute lymphoblastic leukemia and lymphoma patients, *Leukemia,* 17, 1583–1588, 2003.
47. Wahn, V., L-Asparaginase: An essential antineoplastic drug, in *Pharmaceutical Enzymes* (Hrsg. Lauwers/Scharpé), Marcel Dekker, Inc., New York, 1997, pp. S223–S260.
48. Gugliotta, L., et al., Incidence of thrombotic complications in adult patients with acute lymphoblastic leukemia receiving L-asparaginase during induction therapy: A retrospective study, The GIMEMA group, *Eur. J. Hematol.,* 49, 63–66, 1992.
49. Anderson, N., Lokich, J.J., and Tullis, J.L., L-Asparaginase effect on antithrombin-III levels, *Med. Pediatr. Oncol.,* 7, 335–340, 1979.
50. Priest, J.R., et al., The effect of L-asparaginase on antithrombin, plasminogen and plasma coagulation during therapy for acute lymphoblastic leukemia, *J. Pediatr.,* 100, 990–995, 1982.
51. Homans, A.C., et al., Effect of L-asparaginase administration on coagulation and platelet function in children with leukaemia, *J. Clin. Oncol.,* 5, 811–817, 1987.
52. Gugliotta, L., et al., Hypercoagulability during L-asparaginase treatment: The effect of antithrombin III supplementation *in vivo, Br. J. Haematol.,* 74, 465–470, 1990.
53. Barbui, T., et al., L-asparaginase lowers protein C antigen, *Thromb. Haemostas.,* 52, 216, 1984.
54. Vigano D' Angelo, L., et al., L-asparaginase treatment reduces the anticoagulant potential of the protein C system without affecting vitamin K-dependent carboxylation, *Thromb. Res.,* 59, 985–994, 1990.
55. Lee, J.H., Kim, S.W., and Kim, J.S., Sagittal sinus thrombosis associated with transient free protein S deficiency after L-asparaginase treatment: Case report and review of the literature, *Clin. Neurol. Neurosurg.,* 102, 33–36, 2000.
56. Nowak-Göttl, U., et al., Prospective evaluation of the thrombotic risk in children with acute lymphoblastic leukemia carrying the MTHFR TT 677 genotype, the prothrombin G20210A variant and further prothrombotic risk factors, *Blood,* 93, 1595–1599, 1999.
57. Mauz-Körholz, C., et al., Low rate of severe venous thromboses in children with ALL treatment according to the CoALL-92 and -97 protocol, *Klin. Pädiatr.,* 211, 215–217, 1999.
58. Mauz-Körholz, C., et al., Prothrombotic risk factors in children with acute lymphoblastic leukemia treated with delayed *E. coli* asparaginase (CoALL-92 and –97 protocols), *Thromb. Haemostas.,* 83, 840–843, 2000.
59. Nowak-Göttl, U., et al., Thromboembolic events in children with acute lymphoblastic leukemia (BFM protocols): Prednisone versus dexamethasone administration, *Blood,* 101, 2529–2533, 2003.
60. Pui, C.H., et al., Risk factors for hyperglycemia in children with leukemia receiving L-asparaginase and prednisone, *J. Pediatr.,* 99, 46–50, 1981.
61. Alvarez, O.A. and Zimmerman, G., Pegaspargase-induced pancreatitis, *Med. Pediatr. Oncol.,* 34, 200–205, 2000.
62. McLean, R., Martin, S., and Lam-Po-Tang, P.R., Fatal case of L-asparaginase induced pancreatitis, *Lancet,* 2, 1401–1402, 1982.
63. Garnick, M.B. and Larsen, P.R., Acute deficiency of thyroxine-binding globulin during L-asparaginase therapy, *New Engl. J. Med.,* 301, 252–253, 1979.

64. Heidemann, P.H., Stubbe, P., and Beck, W., Transient secondary hypothyroidism and thyroxine-binding globulin deficiency in leukemic children receiving polychemotherapy: An effect of L-asparaginase, *Eur. J. Pediatr.*, 136, 291–295, 1981.

65. Ferster, A., et al., Thyroid function during L-asparaginase therapy in children with acute lymphoblastic leukemia: Difference between induction and late intensification, *Am. J. Pediatr. Hematol. Oncol.*, 14, 192–196, 1992.

66. Graham, M.L., Pegaspargase: A review of clinical studies, *Adv. Drug Deliv. Rev.*, 55, 1293–1302, 2003.

10

Recombinant Factor VIIa

Elisabeth Erhardtsen, Nikolai Brun, Niels Kristian Klausen, Egon Persson, and Per Rexen

CONTENTS

10.1   Introduction

Recombinant activated coagulation factor VII (rFVIIa) has been cloned and expressed in mammalian cells and analyses have shown that the amino sequence of rFVIIa is identical to plasma-derived activated factor VII. The manufacture of rFVIIa does not involve any ingredients of human origin. rFVIIa has been approved worldwide under the trade name NovoSeven® for the treatment of bleeding in hemophilia patients with inhibitors (antibodies) against factor VIII or IX. Owing to its unique mechanism of action, rFVIIa is now under consideration for indications in clinical situations with critical bleeding outside the hemophilia setting, generating a hypothesis that rFVIIa could be a universal hemostatic agent.

10.2   Characteristics of the Enzyme

10.2.1   Mechanism of Action of rFVIIa

Coagulation factor VII (FVII) circulates in the blood: ~1% in the active form (FVIIa) and the remainder as proenzyme or zymogen [1,2]. In contrast, its membrane-bound cofactor, tissue factor (TF), is normally hidden in cell layers of the subendothelium. Blood coagulation is initiated upon vascular injury and the concomitant exposure of TF to blood by the ensuing formation of FVIIa·TF complexes [3] (Figure 10.1A). TF serves as a high-affinity

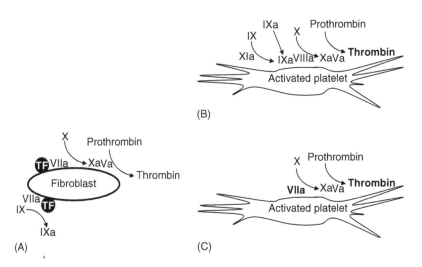

FIGURE 10.1
The normal and pharmacological roles of FVIIa in blood coagulation. (A) Endogenous FVIIa forms a complex with exposed TF on the surface of, for instance, a fibroblast and initiates blood clotting. The resulting small amount of thrombin primes the coagulation system by activating platelets and factors V, VIII, and XI (not shown for simplicity). (B) In the complete hemostatic system, FIXa, generated by either FVIIa·TF or FXIa, forms the Xase complex with FVIIIa on the activated platelet surface. This complex activates FX very efficiently. The resulting FXa forms the prothrombinase complex with FVa, which catalyzes rapid activation of prothrombin leading to a thrombin burst. (C) In hemophilia, Xase is not operational due to the lack of FVIII or FIX. At concentrations far above physiological levels, FVIIa is able to bypass the need for the natural Xase complex and can ameliorate the hemophilic phenotype by generating amounts of FXa sufficient for clinical efficacy.

receptor and allosteric up-regulator of FVIIa, rendering FVIIa biologically active [4,5]. The procoagulant substrates for FVIIa are factors IX (FIX) and X (FX), which are activated in relatively small amounts by FVIIa bound to TF. The activated FX (FXa) in turn generates thrombin to prime the hemostatic system by its local activation of platelets and factors V, VIII, and XI. The activated FIX (FIXa) can move from the TF-bearing cell over to the surface of an activated platelet, where more FIXa is generated by FXIa (Figure 10.1B). The surface of the locally activated platelets then serves as the stage for the propagation phase of the blood coagulation cascade, involving the Xase (FIXa·FVIIIa) and prothrombinase (FXa·FVa) complexes, which results in a burst of thrombin required to catalyze the generation of a fibrin clot.

Under hemophilic conditions, the Xase complex is not operational because either the cofactor FVIIIa (hemophilia A) or the enzyme FIXa (hemophilia B) is missing or neutralized. Consequently, the propagation phase is virtually annihilated. According to one model, pharmacological doses of rFVIIa can overcome this defect by directly and TF-independently activating FX on (FVIIa binds with relatively low affinity to the platelet surface) or in the vicinity of the platelet in sufficient amounts to generate a clinically beneficial amount of thrombin [6–8] (Figure 10.1C). Moreover, it appears that the thrombin formed does not only lead to a fibrin clot but that it also down-regulates fibrinolysis via activation of the thrombin-activatable fibrinolysis inhibitor (TAFI) [9]. Thus, the procoagulant and antifibrinolytic effects of high-dose rFVIIa promote both clot formation and clot stability in the absence of a functional Xase complex. An alternative view of the mechanism of action is that pharmacological doses of rFVIIa, by out-competing endogenous zymogen FVII, assures that TF is saturated with preactivated FVIIa molecules [10]. However, this mechanism could not be confirmed in a system containing cell-associated TF [11]. In addition, recent results show that rFVIIa variants with a selective enhancement of the TF-independent activity have improved potency in a hemophilia setting, suggesting that the TF-dependent component is relatively less important [12,13]. Regardless of the precise nature of the mechanism that best describes the mode of action of rFVIIa, the low affinity of FVIIa for the platelet surface, the low intrinsic (without TF) ability of FVIIa to activate FX, and the need to compete with 10 nM FVII for TF all provide a rationale for the requirement of relatively high therapeutic doses of rFVIIa (>90 μg/kg, which is the currently labeled dose in hemophilia).

10.2.2 Three-Dimensional Structure of FVIIa and its Relation to Function

The architecture of FVIIa is based on domain building blocks. The four domains are (from N- to C terminus, i.e., from the membrane surface) a γ-carboxyglutamic acid (Gla)-rich domain, two epidermal growth factor (EGF)-like domains, and a serine protease domain (Figure 10.2).

The structure of full-length FVIIa has only been determined in complex with TF [14], but the structure of free Gla-domainless FVIIa [15] is very similar to the corresponding portion of TF-bound FVIIa, which is presumably true also for the Gla domain. Bound calcium ions (nine in total) are a physiological and important part of FVIIa, pivotal for TF and membrane binding. The Gla domain binds seven calcium ions and mediates binding to negatively charged phospholipid membranes such as the surface of the activated platelet [7,16]. The first EGF-like domain contains one Ca^{2+}-binding site and contributes most to the affinity for TF [14,17]. The protease domain binds one calcium ion of importance for the enzymatic activity and contains the active site and recognition determinants for FIX and FX. The extensive interface between FVIIa and TF, involving all four domains in FVIIa, explains the tight binding between the two proteins. The high affinity of the interaction is presumably crucial for rapid triggering of the blood coagulation cascade.

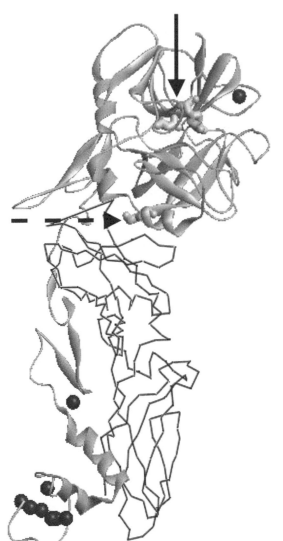

FIGURE 10.2

The structure of the FVIIa·TF complex [14]. The backbone traces of FVIIa and TF are shown as gray ribbon and a black wire, respectively. The nine calcium ions bound to FVIIa are shown as spheres. The Gla and EGF-like domains of FVIIa form a stalk along TF and the protease domain rests on top of TF. The catalytic triad and residue M306 in FVIIa are shown in ball-and-stick representation (marked with a solid arrow and a dotted arrow, respectively, for clarity).

In the complex with membrane-bound TF, FVIIa generates FXa (and FIXa) at a dramatically higher rate than it does in the free form [18]. As the same peptide bond in FX is to be cleaved during activation, free and TF-bound FVIIa presumably position themselves identically relative to FX, but the presence of TF helps to bring enzyme and substrate together. More importantly, TF association also stimulates the enzymatic activity of FVIIa. The mechanism behind the TF-induced increase in activity remains elusive. The differences between free and TF-bound FVIIa are very subtle, both when their available crystal structures [14,15] are compared and when the structural changes induced by TF are monitored spectroscopically [19]. Thus, no conspicuous structural rearrangements appear to occur. Recent work has identified residue M306 in FVIIa as a key mediator of the TF-induced allosteric effect [17,20]. However, the precise route of the allosteric signal from the TF-interactive surface to the active site and the conformational switches are unknown. But it is justifiable to state that interactions between the protease domain of FVIIa and TF unleash the full enzymatic potential, and that the three other domains tether FVIIa to its cofactor and to the membrane surface. In the free form not bound to TF, the form in which we assume that the therapeutic rFVIIa molecule exerts its function, FVIIa has low biological activity and poor membrane affinity. Therefore, high doses of rFVIIa are needed for it to be efficacious in the treatment of bleeding episodes.

10.2.3 Primary Structure of rFVIIa

By activation, the single-chain rFVII is converted to the two-chain form (rFVIIa), consisting of light and heavy chains linked by a disulfide bridge (Figure 10.3). The structural characterization of rFVIIa includes determination of the amino acid sequence as well as determination of the posttranslational modifications. These are γ-carboxylation of glutamic acid in the N-terminal Gla domain, N-linked glycosylation of N145 and N322, and O-linked glycosylation of S52 and S60.

10.2.3.1 Amino Acid Sequence

The amino acid sequence of rFVIIa has been determined by sequence analysis and compared to the sequence of human plasma-derived (pd) FVIIa [21]. After reduction and

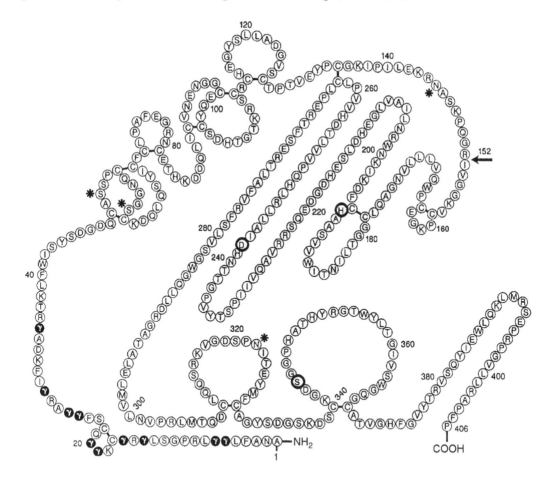

FIGURE 10.3
Human coagulation factor VII (FVIIa). FVIIa is a serine protease of 406 residues. The active two-chain enzyme is generated by specific cleavage after R152 . Posttranslational modifications of the FVII molecule include: (i) γ-carboxylation of ten glutamic acid residues in the N-terminal part of the molecule; (ii) N-glycosylation of asparagine residues in positions 145 and 322; and (iii) O-glycosylation of S52 and S60. γ: γ-carboxyglutamic acid; *: glycosylation sites; →: activation site; O: catalytic site residues.

alkylation of the disulfide bridges, the light and heavy chains were separated. Each of the two chains was subjected to peptide mapping by tryptic digestion and reverse-phase high performance liquid chromatography (HPLC), and the peptide fragments were characterized by N-terminal sequence analysis. The amino acid sequence determined for rFVIIa (Figure 10.3) was identical to the amino acid sequence of pdFVIIa, and in accordance with the sequence deduced from complementary deoxyribonucleic acid (cDNA) [22].

10.2.3.2 γ-Carboxylation

The N-terminal Gla domain of human FVII (Figure 10.3) contains ten glutamic acid residues that can potentially be posttranslationally γ-carboxylated. It has been shown that pdFVIIa is fully γ-carboxylated in all ten possible Gla positions [21]. For rFVIIa, the nine first possible Gla positions are fully γ-carboxylated, while the tenth Gla position (E35) is partially γ-carboxylated. Carboxylation of glutamic acid in position 35 has no effect on the biological activity of rFVIIa [23].

10.2.3.3 O-Linked Glycosylation

The first EGF-like domain of human FVII (Figure 10.3) contains two serine residues that carry O-linked glycosylation [21,24,25]; both O-linked glycosylation sites are fully occupied in rFVIIa. For rFVIIa, three different glycan structures consisting of glucose, glucose–xylose, or glucose–$(xylose)_2$ are found at S52 (Figure 10.4), while a single fucose is found at S60 (Figure 10.4).

The same O-linked carbohydrate structures are found in pdFVIIa with slightly different relative amounts of the three structures linked to S52 [24]. In a study of the functional role of the O-linked glycosylation of FVIIa by use of site-specific mutants, it was suggested that the O-linked glycosylations could provide structural elements that were of importance for the association of FVIIa with the circulating TF pathway inhibitor [26].

10.2.3.4 N-Linked Glycosylation

Human FVIIa contains two potential N-linked glycosylation sites at N145 in the light chain and at N322 in the heavy chain (Figure 10.2), and both sites are found to be fully occupied in rFVIIa. Based on the determination of the carbohydrate composition of pdF-VIIa and rFVIIa, the N-linked glycosylation of the two FVIIa forms is similar, the most pronounced difference being a higher fucose content and a lower sialic acid content of

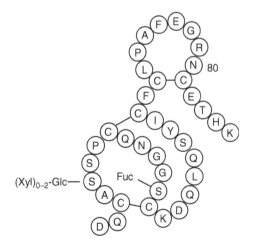

FIGURE 10.4

O-glycosylation. Carbohydrate structures O-linked to S52 and S60 in recombinant factor VII and in plasma factor VII. Glc: glucose; Xyl: xylose; Fuc: fucose.

rFVIIa compared with pdFVIIa [21]. For rFVIIa, the N-linked carbohydrate structures have been structurally characterized [27–29]. A total of 15 carbohydrate structures were found, with the major structures being complex biantennary structures with differences in the number of terminal sialic acid residues (Figure 10.5) [28].

Some of the carbohydrate structures have an *N*-acetylgalactosamine residue at the position where usually a galactose is found. In general, the same carbohydrates were found at both N-glycosylation sites of rFVIIa. However, significant differences were found between the two sites in the relative amounts of the carbohydrate structures, for example the number of structures with *N*-acetylgalactosamine was higher at N322 (30%) than at N145 (7%) [28]. Several of the analytical methods used for the carbohydrate characterization have properties in terms of sensitivity and robustness, making them suitable for routine analysis [27,28]. These methods have been used to document reproducible glycosylation of rFVIIa from batch to batch.

10.3 Manufacturing Process

rFVII is produced in a baby hamster kidney (BHK) cell line, which was genetically modified by transfection with a plasmid construct containing the human gene for FVII as well as promoter and enhancer regions necessary for transcription. The cDNA for the coding region of human FVII was isolated from a liver gene library and characterized as described previously [22]. For details on transfection of BHK cells with human FVII cDNA, see Berkner, et al. [30].

The transfected cells were cloned and a superior clone selected. This clone was used as a progenitor for establishment of the production cell banks. The cell bank system is two tiered with a master cell bank from which working cell banks can be produced. The cell banks are stored in the vapor phase of liquid nitrogen to ensure stability of the cells during

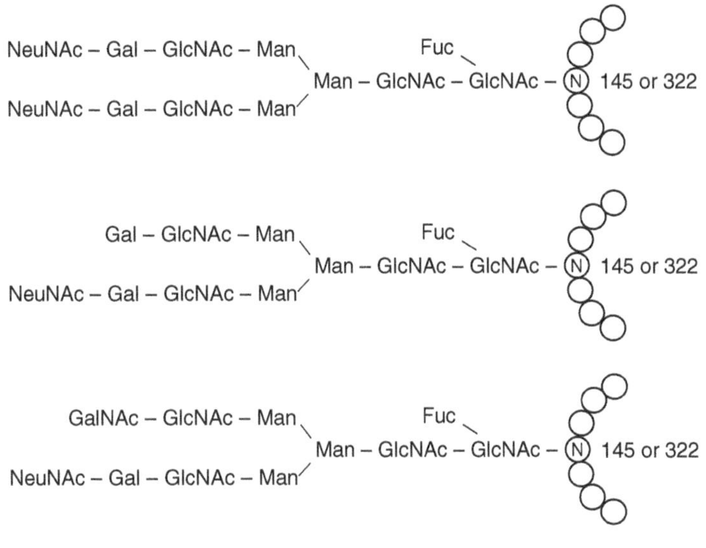

FIGURE 10.5
N-glycosylation. The three major carbohydrate structures N-linked to N145 and N322 in recombinant factor VII. Fuc: fucose; GlcNAc: *N*-acetylglucosamine; Man: mannose; Gal: galactose; GalNAc: *N*-acetylgalactosamine; NeuNAc: *N*-acetylneuraminic acid (sialic acid).

long-term storage. The cell banks are thoroughly tested to ensure the presence of a correct gene construct, sterility, and the absence of mycoplasma and viruses. The cells are capable of stable expression of FVII for several weeks of cultivation and are thus suitable for large-scale production.

Each working cell bank is created from a single vial of the master cell bank, and each rFVIIa production run is initiated by thawing of one working cell bank vial. This ensures that the number of cell generations that has elapsed before each step in the process (e.g., inoculation, harvest, termination) is kept constant for different production runs.

The cells are cultivated in a high cell density bioreactor using microcarriers for cell attachment. After a series of propagation steps (Figure 10.6), the culture medium derived from the BHK cells containing secreted single-chain rFVII is collected by a draw-and-fill process and clarified by centrifugation and filtration before purification. The manufacture of rFVII does not involve any ingredients of human origin.

10.3.1 Activation of Factor VII to Factor VIIa

Activation of FVII to FVIIa involves the specific hydrolysis of a single peptide bond between R152 and I153 (Figure 10.3). This activation is probably carried out *in vivo* predominantly by

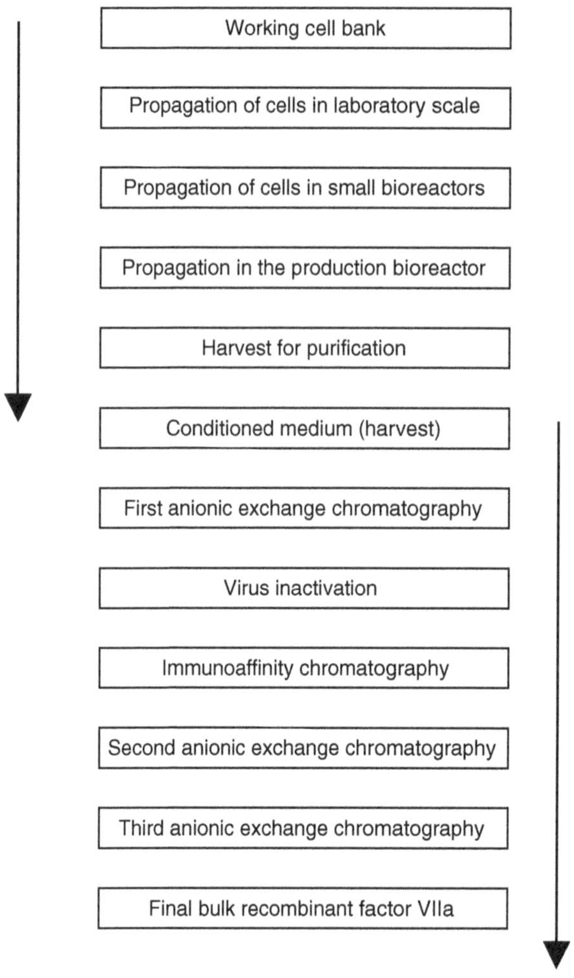

FIGURE 10.6
Flow diagram of the manufacturing process of recombinant factor VIIa.

membrane-bound FXa [31]. In the rFVIIa production process, rFVII (single chain) is converted into rFVIIa (two chain) during the purification process by autocleavage. Sequence analysis has shown that the two-chain form is identical to pdFVIIa. The purification process is optimized so that rFVII is converted into rFVIIa with almost 100% yield [21,32]. The degree of activation seems to depend on the amount of rFVII loaded per volume of ion-exchange material. Single-chain rFVII has no proteolytic activity by itself [33], but trace amounts of rFVIIa could be generated by cellular proteases or proteases released to the medium, and this rFVIIa could initiate the autoactivation process when rFVII and rFVIIa are concentrated on the ion-exchange columns.

10.3.2 Purification

The purification method for rFVII from the cell culture medium has to ensure the removal of non-rFVII proteins and the specific activation of rFVII to rFVIIa as noted above. The following purification procedure (Figure 10.6) was developed to meet these criteria: (1) Culture medium is pH-adjusted and loaded onto a Q-Sepharose FF® column. This step mainly functions to concentrate the protein. (2) Virus inactivation is ensured by treatment with a detergent. (3) rFVII is then loaded on an immunoaffinity column. This step purifies rFVII very efficiently since both the binding of rFVII to the column and the elution of rFVII from the column is specific for the rFVII protein. (4) The final purification and the complete activation of rFVII to rFVIIa are carried out by the use of two anion-exchange chromatography steps. The purification process has been validated with respect to removal of process-related impurities (host cell proteins, host cell DNA, and medium components) as well as inactivation and removal of viruses.

Critical parameters such as residence times, flow, and temperature are controlled within strict limits throughout the manufacturing process. This ensures optimal conditions both for the cell culture and for the product during purification, resulting in consistent high yields and product quality. At critical process steps, important process features are monitored to document that the process is on track. During the fermentation process, the growth and viability of the cells are followed as well as their productivity. At the end of production, the absence of adventitious agents such as bacteria and viruses is documented by vigorous testing of the end of production cells. The efficiency of the purification process is monitored by following the reduction of marker proteins, the degree of activation, and the product yield over each purification step.

The purified and activated rFVIIa bulk drug substance is formulated into a solution of the composition given in Table 10.1. This solution is dispensed into vials and freeze-dried. The final drug product, NovoSeven®, exists in three presentations containing 1.2, 2.4, and 4.8 mg of rFVIIa, respectively.

TABLE 10.1

Final Formulation of Product before Filling and Freeze-drying

	Concentration (mg/mL)
rFVIIa	0.6
NaCl (50 mM)	2.92
Calcium dichloride dihydrate (10 mM)	1.47
Glycylglycine (10 mM)	1.32
Tween 80	0.07
Mannitol	30

10.4   Indications for which Factor VIIa is Approved

rFVIIa was developed for treatment of bleeding in hemophilia patients with inhibitors
(antibodies) against factor VIII or IX. rFVIIa is now approved in 70 countries worldwide.
In the United States, rFVIIa has been approved for the treatment of bleeding episodes in
hemophilia A or B patients with inhibitors to factors VIII or IX. It should be administered
to patients only under the supervision of a physician experienced in the treatment of
hemophilia. This may take place in the home of the patient if needed. In the European
Union, rFVIIa has been approved for bleeding episodes and surgery in patients with
inherited or acquired hemophilia with inhibitors to coagulation factors VIII or IX >10
Bethesda Units (BU), or in patients with antibody titer <10 BU, who are expected to have
a high anamnestic response to factor VIII or IX. Furthermore, home treatment of mild to
moderate bleeding episodes up to 24 h has been approved. In January 2004, the European
Commission approved rFVIIa for the control of bleeding in patients with factor VII deficiency and Glanzmann's thrombasthenia refractory to platelet transfusions (see Sections
10.5.2.3 and 10.5.2.4).

10.5   Developmental History of the Enzyme

10.5.1   Preclinical Development

The hemostatic effect of rFVIIa has been verified in hemophilic dogs and in warfarin-
induced bleeding in rats. rFVIIa (dose range 50 to 220 µg/kg body weight [b.w.]) was able
to correct the cuticle bleeding time in dogs with hemophilia A or B [33,34]. In cases of
warfarin-induced bleeding in rats, the bleeding from the tail cuts was partially normalized
by 50 µg/kg b.w. rFVIIa and fully normalized by 250 µg b.w. rFVIIa [35].

The theoretical lack of systemic activation after rFVIIa treatment has been supported by
preclinical data. Studies in the standard rabbit stasis model, developed as a thrombosis
model in which injury was induced to the vessel wall, have demonstrated that rFVIIa (100
to 1000 µg/kg b.w.) or prothrombin complex concentrate (factor VIII inhibitor bypass
activity [FEIBA]; 50 to 100 U/kg; Immuno, Deerfield, IL) caused clot formation at the site
of injury after 30 min of stasis (restricted blood flow). This reflects the normal pharmacological response to tissue injury. rFVIIa caused no change in platelet count or fibrinogen
concentration even 3 h after administration. Furthermore, no changes were noted in antithrombin levels, nor was there any evidence of generation of soluble fibrin monomers, as
judged by an ethanol gelation test. In contrast, FEIBA caused a significant dose-dependent
decrease in platelets and fibrinogen, suggesting a general activation of the coagulation system. Administration of 100 to 300 µg/kg rFVIIa to rabbits previously exposed to endotoxin
did not result in any significant hematological changes (decreased leukocyte count, platelet
count, or fibrin monomers) compared with rabbits treated with endotoxin alone [36].

Four controlled animal studies examining the effects of rFVIIa after grade IV/V liver
injuries in pigs have been published [37–40]. Generally, the use of rFVIIa in the different
pig studies resulted in measurable changes in the coagulation systems as depicted by the
reduction of prothrombin time (PT) and increased FVII:C activity. Decreased blood loss as
well as increased mean arterial pressure in rFVIIa-treated pigs vs. control groups was
observed. Further, a trend toward decreased mortality and increased time from injury to

death with early use of rFVIIa was noted [38]. None of the studies on pigs demonstrated any evidence of increased thrombotic complications even though high doses of up to 720 µg/kg rFVIIa were administered.

10.5.2   Clinical Development

10.5.2.1   *Pharmacokinetics in Patients*

Pharmacokinetic profiles have been studied in adult and pediatric hemophilia patients, as well as in adults with acquired FVII deficiency (i.e., healthy adult volunteers pretreated with acenocoumarol and patients with liver cirrhosis) [41–45]. The clearance and half-life values (range: 2.4 to 3.2 h) after bolus administration of rFVIIa were in the same range in the adult populations studied. However, pediatric patients with hemophilia have been reported to have a shorter half-life (1.3 h) and higher clearance values than the adults with hemophilia [42,44]. A clinical trial to evaluate this possible difference in half-life and clearance between adults and pediatric patients with hemophilia is in progress.

10.5.2.2   *Hemophilia Patients with Inhibitors*

Therapeutic efficacy and safety of rFVIIa in hemophilia patients with inhibitors have been investigated since 1988 in a number of clinical trials, including the Compassionate Use Study [46–49], the Emergency Use Study [50], the Home Treatment Study [51], and the Surgery Study [52]. The purpose of the Compassionate Use and Emergency programs was to treat patients with life- or limb-threatening bleeds in cases where all other therapeutic alternatives had been exhausted. The multicenter Home Treatment Study [51] documented and emphasized the benefits of early initiation of therapy with rFVIIa, and the Surgery Study [52], a randomized, double-blind, multicenter, dose-finding study, included hemophilia patients with inhibitors who had been scheduled for elective minor or major surgery. All studies showed that treatment with rFVIIa is effective in 80 to 90% of cases and safe in the dose range of 35 to 120 µg/kg, with a recommended dose of 90 µg/kg. The dose should be given as an intravenous bolus dose and repeated after 2 h; when more than two doses are necessary to ensure and maintain hemostasis for minor or moderate bleeds, the dose interval may be prolonged from 2 to 6 h, depending on the size and severity of the bleed. In surgery and treatment of major life- or limb-threatening bleeds, rFVIIa should be given every 2 h for the first 24 h, after which the dose interval may be increased over the next 3 d from 2 to 6 h, depending on the type of surgery performed [53,54].

rFVIIa efficacy is neither influenced by the level of the inhibitor to FVIII or FIX, nor does rFVIIa evoke an anamnestic response in FVIII- or FIX-deficient patients [55]. Therefore, rFVIIa is a suitable treatment for acute bleeding episodes or control of hemostasis during surgery in hemophilia patients with inhibitors, and prior to or during initiation of immune tolerance therapy [56–58].

10.5.2.3   *Glanzmann's Thrombasthenia*

Patients with Glanzmann's thrombasthenia suffer from an abnormality in the glycoprotein (GP) GPIIb/IIIa complex, which results in a failure of the platelet aggregation at the site of injury. An International Registry on rFVIIa and congenital platelet disorders has been initiated [59] in which 11 surgical procedures and 55 bleeding episodes have been reported so far in 28 patients with Glanzmann's thrombasthenia. Data indicate that 9 out of 11 surgical procedures and 37 out of 55 bleeding episodes were treated successfully with rFVIIa.

10.5.2.4 FVII Deficiency

FVII deficiency is a rare coagulation disorder causing spontaneous bleeding in severely affected patients and bleeding after surgery and trauma in mildly affected patients. rFVIIa has been used successfully in FVII-deficient patients during surgery [60,61], in intracerebral bleeding [62], as well as in association with delivery [63–65]. In the open study of Mariani et al. [66], 17 FVII-deficient patients were reportedly treated with rFVIIa with doses ranging from 8.08 to 70.5 µg/kg. The doses were calculated from the dose capable of normalizing PT 15 min after injection; the median dose to normalize the mean PT ratio was 26 µg/kg and that for normalizing the PT (expressed in sec) was 22 µg/kg. Excellent results of all hemarthrosis treated were reported. More than one dose was required in major surgery (four synovectomies, one colonectomy, one craniotomy and one inguinal herniotomy), and for nine of the minor surgeries, more than one dose was necessary to stop bleeding or prevent rebleeding. The outcome was effective in all but one patient, a 2-week-old infant who was accidentally treated for intracranial bleeding with a dose of 800 µg/kg. The infant developed antibodies to FVII, which most likely was the reason for the lack of effect. One more patient with congenital FVII deficiency developed a low-titer transient antibody. As both these patients had been given plasma FVII as well, it has not been possible to define a relationship to rFVIIa [67]. No other reports of antibody generation in relation to rFVIIa administration have been published. No thrombotic events were reported even though in several cases, rFVIIa was used repeatedly and in association with tranexamic acid.

10.5.2.5 Clinical Safety

Since the first approval of rFVIIa in 1996, and until April 15, 2004, approximately 550,000 standard dosages have been administered (one standard dose = one 70-kg patient administered a dose of 90 µg/kg). During this period, 14 spontaneous thromboembolic adverse events were reported in patients with inherited hemophilia A or B. There was no evidence of a dose relationship, and an alternative etiology for thrombosis was identified in the majority of cases. Accordingly, rFVIIa is considered to have a good safety profile in its labeled indication in hemophilia A or B patients with inhibitors, making it possible to proceed with further clinical development in other indications.

10.5.3 Development of rFVIIa as a Universal Hemostatic Agent

Based on the mechanism of action of rFVIIa's generation of thrombin at the site of injury without any systemic effect, a hypothesis has been generated that rFVIIa could be a universal hemostatic agent with the potential to also stop bleeding in patients with otherwise intact hemostatic systems. The hypothesis has been supported by numerous case stories reporting the positive effect of rFVIIa in different bleeding situations such as surgery [68–71], life-threatening bleedings in trauma [72–75], or spontaneous intracranial bleedings [46,62,76]. This has prompted Novo Nordisk to start a number of trials for different indications [77].

10.5.3.1 Results from Finalized Trials Outside the Current Indication

10.5.3.1.1 Patients with Liver Disease

The liver is the principal site of synthesis and clearance of coagulation factors, components of the fibrinolytic system, and anticoagulants. The most frequently encountered hematological abnormalities in patients with liver disease include prolonged PT and hyperfibrinolysis [78,79]. The progressive loss of liver parenchymal cells associated with cirrhosis results in a decreased synthesis of the vitamin K-dependent coagulation factors (FII, FVII [most pronounced], FIX, FX), fibrinogen, and proteins C and S. When bleeding occurs, all these changes may contribute to an impaired coagulation process and thus impaired thrombin generation, and the formation of a less stable fibrin plug that is more easily dissolved by fibrinolytic enzymes.

During major surgical procedures in patients with liver disease, such as orthotopic liver transplantation, bleeding can be an important problem, and excess blood loss is associated with increased morbidity, mortality, and length of stay in the intensive-care unit [80].

A randomized, double-blind, placebo-controlled dose exploratory trial has been carried out in cirrhotic patients undergoing orthotopic liver transplantation to evaluate the hemostatic efficacy of two dose regimens of rFVIIa. One hundred and eighty-three patients were randomized to receive an initial bolus of 60 or 120 µg/kg b.w. rFVIIa or placebo. The product was administered within 10 min prior to first skin cut and repeated every 2 h until 30 min prior to expected start of reperfusion of the transplanted liver. An additional single dose was administered at completion of surgery. Results of this trial (rFVIIa group vs. placebo) indicate that significantly more patients avoided transfusion in the rFVIIa group, significantly less transfusion was seen in patients with normal red blood cell (RBC) levels, and that a similar level of serious adverse events was found in the two groups.

Variceal bleeding is a medical emergency that has a 6-week mortality in the range of 5 to 50%, depending on the severity of the underlying liver disease, mainly because of the high rate of failure to control bleeding during the first days after the initial onset of bleeding [81]. The treatment modalities available for the patient with advanced cirrhosis and active variceal bleeding remains unsatisfactory in terms of a safe and fast correction of the coagulopathy, guarantee of bleeding control, prevention of early rebleeding, and preventing death.

A randomized, double-blind, placebo-controlled trial has been carried out in cirrhotic patients with upper gastrointestinal (UGI) bleeding to evaluate the efficacy of rFVIIa. Two hundred and forty-five patients were randomized to receive eight doses of 100 µg/kg rFVIIa or placebo in addition to pharmacological and endoscopic treatment. The first dose was administered within 6 h after admission (or within 6 h of the index bleeding if the patient was already hospitalized); further doses were administered at 2, 4, 6, 12, 18, 24, and 30 h after first trial product administration. Primary composite endpoints were failure to control UGI bleeding within 24 h postdosing, failure to prevent rebleeding between 24 h and day 5, and 5-d mortality. Significantly fewer patients with severe liver disease (Child-Pugh score B and C) failed on the composite endpoint ($p = 0.03$) and the 24-h-bleeding control endpoint ($p = 0.01$) relative to placebo. rFVIIa did not improve the efficacy of standard treatment in Child-Pugh score A patients. Incidences of adverse events including thromboembolic events were similar between the two groups.

10.5.3.1.2 Surgery

Hepatectomy and prostatectomy are surgical procedures for patients suffering from cancer, and despite refinement of surgical techniques, they are still associated with substantial perioperative blood loss [82,83]. Blood transfusion therapy constitutes a risk factor for cancer recurrence, increased intraoperative morbidity, transmission of infectious disease, alloimmunization, transfusion reactions, and hemolytic reactions [82,84].

In a trial of 185 patients undergoing hepatectomy for hepatic cancer or metastasis to the liver, patients were randomized to receive prophylactically either placebo, 20 or 80 µg/kg of rFVIIa. The proportion of patients requiring perioperative transfusion of RBCs was 30% lower in the 80 µg/kg dose group when compared with placebo, whereas no effect of treatment was evident in the 20 µg/kg dose group. The incidences of any types of adverse events or serious adverse events in the rFVIIa-treated patients were not higher than the incidences reported by patients in the placebo group.

A recent trial in patients undergoing radical retropubic prostatectomy [83] showed that prophylactic administration of a single dose of 20 or 40 µg/kg rFVIIa significantly decreased the number of patients in need of transfusion with RBCs, with a dose of 40 µg/kg rFVIIa completely obviating the need for RBC transfusion.

10.5.3.1.3   *Intracerebral Hemorrhage (ICH)*

Spontaneous ICH constitutes about 15% of all strokes, and has an incidence of about 26 per 100,000 per year. It is the deadliest form of stroke, with a 30 d mortality of 35 to 50%. Currently, no treatment exists for ICH. In either spontaneous (when related to high blood pressure) or traumatic ICH, a significant proportion of the patients exhibit hematoma growth in the hours following the insult [85,86]. Furthermore, a large proportion of the traumatically induced insults lead to systemic disturbances in hemostasis [87]. Since hematoma size has been described as the strongest predictor of outcome in such patients [88], this has been the basis for testing the ability of rFVIIa to halt hematoma expansion if administered immediately after the insult. To date, results from two dose-escalation trials [89,90] have been published demonstrating safety in 88 patients dosed in the range of 5 to 160 µg/kg. Based on these results, a large efficacy trial including 400 patients was initiated. The results were available in June 2004. Overall rFVIIa reduced the hemorrhage growth from a baseline CT scan within 3 hours of onset to 24 hours by more than 50%. Mortality at day 90 was 38% lower in patients receiving active drug compared with placebo, and the proportion of patients with a severe outcome at day 90 was 69% in placebo compared with 52% in the groups who received active drug. The incidence of thromboembolic SAEs increased from 2% in placebo to 7% in the active-drug groups. This increase is however included in the above outcome results indicating a vastly beneficial benefit-risk-ratio [91].

10.5.3.1.4   *Trauma*

Following severe trauma, a number of changes occur, resulting in impaired hemostasis. The loss of circulating blood volume caused by bleeding leads to a decrease in blood pressure. As blood pressure decreases below colloid osmotic pressure, interstitial fluid moves into the vascular space and dilutes the coagulation factors that remain in the circulation. Infusion of resuscitation fluids and blood components that do not contain sufficient amounts of coagulation factors leads to a further dilution [72].

Coagulopathy in trauma patients with severe bleeding is multifactorial and may be caused by depletion of platelets and coagulation factors through extravascular loss, intravascular consumption, and dilution by resuscitation fluids. Acidosis resulting from hypoxemia, anaerobic metabolism, accumulation of lactic acid as well as hypothermia, the result of poor perfusion and transfusions of stored refrigerated blood components, can further worsen coagulopathy [72]. Furthermore, in case of severe tissue damage, fibrinolytic enzymes are released from damaged cells, leading to increased fibrinolysis and disruption of the formed fibrin clots. Conventional means of controlling bleeding are often successful, and include local pressure, ligation, or embolization of specific vessels, fibrin sealants, and transfusion of allogenic blood.

Recently, a randomized prospective placebo-controlled trial [92] evaluating rFVIIa in the treatment of critical bleeding in 283 severely injured penetrating or blunt trauma patients has been finalized. Once a transfusion trigger of >8 units of packed RBC was met, dosing of 200 µg/kg rFVIIa took place followed by a second dose of 100 µg/kg 1 h later, and a third dose of 100 µg/kg 2 h after that. The study showed significant reduction in the number of transfusions needed in the blunt trauma group treated with rFVIIa. No safety concerns were reported with an exactly equal distribution of thromboembolic events in the active and placebo arms, but a trend toward reduction in the incidence of acute respiratory distress syndrome and multiorgan failure was observed.

10.6   Conclusions

rFVIIa is labeled for treatment of bleeding in hemophilia patients with inhibitors and, in Europe, for Glanzmann's thrombasthenia refractory to platelet transfusion and FVII deficiency. Data showing safety and efficacy in other clinical situations with severe bleeding are accumulating, supporting the hypothesis that rFVIIa may become the first universal hemostatic agent for critical bleeding.

References

1. Morrissey, J.H., et al., Quantitation of activated factor VII levels in plasma using a tissue factor mutant selectively deficient in promoting factor VII activation, *Blood*, 81, 734–744, 1993.
2. Wildgoose, P., et al., Measurement of basal levels of factor VIIa in hemophilia A and B patients, *Blood*, 80, 25–28, 1992.
3. Davie, E.W., Fujikawa, K., and Kisiel, W., The coagulation cascade: Initiation, maintenance, and regulation, *Biochemistry*, 30, 10363–10370, 1991.
4. Eigenbrot, C. and Kirchhofer, D., New insight into how tissue factor allosterically regulates factor VIIa, *Trends Cardiovasc. Med.*, 12, 19–26, 2002.
5. Ruf, W. and Dickinson, C.D., Allosteric regulation of the cofactor-dependent serine protease coagulation factor VIIa, *Trends Cardiovasc. Med.*, 8, 350–356, 1998.
6. Hoffman, M., Monroe, D.M., III, and Roberts, H.R., Activated factor VII activates factors IX and X on the surface of activated platelets: Thoughts on the mechanism of action of high-dose activated factor VII, *Blood Coagul. Fibrinolysis*, 9 (Suppl. 1), S61–S65, 1998.
7. Monroe, D.M., et al., Platelet activity of high-dose factor VIIa is independent of tissue factor, *Br. J. Haematol.*, 99, 542–547, 1997.
8. Monroe, D.M., et al., A possible mechanism of action of activated factor VII independent of tissue factor, *Blood Coagul. Fibrinolysis*, 9 (Suppl. 1), S15–S20, 1998.
9. Lisman, T., et al., Inhibition of fibrinolysis by recombinant factor VIIa in plasma from patients with severe hemophilia A, *Blood*, 99, 175–179, 2002.
10. van 't Veer, C., Golden, N.J., and Mann, K.G., Inhibition of thrombin generation by the zymogen factor VII: Implications for the treatment of hemophilia A by factor VIIa, *Blood*, 95, 1330–1335, 2000.
11. Hoffman, M. and Monroe, D.M., The action of high-dose factor VIIa (FVIIa) in a cell-based model of hemostasis, *Semin. Hematol.*, 38 (Suppl. 12), 6–9, 2001.
12. Lisman, T., et al., Enhanced *in vitro* procoagulant and antifibrinolytic potential of superactive variants of recombinant factor VIIa in severe hemophilia A, *J. Thrombos. Haemostas.*, 1, 2175–2178, 2003.
13. Tranholm, M., et al., Improved hemostasis with superactive analogs of factor VIIa in a mouse model of hemophilia A, *Blood*, 102, 3615–3620, 2003.
14. Banner, D.W., et al., The crystal structure of the complex of blood coagulation factor VIIa with soluble tissue factor, *Nature*, 380, 41–46, 1996.
15. Pike, A.C., et al., Structure of human factor VIIa and its implications for the triggering of blood coagulation, *Proc. Natl. Acad. Sci., USA*, 96, 8925–8930, 1999.
16. Persson, E. and Petersen, L.C., Structurally and functionally distinct Ca^{2+} binding sites in the γ-carboxyglutamic acid-containing domain of factor VIIa, *Eur. J. Biochem.*, 234, 293–300, 1995.
17. Dickinson, C.D., Kelly, C.R., and Ruf, W., Identification of surface residues mediating tissue factor binding and catalytic function of the serine protease factor VIIa, *Proc. Natl. Acad. Sci., USA*, 93, 14379–14384, 1996.

18. Bom, V.J.J. and Bertina, R.M., The contributions of Ca^{2+}, phospholipids and tissue-factor apoprotein to the activation of human blood coagulation factor X by activated factor VII, *Biochem. J.*, 265, 327–336, 1990.

19. Freskgård, P.O., Olsen, O.H., and Persson, E., Structural changes in factor VIIa induced by Ca^{2+} and tissue factor studied using circular dichroism spectroscopy, *Protein Sci.*, 5, 1531–1540, 1996.

20. Persson, E., Nielsen, L.S., and Olsen, O.H., Substitution of aspartic acid for methionine-306 in factor VIIa abolishes the allosteric linkage between the active site and the binding interface with tissue factor, *Biochemistry*, 40, 3251–3256, 2001.

21. Thim, L., et al., Amino acid sequence and posttranslational modifications of human factor VIIa from plasma and transfected baby hamster kidney cells, *Biochemistry*, 27, 7785–7793, 1988.

22. Hagen, F.S., et al., Characterization of a cDNA coding for human factor VII, *Proc. Natl. Acad. Sci., USA*, 83, 2412–2416, 1986.

23. Persson, E. and Nielsen, L.S., Site-directed mutagenesis but not γ-carboxylation of Glu-35 in factor VIIa affects the association with tissue factor, *FEBS Lett.*, 385, 241–243, 1996.

24. Bjoern, S., et al., Human plasma and recombinant factor VII. Characterization of O-glycosylations at serine residues 52 and 60 and effects of site-directed mutagenesis of serine 52 to alanine, *J. Biol. Chem.*, 266, 11051–11057, 1991.

25. Nishimura, H., et al., Identification of a disaccharide (Xyl-Glc) and a trisaccharide (Xyl2-Glc) O-glycosidically linked to a serine residue in the first epidermal growth factor-like domain of human factors VII and IX and protein Z and bovine protein Z, *J. Biol. Chem.*, 264, 20320–20325, 1989.

26. Iino, M., Foster, D.C., and Kisiel, W., Functional consequences of mutations in Ser-52 and Ser-60 in human blood coagulation factor VII, *Arch. Biochem. Biophys.*, 352, 182–192, 1998.

27. Klausen, N.K. and Kornfelt, T., Analysis of the glycoforms of human recombinant factor VIIa by capillary electrophoresis and high-performance liquid chromatography, *J. Chromatogr. A.*, 718, 195–202, 1995.

28. Klausen, N.K., Bayne, S., and Palm, L., Analysis of the site-specific asparagine-linked glycosylation of recombinant human coagulation factor VIIa by glycosidase digestions, liquid chromatography, and mass spectrometry, *Mol. Biotechnol.*, 9, 195–204, 1998.

29. Palm, L., Roepstorff, P., and Klausen, N.K., Elucidation of N-linked carbohydrate structures in recombinant human factor VII (rFVIIa) by combination of MALDI–MS and glycosidase digestions, *Proceedings of the XVIII International Carbohydrate Symposium*, July, Milano, Italy, 1996.

30. Berkner, K., et al., Isolation and expression of cDNAs encoding human factor VII, *Cold Spring Harb. Symp. Quant. Biol.*, 51, 531–541, 1986.

31. Butenas, S. and Mann, K.G., Kinetics of human factor VII activation, *Biochemistry*, 35, 1904–1910, 1996.

32. Bjoern, S. and Thim, L., Activation of coagulation factor VII to VIIa, *Res. Discl.*, 269, 564, 1986.

33. Wildgoose, P., Berkner, K.L., and Kisiel, W., Synthesis, purification, and characterization of an Arg152-Glu site-directed mutant of recombinant human blood clotting factor VII, *Biochemistry*, 29, 3413–3420, 1990.

34. Brinkhous, K.M., et al., Effect of recombinant factor VIIa on the hemostatic defect in dogs with hemophilia A, hemophilia B, and von Willebrand disease, *Proc. Natl. Acad. Sci., USA*, 86, 1382–1386, 1989.

35. Diness, V., Lund-Hansen, T., and Hedner, U., Effect of recombinant human FVIIa on warfarin-induced bleeding in rats, *Thromb. Res.*, 59, 921–929, 1990.

36. Diness, V., et al., Recombinant human factor VIIa (rFVIIa) in a rabbit stasis model, *Thromb. Res.*, 67, 233–241, 1992.

37. Jeroukhimov, I., et al., Early injection of high-dose recombinant factor VIIa decreases blood loss and prolongs time from injury to death in experimental liver injury, *J. Trauma-Injury Infect. Crit. Care*, 53, 1053–1057, 2002.

38. Lynn, M., et al., Early use of recombinant factor VIIa improves mean arterial pressure and may potentially decrease mortality in experimental hemorrhagic shock: A pilot study, *J. Trauma-Injury Infect. Crit. Care*, 52, 703–707, 2002.

39. Martinowitz, U., et al., Intravenous rFVIIa administered for hemorrhage control in hypothermic coagulopathic swine with grade V liver injuries, *J. Trauma-Injury Infect. Crit. Care*, 50, 721–729, 2001.

40. Schreiber, M.A., et al., The effect of recombinant factor VIIa on coagulopathic pigs with grade V liver injuries, *J. Trauma-Injury Infect. Crit. Care*, 53, 252–257, 2002.

41. Erhardtsen, E., et al., The effect of recombinant factor VIIa (NovoSeven(TM)) in healthy volunteers receiving acenocoumarol to an International Normalized Ratio above 2.0, *Blood Coagul. Fibrinolysis*, 9, 741–748, 1998.

42. Erhardtsen, E., Pharmacokinetics of recombinant activated factor VII (rFVIIa), *Semin. Thromb. Hemost.*, 26, 385–391, 2000.

43. Lindley, C.M., et al., Pharmacokinetics and pharmacodynamics of recombinant factor VIIa, *Clin. Pharmacol. Ther.*, 55, 638–648, 1994.

44. Hedner, U., et al., Pharmacokinetics of rFVIIa in children, *Haemophilia*, 4, 355, 1998.

45. Girard, P., et al., Population pharmacokinetics of recombinant factor VIIa in volunteers anticoagulated with acenocoumarol, *Thrombos. Haemostas.*, 80, 109–113, 1998.

46. Arkin, S., et al., Activated recombinant human coagulation factor VII therapy for intracranial hemorrhage in patients with hemophilia A or B with inhibitors. Results of the novoseven emergency-use program, *Haemostasis*, 28, 93–98, 1998.

47. Hay, C.R.M., Negrier, C., and Ludlam, C.A., The treatment of bleeding in acquired haemophilia with recombinant factor VIIa: A multicentre study, *Thrombos. Haemostas.*, 78, 1463–1467, 1997.

48. Liebman, H.A., et al., Activated recombinant human coagulation factor VII (rFVIIa) therapy for abdominal bleeding in patients with inhibitory antibodies to factor VIII, *Am. J. Hematol.*, 63, 109–113, 2000.

49. Lusher, J.M., Early treatment with recombinant factor VIIa results in greater efficacy with less product, *Eur. J. Haematol. Suppl.*, 63, 7–10, 1998.

50. Arkin, S., et al., Human coagulation factor FVIIa (recombinant) in the management of limb-threatening bleeds unresponsive to alternative therapies: Results from the NovoSeven(R) emergency-use programme in patients with severe haemophilia or with acquired inhibitors, *Blood Coagul. Fibrinolysis*, 11, 255–259, 2000.

51. Key, N.S., et al., Home treatment of mild to moderate bleeding episodes using recombinant factor VIIa (NovoSeven) in haemophiliacs with inhibitors, *Thrombos. Haemostas.*, 80, 912–918, 1998.

52. Shapiro, A.D., et al., Prospective, randomised trial of two doses of rFVIIa (NovoSeven) in haemophilia patients with inhibitors undergoing surgery, *Thrombos. Haemostas.*, 80, 773–778, 1998.

53. Ingerslev, J., et al., Treatment of acute bleeding episodes with rFVIIa, *Vox Sang.*, 77 (Suppl. 1), 42–46, 1999.

54. Ingerslev, J., Efficacy and safety of recombinant factor VIIa in the prophylaxis of bleeding in various surgical procedures in hemophilic patients with factor VIII and factor IX inhibitors, *Semin. Thromb. Hemost.*, 26, 425–432, 2000.

55. Johannessen, M., Andreasen, R.B., and Nordfang, O., Decline of factor VIII and factor IX inhibitors during long-term treatment with NovoSeven(R), *Blood Coagul. Fibrinolysis*, 11, 239–242, 2000.

56. Brackmann, H.H., et al., Immune tolerance induction: A role for recombinant activated factor VII (rFVIIa)? *Eur. J. Haematol. Suppl.*, 63, 18–23, 1998.

57. Kobelt, R., Swiss treatment concept for the use of rFVIIa in context of immune tolerance therapy, in *Recombinant Factor VIIa. Current and Future Indications*, Scharrer, I. and von Depka Prondzinski, M., Eds., Weller Verlag, Frankfurt/Main, Germany, 2000, p. 50.

58. Manno, C.S., Treatment options for bleeding episodes in patients undergoing immune tolerance therapy, *Haemophilia*, 5 (Suppl. 3), 33–41, 1999.

59. Poon, M.C., et al., Use of recombinant factor VIIa (NovoSeven(R)) in patients with Glanzmann thrombasthenia, *Semin. Hematol.*, 38, 21–25, 2001.

60. Billio, A., et al., Successful short-term oral surgery prophylaxis with rFVIIa in severe congenital factor VII deficiency, *Blood Coagul. Fibrinolysis*, 8, 249–250, 1997.

61. Cobos, E., et al., Use of recombinant factor VIIa for major elective surgery in a patient with factor VII deficiency, retroperitoneal fibrosis and hydronephrosis, *Clin. Appl. Thromb. Hemost.*, 3, 33, 1997.

62. Wong, W.Y., et al., Clinical efficacy and recovery levels of recombinant FVIIa (NovoSeven) in the treatment of intracranial haemorrhage in severe neonatal FVII deficiency, *Haemophilia*, 6, 50–54, 2000.

63. Eskandari, N., Feldman, N., and Greenspoon, J.S., Factor VII deficiency in pregnancy treated with recombinant factor VIIa, *Obstet. Gynecol.*, 99, 935–937, 2002.

64. Jimenez, Y., et al., Continuous infusion of recombinant activated factor VII during caesarean section delivery in a patient with congenital factor VII deficiency, *Haemophilia*, 6, 588–590, 2000.
65. Eskandari, N., Feldman, N., and Greenspoon, J.S., Factor VII deficiency in pregnancy treated with recombinant factor VIIa, *Obstet. Gynecol.*, 99, 935–937, 2002.
66. Mariani, G., et al., Use of recombinant, activated factor VII in the treatment of congenital factor VII deficiencies, *Vox Sang.*, 77, 131–136, 1999.
67. Nicolaisen, E.M., Antigenicity of activated recombinant factor VII followed through nine years of clinical experience, *Blood Coagul. Fibrinolysis*, 9 (Suppl. 1), S119–S123, 1998.
68. Aldouri, M., The use of recombinant factor VIIa in controlling surgical bleeding in non-haemophiliac patients, *Pathophysiol. Haemost. Thromb.*, 32, 41–46, 2002.
69. Kalicinski, P., et al., Quick correction of hemostasis in two patients with fulminant liver failure undergoing liver transplantation by recombinant activated factor VII, *Transplant. Proc.*, 31, 378–379, 1999.
70. Slappendel, R., et al., Use of recombinant factor VIIa (NovoSeven[R]) to reduce postoperative bleeding after total hip arthroplasty in a patient with cirrhosis and thrombocytopenia, *Anesthesiology*, 96, 1525–1527, 2002.
71. Tobias, J.D., Synthetic factor VIIa to treat dilutional coagulopathy during posterior spinal fusion in two children, *Anesthesiology*, 96, 1522–1525, 2002.
72. Martinowitz, U., et al., Recombinant activated factor VII for adjunctive hemorrhage control in trauma, *J. Trauma*, 51, 431–438, 2001.
73. O'Neill, P.A., et al., Successful use of recombinant activated factor VII for trauma-associated hemorrhage in a patient without preexisting coagulopathy, *J. Trauma-Injury Infect. Crit. Care*, 52, 400–405, 2002.
74. Dutton, R.P., Hess, J.R., and Scalea, T.M., Recombinant factor VIIa for control of hemorrhage: Early experience in critically ill trauma patients, *J. Clin. Anesth.*, 15, 184–188, 2003.
75. Kenet, G., et al., Treatment of traumatic bleeding with recombinant factor VIIa, *Lancet*, 354, 1879, 1999.
76. Schmidt, M.L., et al., Recombinant activated factor VII (rFVIIa) therapy for intracranial hemorrhage in hemophilia A patients with inhibitors, *Am. J. Hematol.*, 47, 36–40, 1994.
77. Erhardtsen, E., Ongoing NovoSeven® trials, *Intensive Care Med.*, 28 (Suppl. 2), S248–S255, 2002.
78. Joist, J.H., Hemostatic abnormalities in liver disease, in *Hemostasis and Thrombosis*, Colman, R.W., Hirsh, J., Marder, V.J., and Salzman, E.W., Eds., Lippincott, Philadelphia, 1994, p. 906.
79. Paramo, J.A. and Rocha, E., Hemostasis in advanced liver disease, *Semin. Thromb. Hemost.*, 19, 184–190, 1993.
80. Porte, R.J., Knot, E.A., and Bontempo, F.A., Hemostasis in liver transplantation, *Gastroenterology*, 97, 488–501, 1989.
81. McCormick, P.A. and O'Keefe, C., Improving prognosis following a first variceal haemorrhage over four decades, *Gut*, 49, 682–685, 2001.
82. Cunningham, J.D., et al., One hundred consecutive hepatic resections. Blood loss, transfusion, and operative technique, *Arch. Surg.*, 129, 1050–1056, 1994.
83. Friederich, P.W., et al., Effect of recombinant activated factor VII on perioperative blood loss in patients undergoing retropubic prostatectomy: A double-blind placebo-controlled randomised trial, *Lancet*, 361, 201–205, 2003.
84. Nash, P.A., et al., The impact of pre-donated autologous blood and intra-operative isovolaemic haemodilution on the outcome of transfusion in patients undergoing radical retropubic prostatectomy, *Br. J. Urol.*, 77, 856–860, 1996.
85. Brott, T., Broderick, J.P., and Kothari, R.E.A., Early hemorrhage growth in patients with intracerebral hemorrhage, *Stroke*, 28, 1–5, 1997.
86. Oertel, M., et al., Progressive hemorrhage after head trauma: Predictors and consequences of the evolving injury, *J. Neurosurg.*, 96, 109–116, 2002.
87. Stein, S.C., et al., Association between intravascular microthrombosis and cerebral ischemia in traumatic brain injury, *Neurosurgery*, 54, 687–691, 2004.
88. Broderick, J.P., et al., Guidelines for the management of spontaneous intracerebral hemorrhage: A statement for Health Professionals from a Special Writing Group of the Stroke Council, American Heart Association, *Stroke*, 30, 905–915, 1999.

89. Mayer, S. and Brun, N., Safety and preliminary efficacy of activated recombinant factor VII in acute intracerebral hemorrhage, *Stroke*, 34, 242, 2003.
90. Mayer, S. and Brun, N., Safety and preliminary efficacy of recombinant coagulation factor VIIa in acute intracerebral hemorrhage: US phase IIa study, *Stroke*, 35, 332, 2004.
91. Mayer, S.A., et al., Recombinant activated factor VII for acute intracerebral hemorrhage. *N. Engl. J. Med.*, 352, 777–785, 2005.
92. Boffard, K., NovoSeven® in trauma — Presentation at Late Breaking Session, *6th World Congress on Trauma, Shock, Inflammation and Sepsis — Pathophysiology, Immune Consequences and Therapy*, Munich, Germany, 2004.

11

Factor IX (Protease Zymogen)

Barry M. McGrath

CONTENTS

11.1   Introduction

Coagulation factor IX (FIX) is a zymogen of a vitamin K-dependent serine protease that plays a critical role in the intrinsic blood-clotting pathway. Human FIX (hFIX) is a single-chain glycoprotein of approximately 55 kDa that is synthesized in the liver and is the largest of the vitamin K-dependent proteins. The protease zymogen undergoes extensive post-translational modifications after synthesis, which are required for the normal biological activity of its enzymatic form, activated FIX (FIXa) [1–3]. The serine protease FIXa (EC 3.4.21.22), in the presence of calcium ions, phospholipids, and factor VIII (FVIII), forms an active complex called the tenase complex, which converts factor X (FX) into its activated form, FXa [4]. Subsequent stages of the blood-clotting cascade proceed, culminating in the deposition of fibrin, the structural polymer of the blood clot (see Figure 11.1).

Deficiencies of FIX result in a severe bleeding disorder called hemophilia B [3,5]. Treatments for this life-threatening disorder became available in the latter part of the 20th century

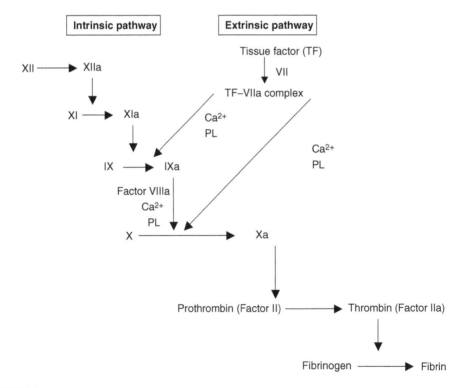

FIGURE 11.1
Schematic diagram of the blood-clotting cascade. This scheme is simplified and omits many details for clarity. PL = phospholipids; TF = tissue factor.

consisting mainly of prothrombin complex concentrates (PCCs) and subsequently with high-purity plasma-derived FIX (pdFIX) products obtained from pooled blood donations [6]. Owing to the incidence of viral transmission associated with these products, serious safety concerns have been raised. Consequently, efforts have been made to develop safer treatments for hemophilia B. Since the late 1990s, an approved recombinant form of FIX has been available in the United States and Europe, which offers the greatest margin of safety among currently available FIX products, and has become the recommended treatment of choice in most developed countries for patients suffering from hemophilia B [1,6,7]. Exciting developments in the area of gene therapy for hemophilia B have been reported recently as well.

11.2 Biochemical Properties and Characterization of FIX

11.2.1 FIX Gene Structure

The complete nucleotide sequence [8] and gene structure [9] for hfIX are known. The gene coding for FIX (*F9*) is found on the X chromosome located at Xq27.1 and is ~33.5 kb in length. Approximately 4% of the gene nucleotide sequence codes for protein and is contained within eight exons, separated by seven introns of varying size (Figure 11.2) [8,9].

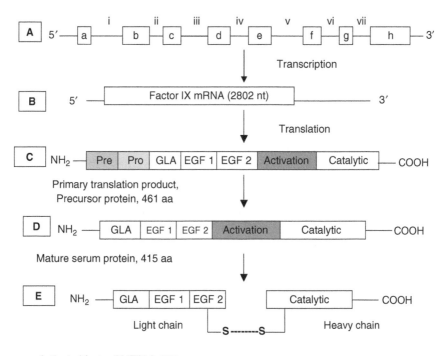

FIGURE 11.2
Schematic diagram outlining (A) the genomic organization of the human *F9* gene. The exons (a–h) and introns are labeled according to the scheme proposed in [9]. (B) FIX mRNA transcribed from *F9*. (C) The 461-aa precursor FIX protein, with its seven structural domains. (D) The 415-aa mature hFIX, found circulating in plasma, consists of five structural domains. (E) The 385-aa activated FIX (FIXa) contains an N-terminal light chain (composed of the Gla and EGF 1 and 2 domains), and is linked via a disulfide bond to the C-terminal heavy chain (containing the catalytic domain). See text for further details. The diagram is not drawn to scale.

The primary transcript of the *F9* gene is ~2802 bases in length, and is made up of a short 5'-untranslated region (29 bases), an open reading frame (ORF) of 1383 bases, and a 3'-untranslated region (1390 bases). The ORF encodes a 461-amino acid (aa) precursor polypeptide, which is modified extensively before release into the bloodstream [3].

The *F9* gene is phylogenetically conserved and shares high homology with the factor VII (*F7*), factor X (*F10*), and protein C genes. The basic exon structure of *F9* is organized in a similar fashion to other coagulation factors such as factor VII (FVII) and FX, and protein C, suggesting that they all evolved from a common ancestral gene by duplication [1,4]. The eight exons of *F9* encode a number of structural domains in the protein, which are identified according to structure and function and are discussed below.

11.2.2 Protein Domain Structure of FIX

hFIX is typically found circulating in plasma at concentrations of approximately 4 to 5 µg/mL [2], and has a half-life of ~24 h [6]. FIX is initially synthesized in the liver as a precursor 461-aa residue polypeptide molecule, 46 aa residues longer at its N terminus than the mature 415-aa FIX found circulating in plasma. The primary translation product of the human *F9* gene consists of a 461 prepropeptide sequence, which consists of seven structural domains (Figure 11.2 and Figure 11.3).

The first FIX protein domain, the 28-aa pre (or signal) sequence (residues −46 to −19) directs FIX for secretion into the blood stream. After translocation of the nascent FIX polypeptide to the lumen of the endoplasmic reticulum (ER), the 28-aa signal sequence is removed [10].

The pro domain (residues −18 to −1) provides a binding domain for γ-carboxylase, which carboxylates glutamic acid residues in the adjacent γ-carboxyglutamic acid (Gla) domain. The 18-aa FIX propeptide domain serves as a recognition signal for γ-glutamyl carboxylase [11], and is removed following carboxylation by a paired aa cleaving enzyme (PACE, also known as furin), a 90-kDa subtilisin serine protease found in the Golgi apparatus [12]. Removal of the propeptide domain, mediated by an endoprotease, is required for FIX activity [13].

Structurally, mature FIX found circulating in blood consists of five main domains (Figure 11.2 and Figure 11.3) [2,3,9,14]. The Gla domain (residues 1 to 40) possesses several Ca^{2+}-binding sites. Binding of phospholipids for the activation of the zymogen occurs in a Ca^{2+}-dependent manner [15]. The Gla domain participates in binding FIX to the tissue factor (TF)–activated factor VII (FVIIa) complex during activation of FIX [16]. The Gla domain has also been shown to bind the FIXa cofactor, activated factor VIII (FVIIIa), in the tenase complex [17].

Following the Gla domain is a short hydrophobic stack (residues 41 to 46), linking the Gla domain to the first epidermal growth factor (EGF 1)-like domain (residues 47 to 83). The EGF 1 region shows extensive homologies to human EGF. The EGF 1 domain contains Ca^{2+}-binding sites, and plays a role in the activation of FIX by activated factor XI (FXIa) during the intrinsic pathway. EGF-1 is also required for activation of FIX by the FVIIa–TF complex during the extrinsic pathway [18]. EGF 1 also serves a structural role in binding the FIXa cofactor, FVIIIa, during FIXa-catalyzed FX activation [14].

The second EGF domain (EGF 2, residues 88 to 127) is connected to the EGF 1 domain by linker residues 84 to 87. These linker residues are thought to contribute to the enhancement of FIXa enzymatic activity, which occurs upon assembly of FIXa with its cofactor, factor VIIIa [19]. The EGF 2 domain is highly conserved (>80% aa identity) among different organisms and plays a role in binding FVIIIa, and is also involved in binding the FIXa substrate, FX [20]. Similar to EGF 1, the EGF 2 domain is also required for activation of FIX by the FVIIa–TF complex during the extrinsic pathway [21].

```
          Signal sequence                Pro sequence
   -46  MQRVNMIMAESPGLITICLLGYLLSAEC   TVFLDHENANKILNRPKR   -1

        Gla domain
        **        *  *  **      **   *   *   *    *
        YNSGKLEEFVQGNLERECMEEKCSFEEAREVFENTERTTE FWKQYV DGDQ    50

                         EGF 1 domain
                    ↓β-OH
        CESNPCLNGGSCKDDINSYECWCPFGFEGKNCE LDVT CNIKNGRCEQFCK    100

        EGF 2 domain
        NSADNKVVCSCTEGYRLAENQKSCEPA VPFPCGRVSVSQTSKLTR AEAVF    150

            Activation peptide
        SO4↓  ↓PO4
        PDVDYVNSTEAETILDNITQSTQSFNDFTR VVGGEDAKPGQFPWQVVLNG    200

               Catalytic domain
        KVDAFCGGSIVNEKWIVTAAHCVETGVKITVVAGEHNIEETEHTEQKRNV    250

               Catalytic domain
        IRIIPHHNYNAAINKYNHDIALLELDEPLVLNSYVTPICIADKEYTNIFL    300

            Catalytic domain
        KFGSGYVSGWGRVFHKGRSALVLQYLRVPLVDRATCLRSTKFTIYNNMFC    350

             Catalytic domain
        AGFHEGGRDSCQGDSGGPHVTEVEGTSFLTGIISWGEECAMKGKYGIYTK    400

        VSRYVNWIKEKTKLT    415
```

FIGURE 11.3

The aa sequence of human factor IX (accession number P00470), showing the main protein domains: (1) The *pre* sequence (residues –46 to –19) and the *pro* sequence (–18 to –1); (2) the *Gla* domain (1 to 40), with 12 glutamic acid (E) residues, marked with an asterisk; (3) the epidermal growth factor (*EGF*) domain 1 (47 to 83), containing aspartic acid (D) at residue 64 which undergoes β-hydroxylation (arrow with a "β-OH" symbol); (4) *EGF*-like domain 2 (88 to 127); (5) the *activation peptide* domain (146 to 180), containing a tyrosine (Y) at residue 155 (in bold) which undergoes sulfation (vertical arrow with "SO_4" symbol), and a serine (S) at residue 158 (in bold), which is phosphorylated (vertical arrow with an "PO_4" symbol); (6) the catalytic domain (181 to 145, with the catalytic core residues H221, D269, and S365 underlined and in italics). Numbering on the right refers to aa residues. The protein domains are indicated in italics, and are separated by spaces in the sequence. The activation peptide (underlined) is cleaved from the polypeptide upon activation of FIX, generating the light chain and the heavy chain, which are subsequently linked together by a disulfide bridge between C132 and C289 (both cysteine residues are underlined and in bold), forming FIXa.

The activation peptide (AP) of FIX (residues 146 to 180) is separated from the EGF 2 domain by a short (19-aa) linker residue of unknown function. Within the AP region, O-linked oligosaccharides are linked to T159 and T169, where they are thought to play a role in the induction of a specific conformation required for zymogen activation [22]. The AP region is cleaved and released from FIX during activation of the protease zymogen.

The last domain of mature hFIX is the C-terminal protease domain (residues 181 to 415). This catalytic domain contains a typical serine protease catalytic triad of S365, H221, and D269 (Figure 11.3), which converts FX into its activated form, FXa [23,24].

11.2.3   FIX Modification

After synthesis of the 461-aa precursor FIX polypeptide, FIX undergoes extensive modification during transit through the ER and Golgi apparatus. The hydrophobic signal sequence (residues –46 to –19) is removed following translocation of the nascent FIX polypeptide to the lumen of the ER. Following removal of the signal peptide, FIX transits to the Golgi apparatus, where extensive additional modifications occur [10].

N-linked glycans, two in the AP domain at N157 and N167, and the O-linked glycans, two in the EGF 1 domain at S53 and S61, and three in the AP domain at T159, T169, and T172 [22,25,26], are attached and processed to branched-chain structures.

Twelve glutamic acid residues, located in the Gla domain, undergo extensive γ-carboxylation by a vitamin K-dependent γ-glutamyl carboxylase in the ER during synthesis of FIX [1,27,28]. The pro domain serves as a recognition sequence for γ-glutamyl-carboxylase-mediated carboxylation of the Gla domain, and is removed following carboxylation. This modification of the Gla domain is required for the correct folding and calcium binding of FIX [15]. FIX also undergoes further posttranslational modification in the formation of 11 disulfide bonds, β-hydroxylation of D64, sulfation of Y155, and the phosphorylation of S158 [1–3].

11.2.4 Activation of FIX Zymogen

The mature, secreted FIX is a 415-aa single-chain glycoprotein with a molecular mass of 55 kDa [2], and consists of five structural domains. It is activated enzymatically by proteolytic cleavage between R145 and A146 (α-cleavage), and also between R180 and V181 (β-cleavage), yielding FIXa, and a 35-aa AP (Figure 11.2). The Arg-Ala and Arg-Val cleavages are directed by FXIa (plus Ca^{2+}) through the intrinsic pathway [28], or via the TF–FVIIa (plus Ca^{2+}) complex of the extrinsic pathway [29]. The products of both activation processes yield a 145-residue N-terminal noncatalytic light chain (containing the Gla and EGF domains), a 235-residue C-terminal catalytic heavy chain, and releases the 35-residue AP. Three possible pathways accounting for the sequence of cleavages by the TF/FVIIa/Ca^{2+} or factor XII (FXII)/Ca^{2+} complexes yielding FIXa have been proposed [30]. The light and heavy chains are then linked together by a disulfide bond between C132 on the light chain and C289 on the heavy chain (Figure 11.2) [2].

11.2.5 Catalytic Activity

The 380-residue FIXa contains a typical serine protease catalytic triad of S365, H221, and D269, all located in the heavy chain of FIXa (Figure 11.3) [23,24]. FIXa (EC 3.4.21.22), a 385-residue polypeptide, interacts with a complex (the tenase complex) composed of FVIII, phoshoplipids, FX, and calcium that are located on the surface of platelet membranes. FIXa binds the light chain of factor VIIIa through its Gla domain [17]. FIXa functions as a protease to cleave the peptide bond between R52 and I53 (on the C terminus of the FX heavy chain) converting it into activated factor X (FXa). FXa then interacts with factors V (FV) and II (FII; prothrombin) to convert FII into FIIa (thrombin). FIIa proteolyzes fibrinogen into fibrin monomers, which undergo polymerization in the final stage of the blood-clotting cascade. These fibrin polymers are stabilized by crosslinking activity of factor XIII (FXIII) in association with thrombin and calcium (Figure 11.1).

11.3 Hemophilia B

11.3.1 The Disease

Hemophilia is an inherited bleeding disorder caused by low concentrations of specific blood-clotting factors, and is the most common coagulation disorder known today [6]. Hemophilia A accounts for almost 80% of all hemophilias, affecting approximately

TABLE 11.1

Classification of Hemophilia

Classification	Concentration of Factor (VIII or IX) (IU/mL)
Severe	<0.01 (<1% of normal)
Moderate	0.01–0.05 (1–5% of normal)
Mild	>0.05–0.40 (5–40% of normal)

Adapted from Bolton-Maggs, P.H.B. and Pasi, K.J., *Lancet*, 361, 1801–1809, 2003.

1 in 10,000 males around the globe, and is caused by a deficiency of clotting FVIII in the circulating blood. Hemophilia B is a congenital blood disorder that arises through mutations of blood coagulation factor FIX. Worldwide, it is estimated that more than half a million people suffer from hemophilia [31]. A deficiency or dysfunction in either FVIII or FIX compromises the activation of FX, such that the ensuing steps of the coagulation cascade are compromised, and fibrin formation is either inefficient or does not occur at all [3]. Both disorders are clinically indistinguishable from each other and diagnosis must be performed by a specific factor assay. Hemophilia is defined by the bleeding tendency of sufferers (Table 11.1). Severe hemophilia is typified by spontaneous joint and muscle bleeding, and episodes of bleeding after injuries, accidents, or surgery. Moderate hemophilia manifests as bleeding into joints and muscles after minor injuries, and excessive bleeding after surgery. Mild hemophilia is characterized by a lack of spontaneous bleeding episodes, with bleeding occurring only after surgery or trauma [5,6]. Approximately one third of all hemophilia B patients fall into each of these categories.

Hemophilia B is a hemorrhagic disorder that results from a deficiency of FIX. It was first described over 50 years ago and was originally named "Christmas disease" after the first patient, a 5-year-old boy named Stuart Christmas, was described with this condition [32,33]. It affects approximately 1 in 30,000 male births [5]. Hemophilia B is an X-linked recessive disorder, with the *F9* gene being located on the long arm of the X chromosome at Xq27.1. Hemophilia B is recessive, carried by females (karyotype 46:XX), and present in males (karyotype 46:XY). Males pass the defective gene on to all of their daughters, but none of their sons. Females have a 50% chance of passing the defective gene to both their sons and daughters. The daughters of affected males become obligate carriers, while sons are normal. As it is an X-linked inherited disease, hemophilia B predominantly affects males, although some cases of female suffering from severe hemophilia have been reported [34]. Instances of female hemophilia may arise through the inheritance of the defective gene from both parents (hemophiliac father and carrier mother), or through inactivation of the X-chromosome (lyonization) [3,6]. There have also been reports of severe hemophilia in females suffering from Turner's syndrome (XO karyotype), and females with congenital androgen insensitivity (testicular feminization with XY karyotype) [1].

Diagnosis of hemophilia B is based on bleeding during infancy, followed by analysis of prothrombin time (PT) and activated partial thromboplastin time (aPTT). A normal PT with a prolonged aPTT suggests hemophilia A or B. Subsequent analysis of FVIII and FIX plasma levels reveals whether the patient suffers from hemophilia A or hemophilia B, respectively [5].

11.3.2   Molecular Basis

The first defects in the FIX coding region identified in hemophilia B patients were gene deletions detected in patients with inhibitory antibodies by Southern blotting [35]. Extensive progress has been made over the past two decades in understanding the molecular basis for hemophilia B (reviewed in [1–3]). A database of mutations observed in diseased patients has been established to offer a view of the spectrum of the numerous and diverse mutations causing hemophilia B [34,36]. Numerous point mutations, deletions, or additions account for the majority of hemophilia B cases. More than 90% of *F9* mutations are point mutations; 5 to 10% are deletions, while some large rearrangements have also been described. In the most recent version (updated December 2003), 2511 patient entries are recorded in the hemophilia B mutation database, and of these, 896 show unique molecular events probably causing the disease through missense, nonsense, or splicing mutations involving all eight exons of FIX, while the remainder of events causing the disease are repeat events. Most of these repeats occur at CG doublets, which are known hotspots for mutation, and usually involve a GC→TG or CA transition [1,36]. Of the patient entries, <1% have developed inhibitors, while 52 are females (either affected or nonsymptomatic carriers).

The distribution of mutations according to the FIX protein domain structure, infers that mutations have been detected in all of the FIX protein domains. Most mutations are observed in the calcium-binding EGF 1 and the catalytic domains, illustrating their importance in FIX activity. The signal peptide and AP domains contain the fewest mutations, probably due to the lack of importance of most of their aa residues in terms of mature protein function. Mutations at 9 of the 12 γ-carboxylglutamyl residues have been observed, underlying their importance in the correct functioning of FIX. Substitutions at every 1 of the 22 cysteine residues in circulating FIX have been detected, which probably compromise the disulfide bridges and could therefore have an effect on the structural integrity of the mature protein.

All mutations described so far affect the FIX coding sequence, with a consequent impact on the translated protein. Certain mutations have been localized to the promoter regions of the *F9* gene, which do not result in a change in the FIX protein structure. These substitutions affect binding of proteins involved in transcription of the gene [34,36]. The resulting phenotype (the hemophilia B Leiden patients) is unusual in that it results in severe FIX deficiency at birth and throughout childhood, an increase in FIX levels from puberty to adolescence, and near-normal FIX levels at adulthood. Usually, complete clinical recovery is observed at adulthood [3,6].

11.4 Treatment of Hemophilia B

Medicinal treatments for hemophilia B began in 1954 with the isolation of antihemophilic factors of bovine and porcine origin, although severe allergic reactions were common with these treatments [37]. The subsequent development of cold-insoluble cryoprecipitate and PCC in 1965 dramatically changed the treatment of hemophiliacs. The most significant advance came in the 1970s with the development of lyophilized concentrates of FVIII (for hemophilia A) and FIX (for hemophilia B), which have transformed the life of many hemophiliacs [4,6].

11.4.1 Early Treatments

Crude FIX-containing concentrates derived from pooled blood donations, the PCCs, became available for hemophilia B treatment over 30 years ago, improving the quality of life and increasing the lifespan of many sufferers. These crude preparations displayed low levels of FIX-specific activity (<5 IU/mg), as they usually contained other clotting factors such as FII, FVII, and FX. The presence of other clotting factors in these preparations frequently resulted in thrombogenic complications such as arterial or venous thromboses, pulmonary emboli, and the development of disseminated intravascular coagulation, when administered repeatedly to control bleeding or when given in large amounts to treat serious bleeding episodes.

11.4.2 High-Purity pdFIX Products

Improvements in methods to separate FIX from crude preparations led to the development of high-purity pdFIX concentrates, which increased the safety profiles of treatments available for hemophilia B. High-purity pdFIX concentrates became available for treatment of hemophilia B in the mid-1970s, and have proven very effective in treating bleeding episodes [1,6].

The use of enzyme replacement therapy (ERT), through administration of PCCs and pdFIX products, to treat hemophilia has no doubt enhanced the quality of life of the numerous recipients over the years, but has come at a considerable cost to many individuals receiving ERT. Numerous incidents from around the globe of HIV and hepatitis virus transmission through contaminated blood-clotting factor concentrates for hemophilia treatment have been reported [6,38–40]. Consequently, viral inactivation steps (Section 11.4.2.1) were introduced in the mid-1980s to eliminate the risk of transmission of HIV and hepatitis diseases. Although HIV, hepatitis viruses, and other enveloped viruses have not been transmitted since the introduction of these viral inactivation steps, concern remains about the possibility of nonenveloped viruses (such as parvovirus and hepatitis A) being transmitted [41,42].

11.4.2.1 *Steps to Increase Safety of Blood-Derived Clotting Factor Products*

The possibility of transmission of infectious agents through blood-derived biologics still remains a major safety concern. Relevant regulatory authorities have initiated measures to address such concerns, and numerous safeguard measures have been introduced to enhance the safety of currently available pdFIX products as described below:

1. *Donor selection.* Plasma used for producing blood factor concentrates is obtained from whole-blood donations (recovered plasma) and from aphaeresis (source plasma). The viral burden entering the plasma pool can be limited by careful selection of donors [41]. Many countries now rely on aphaeresis centers that use carefully screened repeat donors, which constitute an extremely safe pool from which clotting factors are derived [41,43].
2. *Plasma testing.* Screening plasma for HIV, hepatitis (A, B, and C), parvovirus B19, syphillis, and cytomegalovirus is now a routine and standard practice. Traditionally, this was performed using enzyme-linked immunosorbent assay (ELISA) testing, an extremely sensitive method for detecting pathogens [42]. More rapid and sensitive nucleic acid amplification testing (NAT) has been introduced in most North American and European countries since the late 1990s. NAT offers an increased margin of safety for clotting factor concentrates [41], in that it enables detection of hepatitis A and parvovirus, both of which are relatively recalcitrant to many viral inactivation technologies (see below).
3. *Viral inactivation steps.* Heat treatment was first introduced as a virucidal measure in the mid-1980s. Viruses have varying thermal sensitivities, with viruses such as HIV being more susceptible to heat treatment than the hepatitis viruses [41,43]. Heat treatment can result in significant denaturation of the clotting factor protein [41]; furthermore, certain heat treatments (i.e., dry heat treatment)

do not adequately remove viruses such as hepatitis G, implicated in certain types of chronic hepatitis [44]. The addition of solvents (usually tri-*n*-butyl phosphate), in the presence of a nonionic detergent (sodium cholate, Tween 80, or Triton X-100), was introduced as an extra safeguard against possible viral transmission. Solvent/detergent (SD) addition kills most enveloped viruses (such as HIV, hepatitis B virus [HBV], and hepatitis C virus [HCV]) with limited denaturing effects on clotting factors. SD use is limited in its effectiveness against nonenveloped viruses (e.g., parvovirus B19) [43,45]. Most currently available pdFIX products undergo some sort of SD treatment [43].

4. *Increased purification and viral removal.* Partitioning and purification techniques used to separate the desired clotting factor from other plasma components have also been shown to reduce the viral load. Fractionation steps such as cryoprecipitation and chromatographic separation procedures (especially immunoaffinity chromatography), and lyophilisation, have been shown to remove substantial amounts of virus [41,43]. Nanofiltration (NF) of plasma products has been used since the early 1990s to improve the margin of viral safety, and to complement SD addition and/or heat treatment. It was introduced to enhance safety against nonenveloped viruses, and also to provide an additional safeguard against new infectious agents entering the human plasma pool. NF is widely used in industry today for biopharmaceuticals produced from plasma [46]. NF is typically performed by passing the plasma solution through membranes of very small pore size (15 to 40 nm), under conditions that retain viruses in a size-exclusion mechanism and allow 90 to 95% of protein activity to be recovered. NF enables removal of both enveloped and nonenveloped viruses (such as HAV and parvovirus), with nonenveloped viruses being resistant to many other viral inactivation techniques. NF has also been shown to remove effectively added proteinaceous infectious particles (prions) [46,47].

A number of the currently approved high-purity pdFIX products, purification methods, and viral inactivation steps used in their production are highlighted in Table 11.2.

11.4.2.2   *Additional Safety Concerns*

The emergence of transmissible spongiform encephalopathy (TSE) diseases such as bovine spongiform encephalopathy (BSE) in cattle, scrapie in sheep, and Creutzfeldt–Jakob disease (CJD) in humans, caused by abnormal prions, has become a cause for concern due to the associated risk of iatrogenic transmission via blood, blood components, or plasma products [48]. The recent emergence of a new type of TSE, variant CJD (vCJD), caused by a novel type of infectious agent, has become a major cause for concern. In vCJD-infected individuals, associated prions have been detected in tissues such as tonsils, spleen, appendix, and lymph nodes, whereas when tested by comparable methods, these same tissues have been found to be free of any detectable prions in other human prion diseases, such as CJD [49]. This raises the risk of vCJD transmission via blood products. Also, prion-related diseases have proved to be highly recalcitrant to traditional chemical inactivation techniques, although certain physical removal means have proved successful [41,46,49]. A recent report has raised the possibility of vCJD transmission through blood transfusions [50], thereby increasing concerns about the safety of blood-derived plasma products [51]. Currently, there is a paucity of screening methods to detect vCJD and other TSEs [52], in contrast to the numerous methods for detecting numerous viral and bacterial pathogens [42]. Also, contamination of pdFIX products by adventitious viruses and as yet unknown pathogens cannot be ruled out.

TABLE 11.2

Highly Purified pdFIX Concentrates Available for Use in Treating Hemophilia B

Brand	Company	Plasma Source	Fractionation	Viral Inactivation	S.A.*	Comments
Berinin-P = Berinin HS	Aventis Behring, Germany	USA, Austria, Germany: paid and unpaid	DEAE-sephadex, heparin-affinity chromatography	Pasteurization at 60°C, 10 h	146	Antithrombin III, heparin added; no albumin
Immunine	Baxter BioScience, Austria	USA, Austria, Czech Rep., Germany, Sweden: paid aphaeresis	Ion-exchange and hydrophobic interaction chromatography	Polysorbate-80 and vapour heat, 60°C, 10 h, 190 mbar then 80°C, 1 h, 375 mbar	~100	
Hemo-B-RAAS	Shanghai RAAS, China	China: unpaid and paid aphaeresis	Ion-exchange and affinity chromatography	Solvent/detergent, dry heat and NF	>50	No albumin added
Bemofil	Finnish Red Cross BTS, Finland	Finland: unpaid recovered	Ion-exchange and affinity chromatography	Solvent/detergent, 15 nm NF	>110	
Octanyne	Octapharma, Austria	USA, Austria, Germany	Ion-exchange and affinity chromatography	TNBP/polysorbate-80 and NF	50–100	No albumin added
Octanyne F	Octapharma, Austria and France	USA, Austria, Germany, Sweden	Ion-exchange and affinity chromatography	TNBP/polysorbate-80 and NF	>100	No albumin added
Nanotiv	Octapharma, Sweden	Sweden: recovered and aphaeresis	Ion-exchange and heparin ligand chromatography	TNBP/Triton X-100 and NF	190	No albumin added
HIP FIX	SNBTS, Scotland	USA and Germany: unpaid	Ion-exchange and heparin ligand chromatography	TNBP/polysorbate-80; dry heat, 80°C, 72 h	180	Antithrombin III added, no albumin
Mono FIX-VF	CSL Ltd., Australia	Australia, New Zealand, Singapore, Hong Kong: unpaid	Ion-exchange and heparin-affinity chromatography	TNBP/ polysorbate-80 and NF	70	Antithrombin II, heparin added, no albumin
Christmassin-M	Benesis, Japan	Japan: unpaid	Ion-exchange and immunoaffinity chromatography	TNBP/polysorbate-80; dry heat, 60°C, 72 h; 15 nm NF	~170	Albumin added

(Continued)

TABLE 11.2 (Continued)

Brand	Company	Plasma Source	Fractionation	Viral Inactivation	S.A.*	Comments
Aimafix D.I.	Kedrion, Italy	Europe and USA: paid and unpaid	Anion-exchange, DEAE-Sephadex/Sepharose and heparin–affinity chromatography	TNBP polysorbate-80, dry heat, 100°C, 30 min; 35 + 15 nm NF	>100	Antithrombin III, heparin added, no albumin
Betafact	LFB, France	Western Europe, unpaid	DEAE–Sephadex, anion-exchange, affinity chromatography	TNBP/polysorbate-80, 15 nm NF	>110	No albumin added
Faktor IX SDN	Biotest, LFB, France	Western Europe, unpaid	DEAE–sephadex, anion-exchange, affinity chromatography	TNBP / polysorbate-80, 15 nm NF	>110	No albumin added
NOVIX	Grifols, Spain	USA paid, Spain and Czech Rep., unpaid	Precipitation and multiple chromatography	Solvent/detergent, 15 nm NF	>150	No albumin added
Alphanine	Grifols, USA	USA: paid aphaeresis	Ion-exchange, carbohydrate ligand chromatography	TNBP/polysorbate-80, NF	210	No albumin added
Mononine	Aventis Behring, USA	USA: aphaeresis paid	Immunoaffinity chromatography	Sodium thiocyanate and ultrafiltration	>190	
Nonafact	Sanquin, Netherlands	The Netherlands: unpaid	Immunoaffinity chromatography	TNBP/polysorbate-80; NF	200 or more	No albumin added
Novact M	Kaketsuken, Japan	Japan: unpaid	Immunoaffinity chromatography	Dry heat, 65°C, 96 h; 15 nm NF	200	Albumin added
Replenine – VF	Bio Products Lab., U.K.	USA: paid aphaeresis	Metal chelate chromatography	Solvent/detergent; 15 nm NF	200	No albumin added

*Specific activity (factor IX IU/mg) calculated without added albumin (where applicable).

Abbreviations: NF = nanofiltration, TNBP = tri-*n*-butyl phosphate.

Data adapted from Kasper, C.K. and Costa e Silvia, M., *Registry of Clotting Factor Concentrates*, 4th ed., 2003. With updated data kindly supplied by Dr. Carol K. Kasper, Department of Medicine (Hematology), University of Southern California, and Orthopaedic Hospital, Los Angeles, CA.

Thus, it is now widely believed that recombinant products offer the greatest level of safety for hemophiliac patients [1,6,7]. In the United Kingdom (where the highest incidences of vCJD and BSE have been recorded), the Department of Health announced in 2004 that all plasma-derived blood products were to be phased out and replaced with recombinant factor VII (rFVII [for hemophilia A]) and recombinant FIX (rFIX [for hemophilia B]) [53]. However, many developing countries worldwide still rely on pdFIX concentrates and PCCs [54,55]. An overview of rFIX (developed by Genetics Institute, Wyeth, Boston, MA), the only currently approved therapeutic recombinant FIX product available in the European Union and the United States, follows in the next section.

11.5 rFIX

The gene for hFIX was first cloned in 1982 [56,57] and the complete nucleotide sequence for hFIX has been available since 1985 [58]. However, a recombinant version of FIX (trade name BeneFIX®, international nonproprietary name [INN] = nonacog alfa), developed by the Genetics Institute, was not approved for use in the United States and Canada until 1997, and received EU approval only in 1999. The principal reason for this lag in developing an approved therapeutic form of rFIX arose from the numerous technical difficulties that were encountered while trying to replicate *in vivo* posttranslational and glycosylation of FIX, which are essential for forming an active and therapeutically viable form of FIX (reviewed in [1,59]).

11.5.1 Development of an rFIX Production Line

After the gene for hFIX was first cloned, expression systems were examined by numerous academic and industrial groups to develop a biologically active form of hFIX. Expressing a recombinant, biologically active form proved to be a challenge due to the extensive posttranslational modifications required for a functional hFIX protein. In 1985, Anson, et al. [60] reported a biologically active form of rFIX expressed in rat hepatoma cells that had been transfected with an expression plasmid containing hFIX, although the yields of biologically active FIX were quite low (<7%). Higher yields of active rFIX were achieved using baby hamster kidney (BHK) cells [61], human hepatoma (HepG2) cells [62], and Chinese hamster ovary (CHO) cell lines [63].

The ability to express biologically active rFIX in CHO cells proved to be very significant, as this cell line has been extensively characterized and used widely in industry to produce recombinant proteins. In addition, CHO cells, deficient in dihydrofolate reductase (DHFR), have been developed to enable high-level expression of transfected proteins [64].

Subsequent development work was undertaken by the Genetics Institute (now part of Wyeth) to develop an rFIX production line with an expression construct encoding hFIX under conditions that enabled isolation and purification of functional FIX protein. Full-length cDNA coding for hFIX was cloned into an expression vector, pMT2-1X, and transfected into a DHFR-negative CHO cell line. Analysis of candidate cell lines revealed the presence of high levels of biologically active FIX, but approximately 20 to 30% of the produced rFIX contained the 18-aa propeptide domain, which must be cleaved for functional activity of FIX [13]. To circumvent this problem, another expression plasmid, pEA-PACE-SOL, was created, which contains the nucleotide sequence for a truncated, soluble form of the serine protease PACE [12]. Coexpression of this protease allowed the selection of rFIX-producing CHO cell lines, which displayed an increased ability to remove the propeptide sequence from rFIX. The selected cell lines were then adapted for growth in suspension culture in a defined, serum-free medium that lacked any blood or plasma products. They were then further adapted to grow in stirred-tank bioreactors [65].

11.5.2   Cell Banking and Stability of the Cell Line

A cell banking process was established for rFIX that initially involved adapting the rFIX-producing CHO cells to a serum-free medium, with recombinant human insulin as the only protein component. Stable cell lines producing the highest levels of rFIX were used to establish a master cell bank (MCB). A working cell bank (WCB) is then established in the same medium as the MCB. Cells from the WCB are used to prepare individual lots of rFIX by initiating the cell culture process and the associated purification steps. An extended cell bank for postprocess analysis is also established. The MCB, WCB, and the end-of-production (EOP) cells used to synthesize rFIX undergo extensive testing for purity, viral safety, and cellular productivity [59].

The MCB, WCB, and EOP cells are routinely screened for the presence of mycoplasma, bacterial and fungal contaminants, and for the presence of viral contaminants such as porcine and bovine parvovirus, murine viruses, and infectious retroviruses. The CHO cells used in rFIX production have been shown to be poor substrates for the growth of many types of viruses, including adventitious human viruses [65,66]. Electron microscopic examination of the MCB and EOP cells has revealed that they contain A- and C-type retroviral particles, as observed with all CHO cells used in recombinant protein production. These particles are not associated with any evidence of infectivity and have been shown by sequencing and cloning studies to be defective [66].

Additional analyses of the plasmid encoding rFIX, pMT2-1X, and the plasmid encoding PACE-SOL, pEA-PACE-SOL, reveals that the copy number of both plasmids remains the same from rFIX WCB through to rFIX EOP cells. Furthermore, both plasmids remain stably integrated and maintained in the genome of the CHO cell line during inoculum buildup and full-scale production [59,65].

11.5.3   The Manufacturing Process for rFIX

rFIX is manufactured in a series of distinct processes, beginning with the synthesis of rFIX in cultured cells, and followed by a number of purification steps, as described below. The purified product is formulated and packaged ready for use [65].

11.5.3.1   rFIX Production Cell Line

rFIX is synthesized in CHO cells, which provide the capacity for glycosylation and other posttranslational modifications, are adaptable to large-scale culture, and can be grown in the absence of animal- and human-derived raw materials, thereby minimizing the risk of pathogen transmission.

The steps in the rFIX cell culture manufacturing process consist of:

1. Inoculating spinner flasks with vials of cells from the WCB
2. Inoculating a 250 L bioreactor from the spinner flasks
3. Expanding the volume of the cell culture in the 250 L bioreactor
4. Inoculating 2500 L bioreactors from the 250 L bioreactor
5. Growing cells in the 2500 L bioreactors
6. Harvesting the cell culture

7. Separating the cells by microfiltration
8. Concentrating the buffer exchanging the cell-free conditioned medium by a combined ultrafiltration–diafiltration step

Once the cell culture medium has been expanded into the 2500 L bioreactors, a batch of rFIX is produced by growing the cells for ~3 d, until they have reached appropriate cell densities. Approximately 80% of the cell suspension is then removed from the bioreactor, the cells are separated by filtration, and the resulting cell-free conditioned medium is taken through the purification steps (Section 11.5.3.2). The remaining 20% of the cell suspension in the bioreactor is resuspended in fresh medium and acts as the source of cells for the next batch production cycle. This process is repeated for up to 20 batch cycles, at which point the production cycles are terminated. To initiate a new production cycle, cells from the WCB are thawed and the process described above is repeated [59,65].

11.5.3.2 Purification of rFIX

A large-scale purification process that does not require the use of monoclonal antibodies for affinity purification has been developed to avoid any potential risk of introducing viral contaminants. rFIX secreted into the medium of CHO cells is purified in a series of filtration and chromatographic separation procedures that ensure a highly purified, consistent product [59,65], as described below:

1. *Ultrafiltration–diafiltration.* rFIX secreted into the cell-culture medium is concentrated by ultrafiltration and subsequently diafiltered against a Tris–NaCl buffer to remove low-molecular-weight components, and also to provide a consistent buffer matrix for loading onto the first chromatography column [65,67].
2. *Q-Sepharose fast flow (FF) chromatography.* The initial chromatographic process uses Q-Sepharose FF (Pharmacia) to bind rFIX from the previous filtration procedure, and also separates rFIX from impurities in the media. It is operated in pseudo-affinity mode, providing a >90% yield, and averts the use of immunoaffinity procedures and their associated risk of viral contamination [67,68]. rFIX binds to the column resin via charge interactions at pH 8.0. The column is washed with buffer of increasing conductivity to remove impurities. rFIX is eluted from the column by the addition of calcium chloride to the buffer at pH 8.0, inducing a conformational change unique to FIX, causing it to detach from the Q-Sepharose FF column. The majority of impurities (>95%) are removed during this first chromatographic step. The remaining steps provide additional removal of low-level impurities [65].
3. *Matrex cellufine sulfate chromatography.* The eluate from the Q-Sepharose FF chromatography step is purified of any residual impurities introduced during the chromatographic procedure by addition to a column consisting of Matrex Cellufine Sulfate (Amicon), a heparin analog. After loading, the column is washed with Tris–NaCl (pH 8.0) buffer to remove loosely bound contaminants. rFIX is then eluted by increasing the NaCl concentration [65,68].
4. *Ceramic hydroxyapatite purification.* Ceramic hydroxyapatite, a synthetic form of calcium phosphate, consisting of spheroidal macroporous particles with high mechanical strength, is used to separate proteins of varying charge on the basis of specific interactions with the resin. In rFIX purification, ceramic hydroxyapatite is used to provide additional capacity for removal of lower specific activity forms of rFIX, and also provides an elution pool in a buffer appropriate for loading onto the final chromatographic column. The pH of the product pool from the Cellufine chromatographic step is adjusted to pH 7.2 prior to loading. The column is

washed with a low concentration potassium phosphate buffer (0.05 M), and rFIX is eluted by increasing, in a stepwise manner, the potassium phosphate concentration to 0.5 M [65,68].

5. *Chelate-EMD-Cu(II) chromatography.* The final step of the chromatographic process in rFIX purification uses a Chelate-EMD resin, composed of a methacrylate polymer to which transition-state metal ions can be bound. Proteins that interact with the metal ions are retained by the resin. Copper (II) is used as the immobilized metal ion in rFIX purification. The product peak pool from the ceramic hydroxyapatite step is loaded onto the column, which is then washed with potassium phosphate/NaCl solution. rFIX is then eluted with imidazole as the displacer. This chromatographic process enables the removal of trace contaminants, including residual levels of host-cell proteins from the CHO cell line [65,66].

6. *NF.* NF is employed as an additional viral safety procedure. The membrane used (Viresolve-70, Millipore) retains molecules with a molecular weight >70 kDa (e.g., viral particles), while smaller molecules (such as rFIX, molecular mass ~55 kDa) pass through the membrane [66,68]. The NF step employed in rFIX production has been shown to effectively remove many model viruses [66].

7. *Final ultrafiltration–diafiltration.* The final ultrafiltration–diafiltration step is designed to exchange the chelate-EMD-Cu(II) product peak pool buffer with the formulation buffer and also to concentrate rFIX further [59,65].

11.5.4   Quality Control Evaluations

Extensive analysis of rFIX is undertaken in accordance with industry standards for recombinant proteins to assess the (1) identity, (2) purity, (3) potency, and (4) safety and quality of the rFIX product obtained from the cell culture and purification processes (the drug substance) and also of the final formulated enzyme product (Section 11.5.5) [59]. In terms of purity, rFIX consists of both zymogen (mature, inactive FIX) and activated products of the mature zymogen. The cleavage products of both pdFIX and rFIX preparations are similar, with both containing FIX and FIX-related species (such as FIXa), although the amounts in each type of preparation may vary. Any non-FIX species derived from host cells or purification processes (including host cell proteins, carbohydrates, and small molecules) are considered impurities [59].

1. *Identity.* The identity of the rFIX drug substance obtained from the cell culture and purification processes is assessed on the basis of its biological activity, electrophoretic mobility, the Gla content, peptide maps, and carbohydrate fingerprinting. The one-stage clotting assay is used to determine the biological activity of the drug substance. Reduced SDS–PAGE analysis is performed to determine identity. Individual batches are compared to a reference to determine drug substance identity. Anion-exchange HPLC is used to determine the Gla content of the rFIX drug substance. Peptide-mass analysis is routinely used to assess batch-to-batch consistency of the rFIX drug substance during manufacture, and is also used to confirm product identity. N-linked oligosaccharide fingerprint analysis is performed routinely to monitor oligosaccharide content, changes in sialic acid content, and modifications to the expected glycan structure [59].

   SDS–PAGE analysis, under reducing conditions, and assessment of the biological activity of rFIX, are performed on each lot of the final rFIX formulated enzyme product produced, as specifications for the identity of the final enzyme product [59].

2. *Purity.* Size-exclusion chromatography (SEC)–HPLC is used to determine the presence of high molecular weight (HMW) material in the drug substance. SDS–PAGE analysis, under reducing conditions, is used to detect impurities. Reverse-phase (RP)–HPLC is also used to determine impurity levels. All species that are neither zymogen nor zymogen-related are defined as impurities and are quantified [59].

Assessment of the purity of the final enzyme product is performed using a number of techniques. SEC–HPLC is used to determine the amount of HMW components present, and SDS–PAGE analysis is used for the detection of other impurities. In addition, analysis of levels of FIXa is performed in accordance with the method described in the European Pharmacopoeia monograph 554 [69].

3. *Potency.* The activity of the rFIX drug substance is measured by a one-stage clotting assay using FIX-deficient plasma with an international reference material for FIX clotting activity, in accordance with the European Pharmacopoeia monograph 554 [69]. The total protein concentration of the rFIX drug substance is determined by SEC–HPLC, and this technique is also used to determine the level of HMW materials. Extensive endotoxin and bioburden testing are carried out using standard methods [59].

Potency specifications for the final rFIX enzyme product have been established to ensure adequate delivery of the dose of rFIX. The potency (IU/vial) is assessed as for the drug substance (see above), with specifications for the final enzyme product requiring that the estimated potency should neither be less than 80%, nor exceed 125% of the stated potency.

4. *Safety and quality.* The safety of the drug substance is assessed through endotoxin and bioburden analyses. The microbiological quality of the drug substance is also assessed.

The safety of the final rFIX enzyme product (defined as the relative freedom from harmful effect to the patient) [59] is ensured by adhering to the following requirements: freedom from contaminating viable organisms as determined by sterility testing, freedom from pyrogenic substances determined by endotoxin testing, freedom from visible particles, and relative freedom from subdivisible particles.

rFIX product quality is determined by the appearance of the product before and after reconstitution in sterile water, pH, residual moisture, and FIXa. The extensive tests described above for bulk drug substances and finished enzyme products are performed on every lot of rFIX produced. More than 150 different tests are carried out on each lot before rFIX is released for sale [59].

11.5.5 rFIX Formulation

A lyophilized form of rFIX has been formulated that is reconstituted easily in sterile water for injection (SWFI) and which exhibits a high degree of stability [70,71]. The final rFIX product is formulated in nonproteinaceous excipients only, and does not contain any albumin, blood-derived products, or preservatives. The excipients used in rFIX formulation are shown in Table 11.3. Glycine provides for a high-quality cake morphology and good overall stability characteristics. Histidine provides optimal buffering stability near physiological pH and minimizes HMW aggregate formation upon storage in the lyophilized state, and also leads to better cake morphology and better long-term stability. Sucrose reduces the development of aggregates while maintaining the protein's biological activity during storage in the freeze-dried state. Polysorbate-80 is used to inhibit aggregation and provides protection for the protein from freezing-induced damage. The mixture of these components enables easy reconstitution of rFIX in SWFI, and ensures that the final product is

TABLE 11.3

Final Formulation of rFIX

Component	Final Concentration	Function
Glycine	260 mM	High-cake morphology
Histidine	10 mM	Buffering stability
Polysorbate-80	0.0005% (pH 6.8)	Inhibits aggregate formation
Sucrose	1%	Protection in freeze-dried state

Adapted from Bush, L., et al., *Semin. Haematol.*, 35 (Suppl. 2), 18–21, 1998.

stable [59,65,70,71]. The long-term stability of the final rFIX formulation was evaluated and found to exhibit a high degree of stability over a variety of storage conditions. In addition, multiple freeze–thaw cycles do not appear to affect rFIX stability [70]. The final rFIX product is neither composed of, nor exposed to, proteins derived from any animal or human sources, thus minimizing any potential risk of acquiring infectious agents during formulation [66,70,72].

BeneFIX is supplied as a sterile, nonpyrogenic, lyophilized cake for reconstitution with SWFI. It is a single-use product intended for intravenous (i.v.) administration. BeneFIX is available in three dosage strengths (250, 500, and 1000 IU per vial). After reconstitution of the powder in SWFI (5 or 10 mL), the concentration of the finished product is either 100 IU/mL (500 or 1000 IU presentations) or 50 IU/mL (250 IU presentation).

11.5.6 rFIX Biochemical Properties and Characterization

Extensive biochemical characterization of rFIX has been carried out [10,72,73] by assessing the following properties:

1. *Primary structure and posttranslational modifications.* The primary structure of rFIX has been analyzed using N- and C-terminal sequencing, in addition to peptide-mapping and mass spectrometry. The aa sequence of rFIX was found to be identical to the A148 allotype of pdFIX. The molecular mass of rFIX (determined by MALDI–TOF analysis) was found to be ~55 kDa, which is higher than the predicted value of 47 kDa, reflecting the additional mass added by posttranslational modifications [59,72].

   The posttranslational modifications of rFIX have been characterized extensively (Table 11.4). Purified rFIX shows a slightly reduced γ-carboxylation level relative to pdFIX within the Gla domain. All 12 glutamic acid sites are occupied (i.e., γ-carboxylated) in pdFIX, while in ~65% of rFIX examined, 12 sites are occupied, ~35% have 11 sites occupied, and ~5% have 10 sites occupied, resulting in an rFIX average of 11.5 Gla residues per molecule. The 11 and 10 Gla isoforms of rFIX have been shown to be undercarboxylated at residue 40, or at residues 36 and 40, respectively. Posttranslational modification of residues 36 and 40 are not required for FIX activity [74]. The three Gla-isoforms have been shown to exhibit similar clotting activities [74], and also exhibit similar phospholipid binding, endothelial cell binding, and activation of FX via the tenase complex [73].

   Within the EGF-like domains, the carbohydrates structure and content, as determined by peptide mapping and mass spectrometry (MS) (O-linked glycosylation at S53 and S61) are the same in rFIX and pdFIX, with some minor differences. The relative proportion of β-hydroxylation of D64 was slightly less in rFIX than

TABLE 11.4

Comparison of Posttranslational Modifications of Plasma-Derived and Recombinant FIX

	pdFIX	rFIX
Primary structure	A148/T148	A148
Secondary/tertiary structure	Indistinguishable by fluorescence, circular dichroism, or analytical ultracentrifugation	
γ-Carboxyglutamic acid (Gla)		
12 of 12 Gla residues	100%	60%
11 of 12 Gla residues	0%	35%
10 of 12 Gla residues	0%	5%
β-Hydroxyaspartic acid (64)	37%	46%
Carbohydrate		
N-linked glycans		
N157 ⎫	High heterogeneity,	Low heterogeneity,
N167 ⎭	fully sialylated	<fully sialylated
O-linked glycans		
S53	$(Xyl)_{1-2}$-Glc	$(Xyl)_2$-Glc
S61	NeuAcGalGlcNAcFuc	NeuAcGalGlcNAcFuc
T159, T167, T172	Classical, partially filled	Classical, partially filled
Y155 sulfation	>90%	<15%
S158 phosphorylation	>90%	<1%

Reproduced from White, G.C., II, et al., *Thrombos. Haemostas.*, 78, 261–265, 1997. With permission from Blackwell Publishing, Oxford, U.K.

in pdFIX [72]. In the rFIX AP domain, <1% of S158 residues are phosphorylated and <15% of Y155 residues is sulfated, while in pdFIX both residues are almost completely modified [72,73]. The carbohydrate contents (O-linked glycosylation at N157 and N167; and N-linked glycosylation at T159, T169, and T172) in rFIX and pdFIX are comparable.

Despite displaying some posttranslational differences to pdFIX, none of these differences appear to be significant to the biological activity of rFIX. However, rFIX has been shown to have a significantly lower (~30%) recovery than pdFIX products seen in patients receiving ERT [75]. The lower levels of sulfation and phosphorylation observed in rFIX may account for the lower recovery rates [72,73].

2. *Higher order structure.* The higher order structure of rFIX was evaluated using a number of biophysical techniques. MALDI–TOF MS analysis, following proteolytic digestion of rFIX, definitively identified 4 of the 11 disulfide bonds found in FIX and tentatively identified the remaining 7 [73]. All disulfide bond assignments were consistent with the proposed structure for FIX based on sequence homologies for the Gla, EGF-like, and catalytic domains [73], in addition to the porcine-FIX crystal-structure domain [23]. Using fluorescence spectroscopy, circular dichroism spectroscopy, and analytical ultracentrifugation, the secondary and tertiary structures of rFIX were similar to high-purity pdFIX [59,73].

3. *Specific activity.* The specific activity of rFIX was analyzed using a one-clot assay with FIX-dependent plasma and activated partial thromboplastin reagent. The mean specific activity of rFIX was determined to be 260 IU/mg, which is significantly higher than that of some four commercially available pdFIX products [73]. The difference in mean specific activities is consistent with the presence of inactive, HMW material and other non-FIX proteins typically found in pdFIX products [73].

4. *Purity.* The purity of rFIX (defined as the lack of non-FIX-related species and HMW materials) was assessed using a number of analytical techniques including SDS–PAGE, SEC–HPLC, RP–HPLC, and N-terminal sequencing [73]. Nonreducing SDS–PAGE analysis revealed a single major band for rFIX, in contrast to multiple bands typically found in several other high-purity pdFIX preparations [73,76]. N-terminal sequencing of the additional bands found in other pdFIX products revealed the presence of non-FIX proteins, including prothrombin and protein C [73]. Reducing SDS–PAGE revealed some additional secondary bands for pdFIX and rFIX preparations. Further analysis by N-terminal sequencing showed that for rFIX, these bands corresponded primarily to activated light and heavy chains of FIXa [73]. FIXa is typically found at low levels in commercially available pdFIX products and also in rFIX preparations [72,73,76,77].

11.5.7 Clinical Evaluation

11.5.7.1 Preclinical Studies

Preclinical testing of new pharmaceuticals generally includes evaluations of: (1) pharmacokinetic (PK) profiles, (2) toxicological studies, and (3) efficacy, if a suitable animal model is available. In addition, coagulation replacement factors generally require additional assessment to evaluate their thrombogenic potential. rFIX has been comprehensively evaluated in several preclinical studies [78–80].

The efficacy of rFIX was assessed using a canine model of hemophilia B, and was compared to a high-purity pdFIX product, Mononine [78]. Both rFIX and pdFIX produced correction of both whole blood-clotting time (WBCT) and partial thromboplastin time (PTT). In addition, the ability to restore hemostasis after experimentally induced bleeding was assessed. These studies indicated that rFIX was as effective as the high-purity pdFIX in normalizing WBCTs and PTTs, as well as in restoring normal hemostasis after bleeding [78,80].

The PK parameters of rFIX have been evaluated in mice, rats, and dogs [78–80]. PK parameters for rFIX were compared to commercially available pdFIX products, and were found to be similar with respect to elimination half-life, distribution, clearance, and maximum FIX concentrations. The only notable difference was that recovery of rFIX was ~30% lower than recovery of pdFIX [80]. The lower recovery of rFIX relative to pdFIX products is thought to be due to slight differences in posttranslational modifications (Section 11.5.6). rFIX has been evaluated for its mutagenic potential. *In vitro* toxicological studies performed on rFIX included the Ames assay and the human lymphocyte chromosomal aberration assay. No evidence of rFIX mutagenicity was observed in either *in vitro* tests, despite the fact that concentrations of rFIX used were 60 to 100 times in excess of normal circulating levels of FIX [80]. Acute to subchronic *in vivo* toxicological studies were conducted in Swiss ICR and CD-1 mice, Sprague–Dawley rats, and Beagle dogs [78–80]. The only adverse effect reported from these studies was the occurrence of thrombosis and consumptive coagulopathy in mice given high doses (>500 IU/kg/d) intraperitoneally for 1 to 7 d; similar effects have been reported with pdFIX products. It has been suggested that these phenomena are unique to mice, as no similar effects were noted in rabbits, dogs, and humans [80].

Preclinical evaluation of thrombogenic potential is an additional preclinical assessment that needs to be performed for human replacement coagulation factor concentrates. The thrombogenic potential of rFIX was assessed and compared with two pdFIX products and a PCC in rabbits, using a modified Wessler stasis model [80,81]. Only 1 out of 28 rabbits tested with rFIX (at doses of 50 to 1000 IU/kg) developed a thrombus, compared to 7 out of 12 using PCC (50 IU/kg), while 5 out of 18 rabbits tested with the two pdFIX (1000 IU/kg) products developed thrombi. It was concluded that rFIX has very low thrombogenic potential, even at doses up to 1000 IU/kg [80,81].

On the basis of the findings from these extensive preclinical studies, rFIX was considered safe for proceeding with clinical trials in the treatment of hemophilia B [59,80].

11.5.7.2   Clinical Studies

To date, four clinical trials have evaluated the effectiveness of rFIX, three being performed in previously treated patients (PTPs, i.e., patients who had previously received other pdFIX or PCC products), and one in previously untreated patients (PUPs). These clinical trials include: (1) a completed study comparing the PK profiles of rFIX with the PK profiles of a high-purity monoclonal-antibody-purified pdFIX (Mononine), (2) a completed study of rFIX efficacy and safety for the prevention and control of spontaneous bleeding episodes, (3) a completed study in PTPs using rFIX during surgery, and (4) an ongoing study of rFIX in PUPs.

11.5.7.2.1   rFIX PK Profile

A double-blind crossover study of 11 patients with hemophilia B receiving a single 50 IU/kg BeneFIX dose compared the PK profile of rFIX with a high-purity pdFIX [82]. There were no statistically significant differences between the rFIX and pdFIX elimination half-lives or mean residence times. There was, however, a significant difference between rFIX and pdFIX *in vivo* recovery rates. rFIX had a ~28% lower *in vivo* recovery than pdFIX, as reported during preclinical studies in animal models [80]. The lower extent of sulfation and lack of phosphorylation observed in rFIX (Section 11.5.6) may account for the lower recovery of rFIX compared with pdFIX [72,73]. A postlicensing study of BeneFIX has confirmed the reported lower recovery of rFIX in comparison with other pdFIXs in PTPs [83]. Other reports have confirmed that the recovery of rFIX in hemophilia B patients is on average 30% lower than that in pdFIX [71,75,84].

11.5.7.2.2   rFIX Efficacy in Spontaneous Bleeding

The safety and efficacy of rFIX was evaluated in an international multicenter study across North America and Europe in 56 PTPs who had received a monoclonal-antibody-purified pdFIX product [82]. Efficacy was assessed for treatment of a bleeding episode and was rated on a four-point scale: (1) "excellent," where the response is deemed to lead to as much and as rapid an improvement as the best pdFIX-related response; (2) "good," where the response is deemed to lead to as much and as rapid an improvement as most pdFIX-related responses; (3) "moderate," deemed not as good as most pdFIX-related responses; and (4) "no response," where no improvement is observed.

The initial trial assessed a total of 1070 hemorrhages requiring 1514 infusions of rFIX (approximate doses of 50 IU/kg) [82]. Over 80% of the hemorrhages required a single rFIX infusion for resolution, while those hemorrhages that involved more than one infusion were typically in response to a major hemorrhage or complicated bleeding episode. 87% of rFIX infusions were rated by self-assessment or clinical observation as providing an "excellent" or "good" response, with less than 1% reporting "no response."

In a postlicensing follow-up study conducted over a 4 year period, which involved over 2758 infusions to treat 1796 bleeds, all bleeding episodes were resolved, with 81% requiring only a single rFIX infusion. The majority of hemorrhages (~91%) were reported to have an "excellent" or "good" response to rFIX treatment [83].

The safety of rFIX was assessed in PTPs and reported on the basis of the development of neutralizing (inhibitor) and nonneutralizing antibodies to rFIX. One PTP developed a low-level transient FIX inhibitor after 9 months of the study, which was associated with a reduced half-life of rFIX, but did not affect rFIX recovery. The inhibitor was undetectable after month 19 of the study, and the half-life of rFIX subsequently returned to baseline levels. rFIX was not associated with any thrombotic events, any severe adverse reactions, or evidence of any viral transmission. It was concluded that rFIX was safe and effective for the treatment of hemophilia B [83].

11.5.7.2.3   rFIX Efficacy during Surgery

rFIX has been evaluated in 28 PTPs (26 males with severe, moderate or mild hemophilia B and 2 female hemophilia B carriers) undergoing a variety of surgical procedures in 12 investigation sites in the United States and Europe. Efficacy was assessed by evaluating parameters such as blood loss during and after surgery, duration of blood loss, transfusion requirement, and persistence of bleeding. Preoperative bolus administration of rFIX (dose range 25 to 155 IU/kg) and postoperative doses (range 30 to 170 IU/kg), maintained by continuous infusion or pulse replacement regimens, were given to each patient. The initial study, involving 12 PTPs reported that clinical responses were rated as excellent or good in 97% of cases [82]. The completed study, involving 28 PTPs, also rates the responses as excellent or good in 97% of cases. rFIX was well tolerated, with no evidence of thromboembolic events, thrombogenicity, or activation of coagulation [85]. Mild adverse reactions (such as coughing, rash development, headache, sneezing, and local phlebitis) were reported in a number of patients. No evidence of viral transmission was reported. One patient developed a low-level transient FIX inhibitor preoperatively, but required no change in treatment, and the condition was subsequently resolved. rFIX was deemed safe and effective in achieving hemostasis in hemophilia B patients undergoing surgery [85].

11.5.7.2.4   Evaluation of rFIX in PUPs

An ongoing trial (study C4918–21) attempts to evaluate the efficacy and safety of rFIX in PUPs with severe to moderate hemophilia B. PUPs are thought to provide the most effective means of assessing inhibitor formation and evidence of viral transmission, having never previously been exposed to blood or plasma products [82]. Initial reports from this study, involving at least 42 patients, report that 92% of responses were rated as "excellent" or "good" [59]. One patient, an 8-month-old, developed a high titer inhibitor after six doses of rFIX, and is now receiving alternative therapy.

11.5.7.2.5   Additional Studies

Based on the initial reports from the clinical trials outlined above, BeneFIX received approval for use in the United States and Canada in 1997, and in 1999 for use in EU countries. In June 2001, the Committee for Proprietary Medicinal Products (CPMP) expressed concern, following the outcome of a Good Clinical Practice inspection conducted on behalf of the European Medicines Agency (EMEA), about the handling of some of the clinical trials [83] that led to the authorization of BeneFIX. In response, Wyeth (license holders in the United States) and Baxter Healthcare (sole European BeneFIX distributor) have established a registry of all new hemophilia B patients in the European Union receiving treatment with rFIX to gather additional safety information on rFIX. Also, two new clinical trials have been initiated to obtain more data on rFIX efficacy and safety. One of these trials concerns severe hemophilia B patients (PTPs and PUPs) under 6 years of age. The other trial will focus on severely to moderately affected children 12 years and older [86,87]. BeneFIX currently remains the only rFIX product licensed for approval in both the European Union and United States.

11.6 Gene Therapy for Hemophilia B

Gene therapy aims to restore, modify, and enhance cellular functions by the insertion of a functional gene into a target cell. Hemophilia B is widely considered an ideal target for gene therapy [5,6,88–92] for a number of reasons: (1) it is caused by single gene defect; (2) a small (1 to 2%) increase in FIX expression levels can achieve palliation, or at least change the degree of phenotypic severity from severe to moderate; (3) FIX, although normally synthesized in liver cells, can also be produced (albeit to a lesser extent) from other tissues such as fibroblasts, endothelial, and muscle cells, thus enabling the use of different cell types for gene therapy; and (4) several animal models are now available for preclinical testing, including mice [93], dogs [94], and apes [95]. Several different vectors for gene delivery have been developed that can be broadly divided into two categories: viral and nonviral vectors.

11.6.1 Viral Vectors for Hemophilia B Gene Therapy

In recent years, extensive progress has been made in the development of vectors for hemophilia gene therapy, including retroviral (oncoretroviral and lentiviral), adenoviral, and adeno-associated viral (AAV) vectors. Adenoviral and AAV in particular have shown therapeutic potential in hemophilia B animal models. Several of these vector systems have achieved near or actual therapeutic levels of FIX, and have also been shown to result in long-term FIX expression in the animal model (reviewed in [88–92,96]).

Some viral vectors encoding hFIX that showed promising results in preclinical studies using animal hemophilia B models have progressed on to clinical trials in humans (reviewed in [88–92]). Despite the success of these vectors in animal models (i.e., long-term FIX expression at therapeutic levels), reports from human clinical trials employing these vectors have dampened the initial enthusiasm. In particular, expression levels of FIX have remained below therapeutic levels, and overall expression has been transient (summarized in Table 11.5). In an ongoing trial concerning FIX administration to liver cells, reports of vector sequences transiently present in semen have raised additional safety concerns [92].

Viral vectors for gene transfer have been fraught with problems relating to production and safety. The preparation and purification of many viral vectors are difficult to achieve, time-consuming, labor-intensive, cost-prohibitive and not amenable to large-scale industrial manufacture [89]. In addition, doubts persist regarding the safety of viral vectors for gene delivery [5,89]. The theoretical risk of insertional mutagenesis by a viral vector integrating into the host chromosome became a reality in a recent gene therapy clinical trial, when two patients developed leukemia due to insertional mutagenesis [97,98]. Administration of an adenoviral vector to a patient suffering from ornithine transcarbamylase deficiency tragically resulted in the death of that patient [99], reinforcing concerns about the potential toxicity of viral vectors. Thus, the development of nonviral gene-transfer technologies enabling stable chromosomal integration and persistent gene expression *in vivo* is highly desirable.

11.6.2 Nonviral Vectors

Due to the safety and efficacy issues associated with viral vector systems, concerted efforts have been made to develop nonviral vectors for use in hemophilia B gene therapy. Nonviral systems include plasmid-based vectors, naked DNA, and DNA encapsulated within delivery systems.

TABLE 11.5

Summary of Gene Therapy Clinical Trials Completed or Underway for Hemophilia B

Sponsor	Vector	Number of Patients	Method of Vector Delivery	Safety Concerns	hFIX Expression Levels	Status	Ref.
Fudan University, China	Oncoretrovirus	2	Intravenous	None apparent	FIX levels to ~4% of normal at 16 months	Closed	[106]
Avigen Inc., CA, USA	AAV serotype 2	8	Intramuscular	None apparent	<1% to a maximum of 1.4% at 1 year	Closed	[92], [107]
Avigen Inc., CA, USA	AAV serotype 2	6	Bolus infusion into hepatic artery	Vector detected in semen of patients for up to 10 weeks	2–3% transient FIX expression in 2 patients	Open	[92], [108]

Plasmid-based vectors offer some advantages over viral systems: (1) plasmid DNA is relatively easy to produce cheaply on a large scale; (2) plasmids typically display low immunogenicity; (3) plasmids are nonpathogenic; and (4) site-specific integration can be achieved. Until recently, plasmid-based delivery systems typically displayed low-level FIX transient expression. Several plasmid-based vector systems have been reported in recent years that seek to address some of these limitations.

Chen et al. [100], using a linear plasmid encoding hFIX administered intraperitoneally, reported a 10- to 100-fold increase in FIX expression from the mouse liver. hFIX expression persisted for over 9 months. Miao, et al. [101] used circular plasmid DNA encoding hFIX to achieve therapeutic levels (0.5 to 2.0 µg/mL) of FIX from mouse liver cells, with expression still maintained after 18 months. Olivares, et al. [102] used a plasmid vector coding for hFIX, and an associated phage integrase-coding plasmid vector that enables stable integration of the hFIX-encoding plasmid into specific sites in the genome of mouse liver cells. hFIX serum levels increased more than tenfold to ~4 µg/mL, similar to normal FIX levels, and remained stable throughout the 8 months of the experiment. Yant, et al. [103] described the successful use of transposon technology for the nonhomologous insertion of the human *F9* gene into genomes of adult mammals using naked DNA. Using the "Sleeping Beauty" transposase, a plasmid encoding hFIX was inserted into the genome of a hemophilia B mouse model. Therapeutic levels of FIX (~3%) were reported, which would convert a severely affected hemophilia B patient to one with a much milder phenotype, and expression was maintained over 5 months. The Sleeping Beauty system was capable of partial correction of the clotting defect in a small animal model, indicating that this technology may have potential in hemophilia B therapy. The system used is amenable to industrial-scale manufacture and should prove useful in human gene therapy applications [103].

Van Raamsdonk, et al. [104] and Hortelano, et al. [105] report alternative methods for hemophilia B gene therapy. Both reports transduced plasmid coding hFIX sequences into secreting mouse C2C12 myoblasts *ex vivo*, and encapsulated the cells into aliginate microcapsules. Hemophilia B mice were transfected with the microcapsules, and treated mice showed increased plasma FIX levels and displayed partial correction of the clotting defect, although expression of FIX in both reports was short-lived and coincided with the emergence of anti-hFIX antibodies. Administration of an immuno-suppressant reduced the antigenic response against the transgene product and improved efficacy. Improvements in vector construction, to ensure higher levels of FIX production, and an increase in the cell density within each microcapsule, should enable an increase in the effective dose of FIX delivered [104].

11.7 Conclusions

pdFIX products for the treatment of hemophilia have been beset by safety problems, with tragic consequences. Numerous high-purity pdFIX products are currently available that undergo extensive screening and viral inactivation steps, minimizing the risk of viral or pathogen transmission. However, fears about possible prion and adventitious viral transmission from pdFIX products remain. A recombinant form of FIX (BeneFIX) has been used successfully since the late 1990s without any incidence of associated viral transmission. rFIX offers a greater margin of safety than pdFIX products, as neither blood products nor proteins of human or animal origin are added during manufacturing. In the future, gene therapy for hemophilia seems a realistic possibility, with some hemophilia gene therapies undergoing clinical trials. Several viral and nonviral vectors are currently being assessed for their efficacy and safety. However, it could be some years before these types of therapies become widely available.

References

1. Brownlee, G.G. and Giangrande, P.L.F, Clotting factors VIII and IX, in *Recombinant Drug Proteins (Milestones in Drug Therapy)*, Buckel, P., Ed., Birkhäuser Verlag, Basel, Switzerland, 2001, pp. 67–88.
2. Thompson, A.R., Structure, function, and molecular defects of Factor IX, *Blood*, 67, 565–572, 1986.
3. Bowen, D.J., Haemophilia A and haemophilia B: Molecular insights, *J. Clin. Pathol: Mol. Pathol.*, 55, 1–18, 2002.
4. Furie, B. and Furie, B.C., The molecular basis of blood coagulation, *Cell*, 53, 505–518, 1988.
5. Castaldo, G., et al., Haemophilia B: From molecular diagnostics to gene therapy, *Clin. Chem. Lab. Med.*, 41, 445–451, 2003.
6. Bolton-Maggs, P.H.B. and Pasi, K.J., Haemophilias A and B, *Lancet*, 361, 1801–1809, 2003.
7. United Kingdom Haemophilia Centre Doctors' Organisation (UKHCDO), Guidelines on the selection and use of therapeutic products to treat haemophilia and other hereditary bleeding disorders, *Haemophilia*, 9, 1–23, 2003.
8. Yoshitake, S., et al., Nucleotide sequence of the gene for human factor IX (antihemophilic factor B), *Biochemistry*, 24, 3736–3750, 1985.
9. Anson, D.S., et al., Gene structure of human anti-haemophilic factor IX, *EMBO J.*, 3, 1053–1064, 1984.
10. White, G.C., II, et al., Mammalian recombinant coagulation proteins: Structure and function, *Transfus. Sci.*, 19, 177–189, 1998.
11. Bentley, A.K., et al., Defective propeptide processing of blood clotting factor IX caused by mutation of arginine to glutamine at position −4, *Cell*, 45, 343–348, 1986.
12. Wasley, L., et al., PACE/furin can process the vitamin-K dependent pro-factor IX precursor within the secretory pathway, *J. Biol. Chem.*, 268, 8458–8465, 1993.
13. Bristol, J.A., et al., Profactor IX: The propeptide inhibits binding to membrane surfaces and activation by XIa, *Biochemistry*, 33, 14136–14143, 1994.
14. Schmidt, A.E. and Bajaj, S.P., Structure–function relationships in factor IX and factor IXa, *Trends Cardiovasc. Med.*, 13, 39–45, 2003.
15. Freedman, S.J., et al., Structure of the calcium ion-bound γ-carboxyglutamic acid-rich domain of factor IX, *Biochemistry*, 34, 12126–12137, 1995.
16. Kirchhofer, D., et al., The tissue factor region that interacts with factor IX and factor X, *Biochemistry*, 39, 7380–7387, 2000.
17. Blostein, M.D., The Gla domain of factor IXa binds to factor VIIIa in the tenase complex, *J. Biol. Chem.*, 278, 31297–31302, 2003.
18. Perrson, K.E.M., et al., The N-terminal epidermal growth factor-like domain of coagulation factor IX. Probing its function in the activation of factor IX and factor X with a monoclonal antibody, *J. Biol. Chem.*, 277, 35616–35624, 2002.
19. Celie, P.H.N., et al., The connecting segment between both epidermal growth factor-like domains in blood coagulation factor IX contributes to stimulation by Factor VIIIa and its isolated A2 domain, *J. Biol. Chem.*, 277, 20214–20220, 2002.
20. Chang, Y-J., et al., Identification of functionally important residues of the epidermal growth factor-2 domain of factor IX by alanine-screening mutagenesis, *J. Biol. Chem.*, 277, 25393–25399, 2002.
21. Hertzberg, M.S., Facey, S.L., and Hogg, P.J., An Arg/Ser substitution in the second epidermal growth factor-like module of factor IX introduces an O-linked carbohydrate and markedly impairs activation by factor XIa and factor VIIa/Tissue factor, *Blood*, 94, 156–163, 1999.

22. Agarwala, K.L., et al., Activation peptide of human factor IX has oligosaccharides *O*-glycosydically linked to threonine residues at 159 and 169, *Biochemistry*, 33, 5167–5171, 1994.

23. Brandstetter, H., et al., X-ray structure of clotting factor IXa: Active site and module structure related to Xase activity and hemophilia B, *Proc. Natl. Acad. Sci., USA*, 92, 9796–9800, 1995.

24. Hopfner, K.-P., et al., Coagulation factor IXa: The relaxed conformation of Tyr99 blocks substrate binding, *Structure*, 7, 989–996, 1999.

25. Harris, R.J., et al., Identification and structural analysis of the tetrasaccharide NeuAcα(2→6)Galβ(1→4)GlcNAcβ(1→3)Fucα1→*O*-Linked to serine 61 of human factor IX, *Biochemistry*, 32, 6539–6547, 1993.

26. Nishimura, H., et al., Identification of a disaccharide (Xyl-Glc) and a trisaccharide (Xyl$_2$-Glc) *O*-glycosydically linked to a serine residue in the first epidermal growth factor-like domain of human factors VII and IX and protein Z and bovine protein Z, *J. Biol. Chem.*, 264, 20320–20325, 1989.

27. Soriano-Garcia, M., et al., The Ca^{2+} ion and membrane binding structure of the Gla domain of Ca-prothrombin fragment 1, *Biochemistry*, 31, 2554–2566, 1992.

28. Di Scipio, R.G., Kurachi, K., and Davie, E.W., Activation of human factor IX (Christmas factor), *J. Clin. Invest.*, 61, 1528–1538, 1978.

29. Østerud, B. and Rapaport, S.I., Activation of factor IX by the reaction product of tissue factor and factor VII: Additional pathway for initiating blood coagulation, *Proc. Natl. Acad. Sci., USA*, 74, 5260–5264, 1977.

30. Gailani, D., Activation of factor IX by factor Xia, *Trends Cardiovasc. Med.*, 10, 198–204, 2000.

31. www.wfh.org; The World Federation of Hemophilia (WFH) organisation, based at 1425 René Lévesque Blvd. W., Suite 1010, Montréal, Québec, H3G 1T7 Canada. See also links within this site for list of approved therapeutics and manufacturers, and for links to national haemophiliac societies around the world.

32. Biggs, R., et al., Christmas Disease, a condition previously mistaken for haemophilia, *Br. Med. J.*, 2, 1378–1382, 1952.

33. Aggeler, P.M., et al., Plasma thromboplastin component (PTC) deficiency: A new disease resembling haemophilia, *Proc. Soc. Exp. Biol. Med.*, 79, 692–694, 1952.

34 Green, P.M., et al., Haemophilia B: Database of point mutations and short additions and deletions: Twelfth edition, Last updated, Dec. 2003, (www.kcl.ac.uk/ip/petergreen/intro.html).

35. Giannelli, F., et al., Gene deletions in patients with haemophilia B and anti-factor IX antibodies, *Nature*, 303, 181–182, 1983.

36. Giannelli, F., et al., Haemophilia B: Database of point mutations and short additions and deletions, Eighth edition, *Nucleic Acid Res.*, 26, 265–268, 1998.

37. Biggs, R., Thirty years of haemophilia treatment in Oxford, *Br. J. Haematol.*, 13, 452–463, 1967.

38. Darby, S.C., et al., on behalf of the UK Haemophilia Centre Directors' Organisation, Mortality before and after HIV infection in the complete UK population of haemophiliacs, *Nature*, 377, 79–82, 1995.

39. Darby, S.C., et al., on behalf of the UK Haemophilia Centre Directors' Organisation, Mortality from liver cancer and liver disease in haemophiliac men and boys in UK given blood products contaminated with hepatitis C, *Lancet*, 350, 1425–1431, 1997.

40. Rosenberg, P.S. and Goedert, J.J., Estimating the incidence of HIV infections among persons with haemophilia in the United States of America, *Stat. Med.*, 17, 155–168, 1998.

41. Teitel, J.M., Viral safety of haemophilia treatment products, *Ann. Med.*, 32, 485–492, 2000.

42. Strong, D.M. and Katz, L., Blood-bank testing for infectious diseases: How safe is blood transfusion? *Trends Mol. Med.*, 8, 355–358, 2002.

43. Kasper, C.K., Concentrate safety and efficacy, *Haemophilia*, 8, 161–165, 2002.

44. Alonso-Rubiano, E., et al., Hepatitis G virus in clotting factor concentrates, *Haemophilia*, 9, 110–115, 2003.

45. Flores, G., et al., Seroprevalence of parvovirus B19, cytomegalovirus, hepatitis A virus and hepatitis E virus antibodies in haemophiliacs treated exclusively with clotting-factor concentrates considered safe against human immunodeficiency and hepatitis C viruses, *Haemophilia*, 1, 115–117, 1995.

46. Burnouf, T. and Radosevich, M., Nanofiltration of plasma-derived biopharmaceuticals, *Haemophilia*, 9, 24–37, 2003.

47. Tateishi, J., et al., Scrapie removal using Planova® virus removal filters, *Biologicals*, 29, 17–25, 2001.

48. Foster, P.R., Prions and blood products, *Ann. Med.*, 32, 501–513, 2000.

49. Hill, A.F., et al., Investigation of variant Creutzfeldt-Jakob disease and other human prion diseases with tonsil biopsy samples, *Lancet*, 353, 183–189, 1999.

50. Llewelyn, C.A., et al., Possible transmission of variant Creutzfeldt-Jakob disease by blood transfusion, *Lancet*, 363, 417–422, 2004.

51. Aguzzi, A. and Glatzel, M., vCJD tissue distribution and transmission by transfusion – A worst-case scenario coming true? *Lancet*, 363, 411–412, 2004.

52. Aguzzi, A. and Polymenidou, M., Mammalian prion biology: One century of evolving concepts, *Cell*, 116, 313–327, 2004.

53. www.haemophilia.org.uk; The UK Haemophilia Society, based at Chesterfield House, 385 Euston Road, London NW1 3AU, UK.

54. Kasper, C.K. and Costa e Silvia, M., Registry of Clotting Factor Concentrates, 4th ed., 2003. Published by the WFH and available at the url: http://www.wfh.org/content_documents/FF_monographs/FF6_factorregistry2003.pdf

55. Farrugia, A., Plasma for fractionation: Safety and quality issues, *Haemophilia*, 10, 334–340, 2004.

56. Choo, K.H., et al., Molecular cloning of the gene for human antihaemophilic factor IX, *Nature*, 299, 178–180, 1982.

57. Kurachi, K. and Davie, E.W., Isolation and characterization of a cDNA coding for human factor IX, *Proc. Natl. Acad. Sci., USA*, 79, 6461–6464, 1982.

58. Yoshitake, S., et al., Nucleotide sequence of the gene for human factor IX (antihemophilic factor B), *Biochemistry*, 24, 3736–3750, 1985.

59. Edwards, J. and Kirby, N., Recombinant Coagulation Factor IX (BeneFIX®), in *Biopharmaceuticals, An Industrial Perspective*, Walsh, G. and Murphy, B., Eds., Kluwer Academic Publishers, The Netherlands, 1999, pp. 73–108.

60. Anson, D.S., Austen, D.E.G., and Brownlee, G.G., Expression of active human clotting factor IX from recombinant DNA clones in mammalian cells, *Nature*, 315, 683–685, 1985.

61. Busby, S., et al., Expression of active human factor IX in transfected cells, *Nature*, 316, 271–273, 1985.

62. de la Salle, H., et al., Active γ-carboxylated factor IX expressed using recombinant DNA techniques, *Nature*, 316, 268–270, 1985.

63. Kaufman, R.J., et al., Expression, purification and characterisation of recombinant γ-carboxylated factor IX synthesized in Chinese hamster ovary cells, *J. Biol. Chem.*, 261, 9622–9628, 1986.

64. Chasin, L. and Urlaub, G., Isolation of Chinese hamster ovary cell mutants deficient in dihydrofolate reductase activity, *Proc. Natl. Acad. Sci., USA*, 77, 4216–4220, 1980.

65. Harrison, S., et al., The manufacturing process for recombinant factor IX, *Semin. Haematol.*, 35, 4–10, 1998.

66. Adamson, S.R., et al., Viral safety of recombinant factor IX, *Semin. Haematol.*, 35, 22–27, 1998.

67. Bonam, D., et al., Purification of recombinant factor IX by pseudoaffinity anion exchange chromatography, *Blood*, 86(Suppl. 1), 865a, 1995.

68. Foster, W.B., et al., Development of a process for purification of recombinant human factor IX, *Blood*, 86(Suppl. 1), 870a, 1995.

69. European Department for the Quality of Medicines, Freeze-dried human coagulation factor IX, European Pharmacopoeia, 554, Strasbourg, France, 1987.

70. Bush, L., et al., The formulation of recombinant factor IX: Stability, robustness, and convenience. *Semin. Haematol.*, 35(Suppl. 2), 18–21, 1998.

71. Chowdary, P., et al., Recombinant factor IX (BeneFIX®) by adjusted continuous infusion: A study of sterility, stability and clinical experience, *Haemophilia*, 7, 140–145, 2001.

72. White, G.C., II, Beebe, A., and Nielsen, B., Recombinant Factor IX, *Thrombos. Haemostas.*, 78, 261–265, 1997.

73. Bond, M., et al., Biochemical characterisation of recombinant factor IX, *Semin. Haematol.*, 35, 11–17, 1998.

74. Gillis, S., et al., γ-carboxyglutamic acids 36 and 40 do not contribute to human factor IX function, *Protein Sci.*, 6, 185–196, 1997.

75. Ewenstein, B., et al., Pharmacokinetic analysis of plasma-derived and recombinant FIX concentrates in previously treated patients with moderate or severe hemophilia B, *Transfusion*, 42, 190–196, 2002.

76. Limentani, S.A., Gowell, K.P., and Deitcher, S.R., *In vitro* characterisation of high purity Factor IX concentrates for the treatment of haemophilia B, *Thrombos. Haemostas.*, 73, 584–591, 1995.

77. Gray, E., et al., Measurement of activated factor IX in factor IX concentrates: Correlation with *in vivo* thrombogenicity, *Thrombos. Haemostas.*, 73, 675–679, 1995.

78. Brinkhous, K.M., et al., Recombinant human factor IX: Replacement therapy, prophylaxis, and pharmacokinetics in canine hemophilia B, *Blood*, 88, 2603–2610, 1996.

79. Keith, J.C., Jr., et al., Evaluation of recombinant human factor IX: pharmacokinetic studies in the rat and the dog, *Thrombos. Haemostas.*, 73, 101–105, 1995.

80. Schaub, R.G., et al., Preclinical studies of recombinant factor IX, *Semin. Hematol.*, 35(Suppl. 2), 28–32, 1998.

81 Ferranti, T.J., et al., Recombinant human factor IX has low thrombogenicity in the Wessler stasis model, *Thrombos. Haemostas.*, 73 (Abstr.), 1014, 1995.

82. White, G.C., II, et al., Clinical evaluation of recombinant factor IX, *Semin. Hematol.*, 35(Suppl. 2), 33–38, 1998.

83. Roth, D.A., et al., Human recombinant factor IX: Safety and efficacy studies in hemophilia B patients previously treated with plasma-derived factor IX concentrates, *Blood*, 98, 3600–3606, 2001.

84. Morfini, M., Pharmacokinetics of factor VIII and factor IX, *Haemophilia*, 9(Suppl. 1), 94–100, 2003.

85. Ragni, M.V., et al., Use of recombinant factor IX in subjects with haemophilia B undergoing surgery, *Haemophilia*, 8, 91–97, 2002.

86. Haase, M., Human recombinant factor IX: Safety and efficacy studies in hemophilia B patients previously treated with plasma-derived factor IX concentrates, *Blood*, 100, 4242, 2002.

87 Marder, H. and Ewenstein, B.M., Human recombinant factor IX: Safety and efficacy studies in hemophilia B patients, *Blood*, 100, 4242–4243, 2002.

88. Liras, A., Gene therapy for haemophilia: The end of a 'royal pathology' in the third millennium?, *Haemophilia*, 7, 441–445, 2001.

89. Nathwani, A.C., Davidoff, A.M., and Tuddenham, E.G.D., Prospects for therapy of haemophilia, *Haemophilia*, 10, 309–318, 2004.

90. Walsh, C.E., Gene therapy progress and prospects: Gene therapy for the hemophilias, *Gene Therapy*, 10, 999–1003, 2003.

91. Monahan, P.E. and White, G.C., II, Hemophilia gene therapy: Update, *Curr. Opin. Hematol.*, 9, 430–436, 2002.

92. High, K.A., Clinical gene transfer studies for hemophilia B, *Sem. Thrombos. Hemostas.*, 30, 257–267, 2004.

93. Lin, H.F., et al., A coagulation factor IX-deficient mouse model for human hemophilia B, *Blood*, 90, 3962–3966, 1997.

94. Evans, J.P., et al., Canine hemophilia B resulting from a point mutation with unusual consequences, *Proc. Natl. Acad. Sci., USA*, 86, 10095–10099, 1989.

95. Lozier, J.N., et al., The Rhesus macaque as an animal model for hemophilia B gene therapy, *Blood*, 93, 1875–1881, 1999.

96. Lillicrap, D., Hemophilia gene therapy: It's a matter of expression, *Blood*, 103, 5–6, 2004.

97. Hacein-Bey-Abina, S., et al., LMO2-associated clonal T cell proliferation in two patients after gene therapy for SCID-X1, *Science*, 302, 415–419, 2003.

98. Hacein-Bey-Abina, S., et al., A serious adverse event after successful gene therapy for X-linked severe combined immunodeficiency, *New Engl. J. Med.*, 348, 255–256, 2003.

99. Raper, S.E., et al., Fatal systemic inflammatory response syndrome in a ornithine transcarbamylase deficient patient following adenoviral gene transfer, *Mol. Genet. Metab.*, 80, 148–158, 2003.

100. Chen, Z.Y., et al., Linear DNAs concatemerize *in vivo* and result in sustained transgene expression in mouse liver, *Mol. Ther.*, 3, 403–410, 2001.

101. Miao, C.H., Ye, X., and Thompson, A.R., Long-term and therapeutic-level hepatic gene expression of human factor IX after naked plasmid transfer *in vivo*, *Mol. Ther.*, 3, 947–957, 2001.

102. Olivares, E.C., et al., Site-specific genomic integration produces therapeutic Factor IX levels in mice, *Nat. Biotechnol.*, 20, 1124–1128, 2002.
103. Yant, S.R., et al., Somatic integration and long-term transgene expression in normal and haemophilic mice using a DNA transposon system, *Nat. Genet.*, 25, 35–41, 2000.
104. Van Raamsdonk, J.M., et al., Treatment of hemophilia B in mice with nonautologous somatic gene therapeutics, *J. Lab. Clin. Med.*, 139, 35–42, 2002.
105. Hortelano, G., et al., Sustained and therapeutic delivery of factor IX in nude hemophiliac mice by encapsulated C2C12 myoblasts: Concurrent tumorigenesis, *Haemophilia*, 7, 207–214, 2001.
106. Qui, X., et al., Implantation of autologous skin fibroblast genetically modified to secrete clotting factor IX partially corrects the hemorrhagic tendencies in two hemophilia B patients, *Chin. Med. J.*, 109, 543–552, 1996.
107. Manno, C.S., et al., AAV-mediated factor IX gene transfer to skeletal muscle in patients with severe hemophilia B, *Blood*, 101, 2963–2972, 2003.
108. High, K.A., et al., Immune responses to AAV and to factor IX in a phase I study of AAV-mediated liver-directed gene transfer for hemophilia B, *Blood*, 102, 154a–155a, 2003.

12

α-L-*Iduronidase: The Development of Aldurazyme (Laronidase)*

Emil Kakkis

CONTENTS

12.1 Introduction and Overview

Aldurazyme® (laronidase) is a form of recombinant human α-L-iduronidase (rhIDU) developed as an enzyme replacement therapy (ERT) for the rare recessive genetic disorder, mucopolysaccharidosis I (MPS I) [1]. The α-L-iduronidase enzyme (EC 3.2.1.76) is normally located and active in the lysosome, where it participates in the sequential enzymatic degradation process of certain glycosaminoglycans (GAGs). Patients with MPS I are genetically deficient in α-L-iduronidase and accumulate undegraded GAG chains within lysosomes, leading to a profound and pervasive lysosomal storage disorder (Figure 12.1).

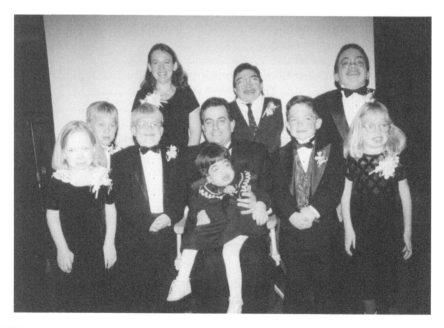

FIGURE 12.1
MPS I patients. A group of nine MPS I patients from the first clinical study of Aldurazyme with the author. The patients cover the spectrum of severe Hurler (patient sitting with the author) to Scheie (tall woman in the back).

The disorder causes substantial disease in every organ and body system, its severe form leading to death by the age of 10 years. The development of an ERT for these patients is based on the seminal discoveries in the 1960s and 1970s that elucidated the critical role of exogenous enzyme uptake and targeting to lysosomes via the mannose 6-phosphate receptor (M6PR) in the "correction" of the defect in Hurler fibroblasts [2–5]. The translation of those early discoveries to the therapeutic known as Aldurazyme required 30 years of research on the biochemistry, cell biology, and molecular biology of the enzyme and MPS I disease [6].

The specific development of Aldurazyme began with the cloning of the human α-L-iduronidase cDNA in 1991 that allowed the development of recombinant Chinese hamster ovary (CHO) cells that overexpress and secrete the human α-L-iduronidase enzyme [7–9]. With these recombinant enzyme-producing cells, microcarrier-based culture processes were developed, and standard column chromatography was designed to purify the enzyme. This product was used to study ERT in the canine MPS I model to establish the dose and efficacy of enzyme therapy in the resolution of lysosomal storage in diverse tissues [10,11]. Based on these preclinical studies, a phase-1 open-label clinical study in ten MPS I patients was performed. The study demonstrated a reduction in measures of lysosomal storage and some clinical benefit was also observed [12]. This study was not sufficient to allow registration of the product and was followed by a randomized, double-blind, placebo-controlled, phase-3 study conducted in 45 MPS I patients. The study demonstrated improvement in the primary endpoints of respiratory function and walking distance [13].

The study results and a set of product briefing documents were reviewed at a meeting of the Endocrinologic and Metabolic Advisory Committee convened by the Food and Drug Administration (FDA) on January 15, 2003. The committee voted 12 to 0 that the data on both the respiratory and walk-test endpoints represented clinically meaningful benefit. Following this advisory committee vote, Aldurazyme was approved on April 25, 2003 by the FDA in the United States. In the United States, the label indication reads:

> ALDURAZYME is indicated for patients with Hurler and Hurler-Scheie forms of Mucopolysaccharidosis I (MPS I) and for patients with the Scheie form who have moderate to severe symptoms. The risks and benefits of treating mildly affected patients with the Scheie form have not been established.

> ALDURAZYME has been shown to improve pulmonary function and walking capacity. ALDURAZYME has not been evaluated for effects on the central nervous system manifestations of the disorder.

In the European Union, a positive opinion from the Committee for Proprietary Medicinal Products (CPMP) was received on February 21, 2003. The European Medicines Agency (EMEA) formally approved Aldurazyme on June 11, 2003. The label indication in the European Union reads:

> Aldurazyme is indicated for long-term enzyme replacement therapy in patients with a confirmed diagnosis of Mucopolysaccharidosis I (MPS I; α-L-iduronidase deficiency) to treat the non-neurological manifestations of the disease.

Following these approvals, Aldurazyme was launched in the United States and the European Union in May and June 2003, respectively. Regulatory filings for the product continue worldwide and MPS I patients in more than 20 countries now receive Aldurazyme ERT. The complete prescribing information is given in the package insert for Aldurazyme.

12.2 Biochemistry and Genetics of Recombinant α-L-Iduronidase

rhIDU is produced using a cDNA copy of the human α-L-iduronidase mRNA message that is overexpressed in recombinant CHO cells [7–9]. The cDNA codes for a protein of 653 amino acids containing six potential N-linked oligosaccharide sites, all of which are utilized (Figure 12.2). The recombinant enzyme undergoes signal peptide cleavage and posttranslational addition of the N-linked oligosaccharide chains as well as mannose 6-phosphate addition. About 50% of the overexpressed enzyme is trafficked directly to the lysosomes, as usually occurs during α-L-iduronidase synthesis at normal levels [9]. The other half of the enzyme is secreted into the media where it may be recovered for purification. The secreted enzyme can be taken up by cells via the M6PR and transported in vesicles that ultimately fuse with primary lysosomes, similar to the process for endogenous enzyme [9,14]. Under the acidic conditions of the lysosome, the enzyme acts to cleave terminal iduronic acid residues from the GAGs, heparan sulfate and dermatan sulfate, as part of a sequence of steps involving numerous lysosomal hydrolases and other enzymes [1].

12.2.1 Enzyme Composition, Synthesis, and Biochemical Action

12.2.1.1 Protein and Gene Sequence and Structure

The coding sequence of human α-L-iduronidase encodes a 653-amino acid protein derived from a gene consisting of 14 exons and covering about 20 kb of sequence on chromosome 4p, close to the Huntington disease locus [15]. The published sequence is one of the many polymorphic forms of the iduronidase enzyme that are found in the human population [16]. The sequence used in the production of Aldurazyme contains one of these polymorphisms, in which a glutamine at position 33 (or position 8 in the mature protein) is replaced

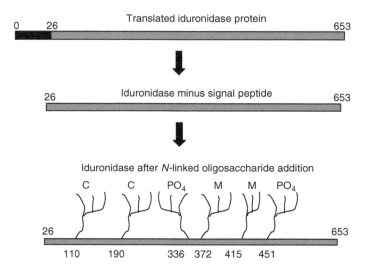

FIGURE 12.2
Iduronidase protein structure and processing. The iduronidase protein is initially synthesized as a 653-amino acid polypeptide and the 25-amino acid signal sequence is clipped off during translation. The protein has six N-linked oligosaccharides added during translation. After carbohydrate addition, the sugars undergo trimming and additions leading to complex or hybrid chains (C), high-mannose 5-9 chains (M), and phosphorylated high-mannose chains (PO₄).

with histidine, a polymorphism present in about 9% of the Caucasian population [16]. There is no known effect of this polymorphism on enzyme activity or stability, although other polymorphisms may affect residual activity of mutant iduronidase proteins, which may account for some heterogeneity between patients with similar mutations.

After synthesis in the rough endoplasmic reticulum, the signal peptide is cleaved. Although the processing step is not well defined for normal α-ʟ-iduronidase due to the difficulties in analyzing the very low normal levels of endogenous protein, the recombinant protein has A26 at its N terminus (Figure 12.2). This N terminus is not well predicted by the von Heijne rules for signal peptide cleavage and so it is not clear if further trimming occurs after the initial signal peptide cleavage [17]. After transport to the lysosome, further clipping of the N terminus can occur and so the terminal amino acids from purified native human α-ʟ-iduronidase may not reflect the original N-terminal cleavage site [7,9]. After transport to the lysosome, recombinant α-ʟ-iduronidase also undergoes an additional N-terminal cleavage that is documented by pulse–chase studies, but it is not clear whether this clip leads to the dissociation of the clipped peptide from the protein, or whether this N-terminal piece remains associated with the enzyme [9].

The complete tertiary structure for α-ʟ-iduronidase has not been determined by X-ray crystallography, although there are structure models proposed using predictive rules based on primary enzyme sequence [18]. The tertiary structure of the protein is active as a monomer in solution in normal salt conditions. No consistent higher-order structure has been described or appears to be required for enzyme activity, unlike β-glucuronidase, for example, which exists normally as a homotetramer and needs to be a homodimer to attain enzyme activity.

12.2.1.2 N-Linked Carbohydrate Structure

There are six Asn-X-Ser/Thr recognition sites for the addition of N-linked oligosaccharides in the α-ʟ-iduronidase protein, and based on analysis and mutagenesis experiments, all sites are used and oligosaccharide addition at all sites are likely required for optimal enzyme folding and activity [9,19]. The sites for addition are site 1 (N110), 2 (N190), 3 (N336), 4 (N372), 5 (N415), and 6 (N451). The pattern of the predominant oligosaccharide type on each was elucidated by Zhao, et al. [19], using a variety of techniques including peptide mapping and matrix-assisted laser desorption ionization–time-of-flight (MALDI–TOF) (Figure 12.2). Sites 3 and 6 have the mannose 6-phosphate chains added, whereas sites 4 and 5 are predominantly high-mannose and sites 1 and 2 are predominantly complex or hybrid type. No O-linked sugars were identified on recombinant α-ʟ-iduronidase. It is not possible to determine precisely whether these identified sugar structures are comparable to those originally found on native α-ʟ-iduronidase, although the larger apparent molecular mass of the recombinant product suggests that the native lysosomal form of the enzyme shows some degradation or differences in the charge (less sialic acid or phosphate) of its oligosaccharide chains presumably due to postlysosomal trimming.

Further analysis of the sugar structures on recombinant α-ʟ-iduronidase have been undertaken by fluorescence-assisted carbohydrate electrophoresis (FACE) [20]. The analysis demonstrates that a substantial fraction of all oligosaccharides contain phosphate and that the *bis*-phosphorylated mannose 7 structure comprises about 11 to 20% of all oligosaccharides found at all sites [21]. This FACE data, combined with the high binding fraction to M6PR columns and the high affinity in the uptake assay showing that essentially all enzyme binds, indicate that a very high fraction (> 90%) of recombinant α-ʟ-iduronidase is phosphorylated. The FACE assay is used during both process development and product release to ensure that sufficient levels of the *bis*-phosphorylated mannose-7 structure is present on the enzyme.

12.2.1.3   *Intracellular Trafficking and Uptake Via M6PR*

After synthesis and initial carbohydrate transfer from the dolichol phosphate carrier, endogenous and recombinant α-L-iduronidase undergo the trim backprocessing typical for glycoproteins leaving high-mannose chains. For certain chains on the protein, a special two-step glycosylation reaction attaches the *N*-acetylglucosamine residue via the phosphate, and then cleaves off the sugar uncovering the phosphate group. Other chains undergo further glycosylation to complex or hybrid structures. In the Golgi, the exposed mannose 6-phosphate residues bind to the small cation-dependent M6PR, which leads to the trafficking of the protein through vesicular transport to deliver the enzyme to primary lysosomes. The enzyme then resides in the lysosome and is relatively resistant to the low pH and proteolytic environment, with a half-life of about 4 to 5 d for recombinant enzyme in Hurler fibroblasts [9]. For overexpressed recombinant α-L-iduronidase, about 50% of the enzyme is secreted into the medium compared with only trace secretion in normal cells.

Once outside the cells, the recombinant α-L-iduronidase with mannose 6-phosphate can be rapidly and efficiently taken up via the larger cation-independent M6PR present on the cell surface of CHO cells or other cell types. For uptake into Hurler fibroblasts, the *bis*-phosphorylated chains interact with high affinity with the overall half-maximal uptake occurring at ~1 nM. Once bound to the surface of cells, the M6PR endocytoses the enzyme and rapidly recycles to the surface. The process is efficient and rapid and can lead to manyfold normal levels of enzyme in Hurler fibroblasts within an hour of exposure to saturating concentration of enzyme. This uptake constant can be measured by assessing the accumulation of recombinant α-L-iduronidase in extracts of the Hurler cells, after exposing plates of Hurler cells to different concentrations of the enzyme. A plot of enzyme activity in the medium vs. enzyme activity in the extract shows receptor saturation as expected (Figure 12.3). By performing a Michaelis–Menten-type kinetic analysis of the uptake data using a double-reciprocal plot, and calculating the K_M from the slope and V_{max} (1/Y intercept), a K_{uptake} value can be determined (Figure 12.3). This value is an accurate estimation of the uptake affinity for the enzyme although it is not technically a true K_D since no equilibrium state is reached. This uptake assessment is used as a test of enzyme quality and potency during process development and release testing of the Aldurazyme product for commercial use.

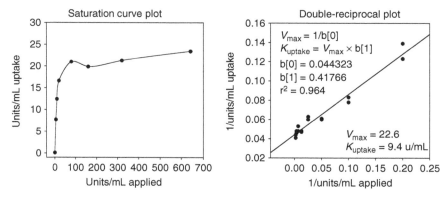

FIGURE 12.3
Uptake curve and Michaelis–Menten double-reciprocal plot. On the left is shown the uptake activity in Hurler cells as a function of medium concentration of iduronidase. Note that the activity in the cells rises and the reaches a plateau when the receptor-mediated uptake reaches saturation. On the right is a double-reciprocal plot of the uptake data that shows a linear relationship. From the intercept, V_{max} can be calculated and from the V_{max} and slope, the apparent K_M can be determined, shown here in enzyme units/mL.

12.2.1.4 Biochemical Function in GAG Metabolism

Recombinant α-ʟ-iduronidase is only one of many enzymes required for the sequential breakdown of two GAGs, heparan sulfate and dermatan sulfate. After uptake into Hurler fibroblasts, the enzyme works very efficiently to degrade GAG stored in the lysosomes. Complete clearance and normalization of stored GAG can occur with only a few percent of normal α-ʟ-iduronidase levels. If the GAGs are labeled using $^{35}SO_4$, and the cell extracts treated with boiling 80% ethanol, only GAGs remain insoluble and can be precipitated and purified [9]. Using $^{35}SO_4$ labeling and the extraction procedure, Hurler cell GAG accumulation can be studied *in vitro*. When Hurler cells are labeled with $^{35}SO_4$ and incubated with enzyme at different concentrations, the half-maximal correction of abnormal GAG accumulation occurs at a very low enzyme level of about 1 pM, or 1/1000th of the uptake constant of 1 nM. This result indicates the high potency and efficiency of the uptake process, and the ability of exogenous α-ʟ-iduronidase to act in concert with other endogenous enzymes to cleave accumulated GAG back to normal levels.

12.3 Clinical Deficiency of α-ʟ-Iduronidase and MPS I

The clinical manifestations for MPS I are pervasive and complicated, and there is no family history for the vast majority of families since it is inherited as an autosomal-recessive disease [1]. Its diagnosis in a child can take several years at times, and the management of these patients for the most part, consists of symptomatic care. When the enzyme levels of patients are analyzed, it is clear that all patients, independent of the severity of the disease, are deficient in α-ʟ-iduronidase to levels below the usual detection limits of clinical assays. Using highly sensitive assays, it is possible to detect very tiny amounts of enzyme of less than 1% normal in patients with milder disease. The trace enzyme activity observed is consistent with the molecular genetics; mutations that allow a small amount of normal enzyme or a small amount of residual activity lead to a milder phenotype [22]. These tiny amounts of enzyme are just sufficient to substantially change the course of the illness. This fact is one of the reasons why the disease was originally targeted as a good candidate for ERT.

12.3.1 Clinical Characteristics of MPS I

The presentation of an MPS I patient for diagnosis can occur at any time from birth to adulthood, depending on the severity of the disease [1]. Most Hurler and Hurler-Scheie patients present with one or more of a variety of clinical problems within the first few years of their life. Patients can show signs of developmental delay and experience frequent respiratory and ear infections, cardiac disease, enlarged liver and spleen, joint stiffness, excessive head growth, hernias, and malformation of the spine. Within a few years time, the patients will usually manifest, to varying degrees, medical problems in every body system.

The patients may grow rapidly during the first year of life, but thereafter will exhibit a failure to thrive and will, in general, be well below the 5th percentile in height and often in weight. Their facial appearance will gradually coarsen due to storage of GAG within the bones and connective tissues, and their enlarging tongue will often protrude. Progressive storage in the brain in the severe Hurler form will lead to declining developmental function and an IQ below 50 by age 3.

MPS I patients suffer recurring sinus, ear, and pulmonary infections that may require hospitalization for an illness that in a normal child would present as a simple cold. Their airway and breathing are compromised owing to storage of GAG in the tongue, airway, and lymph nodes, as well as owing to an abnormal ribcage and the enlarged liver and spleen that push up on the diaphragm. Their heart can experience difficulties both from valvular thickening and regurgitation as well as from coronary artery disease and pulmonary hypertension. Young, severely afflicted patients can die from coronary artery obstruction, whereas older, intermediately and mildly afflicted patients may have more problems with mitral and aortic valve disease.

Storage of GAG within the periarticular tissues and the synovium, along with bony malformation, leads to joint stiffness and pain, almost like rheumatoid arthritis in some patients. The joint stiffness can be profound, leading to difficulty performing the tasks of everyday living such as washing, combing one's hair, bending, and tying one's shoe. Many patients cannot lift their arms high enough to scratch their ear or touch their head.

The diverse problems are usually managed by symptomatic treatments, such as surgery to stabilize the spine, frequent antibiotics for infections, or oxygen therapy for respiratory insufficiency, but in general, these treatments do not prevent the inexorable decline and death of these patients. At the severe end of the spectrum, death occurs in almost all cases by age 10, and at the moderate and less severe end of the spectrum, by the teenage years and 20s, for the most part. Some young severe Hurler patients undergo bone marrow transplantation (BMT) when they are below age 2, which has been shown to improve their physical condition and possibly stabilize their declining brain function. The procedure has substantial morbidity and mortality, and a better treatment alternative is desirable.

12.3.1.1 Pathophysiology of MPS I

The pathophysiology of MPS I is based on the storage of GAG, but the exact mechanism behind how storage causes the clinical manifestations of the disease is not always clear; they may be due to diverse mechanisms, depending on the patient and the tissue. GAG itself is not toxic, but the distortion of cells and the dysfunction or death and lysis of cells with excessive storage in all likelihood plays an important role. The presence of excessive GAG within the extracellular space may also alter development and physiology, although clear and direct proof of this is limited. In the brain, the excessive activation of macrophages with lysosomal storage may lead to the injury of neurons and contribute to the neurological decline of patients. The deformation and malformation of bone structure is cause by the storage within the cells that make or remodel the bone, leading to misshapen and weak bone. The storage in the airway epithelium and soft tissues like the tonsil, blocks the airway and is a more direct example of the swelling and tissue engorgement that underlies MPS disease. The physical effects of storage also have direct clinical effects on patients, for example, the enlarged liver and spleen inhibit breathing, and cause difficulty while bending and significant discomfort.

12.3.1.2 Manifestations of the Spectrum of MPS I Disease

The broad range of severity, both in overall disease status as well as in individual components of the disease, leads to a very heterogeneous population of patients in varying stages of disease progression within the various body systems. At the severe end of the disease spectrum, Hurler patients have severe developmental problems, whereas Hurler-Scheie patients show little or no mental retardation but may experience learning disabilities. Scheie patients do not lose intellectual function, in general. Hurler patients can experience cardiac failure due to stiffening of the heart as well as coronary artery disease. Their valvular disease does not progress fast enough in most cases to be the primary cardiac problem. In contrast, intermediate and milder patients have valvular disease problem as their dominant cardiac problem, often beginning at age 8 to 10, and continuing through their teenage years and twenties. Progressive joint stiffness begins at a young age and is most severe in the interme-diate patients, leading to substantial loss of the ability to care for themselves.

From the perspective of drug design and development, the heterogeneous nature of MPS I makes designing clinical studies difficult. The heterogeneity of its manifestations within different body systems, even among patients of similar overall severity, makes choosing entry criteria and designing endpoints that are meaningful to a sufficient num-ber of patients particularly challenging.

12.3.2　Molecular Genetics and Mutations

The molecular genetics of MPS I were finally approachable once the gene was cloned in 1991. Since then, more than 100 mutations have been identified and there are a few impor-tant outcomes of these studies relating genotype to phenotype [22].

12.3.2.1　Mutations in α-ʟ-*Iduronidase in MPS I*

Within the Caucasian population, the Q70X and W402X mutations are two mutations that may account for about half the alleles and result in premature termination of mRNA and failure to produce any enzyme ("null mutation") [22]. Homozygotes or compound hetero-zygotes of these alleles show no α-ʟ-iduronidase activity and display severe MPS I or Hurler syndrome. Within other populations, other mutations dominate. Patients who have at least one mutation that allows significant residual enzyme in amounts as low as 0.1 to 1% of normal can have much reduced clinical symptoms. A variety of these mild mutations are known. One such interesting mutation is a Scheie mutation that involves the creation of a novel and preferred splice site in an intron [23]. The result is the predominant missplicing of the message and, therefore, a frame-shift termination; however, the normal splice site still remains and can allow a tiny amount of normal spliced mRNA and a trace of activity from a tiny amount of normal α-ʟ-iduronidase enzyme. It is also clear that patients with the same genotype may have substantially different courses, even within the same family, and so α-ʟ-iduronidase genotype is not completely predictive of outcome.

12.3.2.2　Polymorphisms

The α-ʟ-iduronidase coding sequence has many polymorphisms that have a modest effect on the normal enzyme in general. These polymorphisms and their effects may be more profound in patients with another mutation on the same allele, leading to a difference in the compound mutated α-ʟ-iduronidase enzyme [16]. It is not clear to what degree patient heterogeneity relates to these other polymorphic changes that can occur in compound alleles, but there is information that suggests these secondary polymorphisms can affect mutant enzyme stabil-ity or activity. The version of α-ʟ-iduronidase in Aldurazyme has a common polymorphism at position 8 in the mature protein, where a glutamine is changed to a histidine.

12.4　Early Development of ERT

12.4.1　Discovery of Correction: *In Vitro* Uptake and Treatment of MPS I

In 1969, Frantantoni and Neufeld discovered that secretions of normal cells and normal human urine contained "corrective factors" that, when added to Hurler fibroblasts, could correct the metabolic defect behind the GAG accumulation [3]. Although they did not know initially that this factor was an enzyme, it was clear that it was a diffusible factor and that it was very potent at very low concentrations. By 1971, the identity of the corrective factor for MPS I was determined to be α-L-iduronidase [4], which was modified in some manner that made it distinct on heparin chromatography from noncorrective enzyme [24]. In 1977, Kaplan, et al. [25] determined that the modification that allowed for α-L-iduronidase to be corrective was a mannose 6-phosphate moiety on the N-linked high-mannose carbohydrates. Even with both the identity of the enzyme and the reason for its corrective properties known, the ability to test ERT in MPS I was limited by the lack of available sources of appropriately modified enzyme. Enzyme from tissue sources lacked mannose 6-phosphate and was not corrective. In addition, the native enzyme was present in vanishingly small quantities in tissues. It took considerable effort and several years to purify 5 μg of native canine iduronidase in order to microsequence and clone the enzyme [26]. The development and study of ERT would have to wait for a recombinant enzyme source.

12.4.2   Rationale for Enzyme Therapy in MPS I

The rationale of ERT was proposed as a concept by Hers in 1964 [27], but was first practically developed for Gaucher's disease after more than 20 years of effort from the laboratory of Roscoe Brady and colleagues [28]. His group showed that a modified form of purified placental glucocerebrosidase (Ceredase®, alglucerase for injection) could be administered to human Gaucher patients and successfully reduce the organomegaly, anemia, and thrombocytopenia associated with that disorder [see Chapter 6]. The placental form was targeted to the mannose receptor by sequential deglycosylation, leaving the high-mannose core oligosaccharides that were shown to enhance targeting to macrophages, the cell type with the most storage in Gaucher patients. The basic concepts of enzyme infusion and carbohydrate receptor-mediated uptake, as well as the commercial success of Ceredase and the recombinant version Cerezyme® (imiglucerase for injection), provided an important model and rationale for treating MPS I. In contrast to Ceredase, treatment of MPS I required the development of recombinant enzyme sources, and α-L-iduronidase required targeting and uptake into a broader array of tissue types via the M6PR.

Based on the success with Ceredase and the early work of Neufeld and coworkers demonstrating *in vitro* uptake and correction, the possibility of enzyme therapy for MPS existed. Following the cloning of the cDNA for the enzyme, recombinant production was possible and was developed. Although early preclinical studies in the canine model of MPS I showed early success, it became more difficult for the work to receive investment from industry. In 1997, BioMarin Pharmaceutical Inc. first decided to invest in the development of what would become Aldurazyme. Later, in September 1998, Genzyme Corporation joined BioMarin in codeveloping Aldurazyme as part of a 50:50 joint venture.

12.4.3   Early Production of rhIDU

A series of expression vectors for human α-L-iduronidase were created using the human cDNA for the enzyme and a variety of common expression elements. Based on a series of transient and stable cell lines, a recombinant cell line was developed using the DUX B11 strain of CHO cells [9]. The recombinant cell line was studied *in vitro* and was found to produce α-L-iduronidase at the level of 0.6 to 2.4% of the total cellular protein, and to secrete the enzyme at levels 3000- to 7000-fold higher than the background secretion in normal cells. Although the production was impressive compared with natural sources, the amount of enzyme produced was still relatively limited; although many clones were screened, achieving a higher level of production was not possible. The key finding however, was that the enzyme produced was properly glycosylated and had high uptake in Hurler fibroblasts in culture with a K_{uptake} of about 1 nM. This finding was a prerequisite before proceeding further in the development of a recombinant enzyme for ERT. The early production process utilized a gelatin macroporous microcarrier (Cultisphere G) initially and later a dextran solid microcarrier with modified surface charge (Cytodex 2; Pharmacia). The cells were grown in cell culture flasks using 10% fetal bovine serum (FBS)-supplemented DME/F12 medium (Dulbecco's modified Eagle Medium mixed in 1:1 ratio with F12 medium). Once the cells reached near-confluence, the cells were harvested from the flasks and inoculated into a 5 L wand-stirred microcarrier flask. After the cells reached near-confluence on the microcarrier beads at 4 to 5 d, we began removing and replacing 3 to 4 L with DME/F12 containing 2% FBS (production medium) every 12 h. The culture was controlled for temperature and stir rate, but not for oxygen, carbon dioxide, or pH; it lasted less than 20 d. The harvested medium was purified over a sequence of columns including concanavalin A–Sepharose, heparin–CL4B Sepharose and finally, two passes over Sephacryl S-200. The yield from the purification process was about 25%.

12.4.4 Studies of ERT in Canine MPS I

With the production of milligram quantities of high-uptake rhIDU, studies of enzyme replacement in the canine model of MPS I were possible. A series of studies were undertaken, beginning with single dose injections in the fall of 1992, followed by limited studies in a small number of dogs with doses from 0.1 to 0.5 mg/kg and time frames of 2 weeks to 15 months [10,11]. An initial serious problem with recurrent dosing was the occurence of anaphylactoid reactions within seconds after bolus administration. These reactions were due to acute complement activation and profound complement consumption secondary to antibody formation to the infused enzyme. A slower infusion method was developed that mitigated these reactions. The final infusion method required that about 2.5% of the enzyme be infused slowly in the first hour, followed by the rest of the enzyme in the second hour or over an even longer period of time depending on the dose. This slow infusion period appeared to protect the dogs from anaphylactoid reactions when the full rate infusion was provided in the second hour. This method was also used in the first human clinical trial, and despite the fact that four patients showed biochemical evidence of complement consumption, no or minimal clinical symptoms were documented [12].

To summarize the canine studies both in published and unpublished work, rhIDU was shown to circulate with a half-life of about 19 min and to be distributed to a wide variety of cell types, although uptake by the liver was by far the greatest and accounted for about 50% of the total recovered enzyme activity. Based on 3-month studies at a low dose of 0.1 mg/kg, adequate uptake of enzyme and clearance of storage was achieved in some tissues such as liver, spleen, and renal glomerulus, but other tissues such as cartilage, muscle, and renal tubules were not adequately treated, and urinary GAG excretion did not decline substantially. A study in two sibling canines was performed, with one canine receiving weekly enzyme infusions of 0.1 mg/kg for 13 months and the control canine receiving no treatment. The treated canine showed a reduction in liver, spleen, and renal glomerulus storage and also some storage reduction within the renal tubules and the synovial tissue from the joints. This canine also had a greater than 50% decrease in urinary GAG excretion, unlike the canines treated for 3 months. A higher dose treatment of 0.5 mg/kg five times over a 2-week period achieved better enzyme distribution than the 0.1 mg/kg dose, and this dose was studied further.

Subsequent studies in two canines using the higher dose of 0.5 mg/kg once per week over a 15-month period demonstrated a ~70% reduction in urinary GAG excretion, and substantial enzyme uptake and substantial reduction in storage in a wide variety of cell types from 50 to 70% or greater. Even higher doses of 2.0 mg/kg/week did not result in a substantial further reduction in tissue GAG levels.

With the infusions of the higher dose enzyme, a substantial immune response developed in the canines. The antibodies did prolong clearance of the enzyme from the circulation but did not prevent effective reduction of lysosomal storage in the canine model. The IgG response did not neutralize enzyme activity, although it may have interfered with enzyme uptake to some unknown degree. There was no consistent evidence of immune complex disease in these canines.

Together, the MPS I dog studies allowed the determination of a reasonable dose, the infusion method to prevent acute clinical complement reactions, and the expected benefits. They also established the challenges ahead for human enzyme therapy. Although Aldurazyme has been approved, continued studies of the improvement and maximization of its benefits are ongoing.

12.5 Manufacturing of Aldurazyme for the Commercial Market

Following an initial clinical study with enzyme produced from a process improved from the one used in canines, a further improved process was implemented before phase 3 studies. The process described below is the improved process used in phase 3. The information provided is limited for proprietary reasons.

12.5.1 Cell Culture and Perfusion Process

A modified microcarrier-based cell culture process was developed at the 110-L scale in which recombinant CHO cells are grown via spinner flasks and then inoculated into the production vessels in FBS-containing serum with microcarriers that are different from those used previously (Figure 12.4). The cells are grown until they reach an appropriate density, and then a variable rate perfusion is begun with protein-free medium. The 110-L reactors are controlled in the usual fashion for oxygen, temperature, pH, and stir rate. After washout of serum in the medium, harvest collection begins. The collected harvest is stored at 4°C until preparation for purification.

12.5.2 Purification of Highly Purified High-Uptake rhIDU

Purification of the harvested culture fluid begins with acidification of the load and filtration of the harvest fluid (Figure 12.4). The cleared supernatant is loaded onto Blue-Sepharose FF resin, washed, and eluted with high salt. The eluate is loaded onto a Cu^{2+} chelation Sepharose column, and eluted under acidic conditions with pH 3.7 and 10% glycerol. This step was found to reduce CHO cell proteins. The pH 3.7 eluate is held as a viral reduction step, then the pH and salt level are raised and the fraction loaded onto phenyl-Sepharose HP for the final chromatography step. The enzyme is finally diafiltrated and concentrated into a formulation buffer (100 mM sodium phosphate buffer, pH 5.8, containing 150 mM NaCl), passed through DNA and viral retentive filters, and then 0.001% polysorbate-80 is added. The overall yield from the purification is about 40% and provides an enzyme of 99% or greater purity.

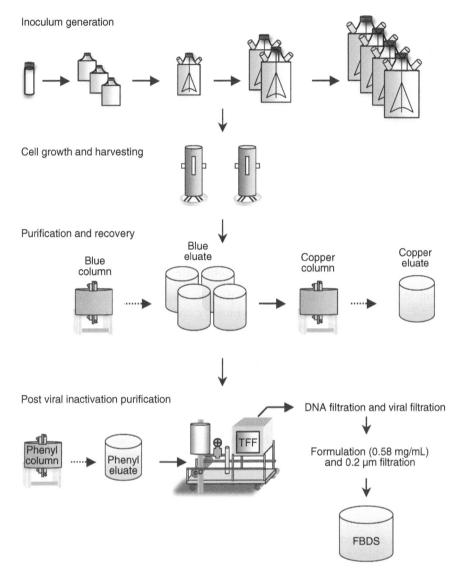

FIGURE 12.4
Cell culture and purification for Aldurazyme. The recombinant CHO cells are grown in 110-L continuous microcarrier-based cultures with continuous perfusion of production medium. The purification for Aldurazyme has three chromatography steps as shown: Blue-Sepharose FF, copper-chelating Sepharose and phenyl-Sepharose HP. The final container shown is the formulated bulk drug substance (FBDS).

12.6 Quality Control System and Assays

The control system for Aldurazyme is consistent with industry standards for recombinant proteins. An appropriate set of in-process analyses are performed to assure freedom from adventitious agents such as mycoplasma and virus. In-process controls for bioburden, endotoxin, purity, and activity of product are tested at multiple steps during purification. A set of release assays is performed on each lot to assess the enzyme product for identity, safety, purity, potency, and composition. Particular attention in release testing is paid to glycosylation, uptake into Hurler cells, and CHO protein impurities. The details of this control system will be limited to some of the basic release testing performed on the product, as noted below.

12.6.1 Purity and Safety

Analysis of purity is performed using several techniques. A silver-stained protein SDS–PAGE gel analysis of the sample is compared with the reference standard. For the quantitative assessment of host cell protein impurities, an antibody reagent was created that reacts with host cell proteins. The reagent is used in an ELISA assay to assess and quantify, using internal CHO protein controls, the quantity of CHO protein in each batch. The control of CHO impurities may be important in reducing clinical allergic reactions. A reverse-phase HPLC assay is also used to assess for the presence of impurities. Endotoxin and sterility are assayed using standard validated methods.

12.6.2 Characterization of Protein and Carbohydrate

The protein structure is assessed both by protein electrophoresis, as already noted in Section 12.6.1, and by peptide mapping, to identify and verify the presence of the peptide components of the protein. Size exclusion chromatography is performed by HPLC to assess the soluble molecular mass of the protein and to search for the presence of aggregates.

The structure of the carbohydrates is verified using a FACE assay in which all the N-linked sugars are removed using N-glycanse F (PNGase-F), and the sugar chains modified with a fluorescent charged tag and then fractionated on a special gel. The pattern of bands is highly specific and the *bis*-phosphate–mannose-7 structure is quantified on the gel. This gives an assessment of the potential affinity to bind the M6PR. The sialic acid content is also quantified using a standard chemical method. The overall charge heterogeneity is assessed using isoelectric focusing gels.

12.6.3 Activity and Potency

The activity of the enzyme is assessed using an artificial substrate, called 4-methylumbelliferyl-iduronide, and compared with specification. The uptake potency of the enzyme is performed using Hurler fibroblasts exposed to a series of concentrations of the enzyme and doing a Michaelis–Menten-type analysis (Figure 12.3).

12.7 Clinical Development of Aldurazyme

The clinical development of Aldurazyme was initiated in December 1997, and it represented the first industry-sponsored ERT study in any MPS disorder. However, investigator-initiated clinical studies and reports on the result of BMT did not adequately establish the clinical variation or quantitative clinical endpoints that might be of use in the study of a novel therapeutic. The lack of significant quantitative information on both the disease and clinical measures, and the rarity and variability of disease expression made the establishment of a clinical development program particularly difficult.

To establish the possible clinical problems appropriate for study, MPS I disease and known clinical evaluations used in MPS I were reviewed. The potential medical problems that seemed most appropriate for study included the enlarged liver and spleen, the joint stiffness, the airway problems with associated sleep apnea, respiratory insufficiency, the diverse cardiac problems, recurrent infections, and the eye disease. Other compound clinical problems that were studied, but with more difficulty, included the fatigue/malaise, severe headaches, the enlarged tongue, and signs of cord compression. Besides clinical measures, the elevated level of GAG in the urine, which reflects excessive renal distal tubular storage, is commonly used as a screen for MPS disease as well.

To establish the possible treatment effects that could be measured in the initial clinical study, the data from the preclinical studies in the MPS I dog with rhIDU, the reports of BMT in MPS I, and the first published clinical study of Ceredase in Gaucher's disease were reviewed. Based on the data from the MPS I dogs undergoing enzyme therapy, both liver storage and urinary GAG were found to be effective measures of lysosomal storage that did accurately reflected the storage in diverse tissues. These measures of storage did decline sharply within weeks of initiating enzyme therapy, suggesting that even a few doses of rhIDU were sufficient to reduce storage *in vivo*. These data were corroborated by the data from MPS I patients posttransplantation that showed a quantitative result in one patient and other qualitative clinical reports of liver-size reduction. Urinary GAG excretion did decrease after BMT, although the actual published clinical data were limited. The data from MPS I dog studies also showed substantial clearance of the synovial engorgement consistent with apparent effects of improved mobility in an MPS I dog after therapy for 1 year. The improvement in joint mobility was also qualitatively noted in BMT. The improvement in lymphoid storage in dogs suggested that the soft tissues storage that blocks the airway might improve, and data from BMT showed improvement in sleep apnea. The changes in cardiac disease in the dog were limited and the long time frame for cardiac disease progression and its irreversibility, especially for valve disease, made this measure less useful for clinical studies. Based on these and other information, the first clinical endpoints were established.

Business, regulatory, and clinical strategy also shaped the design of the first clinical study. The program focused on achieving a significant clinical efficacy and safety result in the first study. Given that the enzyme was a recombinant form of the natural human protein, it was potentially reasonable to treat the compound differently from a new chemical entity. Given the rarity of the disorder (an incidence of ~1:80 to 100,000 births), the young age of the patients, and the intravenous infusions required per week, it was initially thought that a small open-label study comparable to that used for the approval of Ceredase (12 patients, open label) was possible. Given that Ceredase was approved on that single open-label study, the regulatory strategy was to replicate this strategy for the use of rhIDU to treat MPS I.

12.7.1 Phase 1 Open-Label Study in Ten MPS I Patients

12.7.1.1 *Study Objectives and Design*

The first study of Aldurazyme was designed as an open-label study of weekly intravenous infusions of rhIDU at a dose of 0.58 mg/kg in 6 to 10 patients of age 5 years or greater and representing a wide range of disease severity [12]. Given the open-label design, only objectively measured clinical endpoints were proposed, and the analysis was based on comparing pretreatment with posttreatment measurements for the various endpoints. The primary endpoint variables were quantitative measures of storage, including liver or spleen size and urinary GAG excretion. Liver or spleen size is enlarged in MPS I due to storage, and a reduction in organ size was measured by MRI. Urinary GAG excretion is elevated in MPS I patients, and a reduction in urinary GAG excretion would represent a reduction in renal storage. Secondary endpoint variables included sleep apnea, shoulder, knee, and elbow maximum range of motion, cardiac evaluations (a scoring system of history, physical, echocardiography findings, and the New York Heart Association

[NYHA] classification), and eye disease. In prepubertal patients, height and weight growth velocity were also studied. Safety evaluations included the standard clinical laboratory studies, adverse event monitoring, assessments for antibodies to rhIDU, and complement activation.

12.7.1.2   Study Results in Reducing Lysosomal Storage

Liver size decreased sharply by the first assessment at 6 weeks with 6 of 10 patients reaching a normal liver size. By 52 weeks, 9 of 10 patients had a normal liver size with a mean decrease of 25% in size. Spleen size also reduced rapidly, reaching a 20% reduction at 52 weeks. The reductions in liver and spleen size were maintained over 104 weeks. Urinary GAG excretion decreased rapidly within a few weeks of initiating infusions, reaching 63% reduction in 26 weeks, and 72% reduction in 52 weeks. By 104 weeks, the mean urinary GAG excretion was within the normal range for the group of patients, although levels in certain individual patients were still above normal. Overall, the study showed that lysosomal storage, as determined by organ size or urinary GAG excretion, rapidly declines with rhIDU infusions.

12.7.1.3   Study Results in the Clinical Manifestations

Evaluation of range of motion showed that there were improvements in shoulder flexion, elbow extension, and knee extension that increased with time over 104 weeks. Sleep apnea declined 61% by 26 weeks, and the three patients with the most clinically severe sleep apnea all improved. NYHA classifications improved at least one class in all patients by 52 weeks. Visual acuity improved in the three patients with the worst vision. Height and weight growth velocity increased 85 and 131%, respectively, in the six prepubertal patients.

12.7.1.4   Safety

Hypersensitivity responses were observed in some patients during infusions but, in general, these responses declined or resolved with continued weekly therapy. One patient had several recurrences of fever and chills and four others had recurrent episodes of urticaria (hives) and, on occasion, symptoms of angioedema (swelling in the tongue or throat). No clinically significant adverse laboratory results were observed in the patients. All patients developed antibodies to the rhIDU; the titers peaked by 12 to 26 weeks and declined with time over 52 and 104 weeks. Further evaluations of these patients using epitope scanning technology confirmed that the patients tolerated all iduronidase epitopes over a 104-week period [29]. Complement activation was observed in four patients when comparing pre- and postinfusion specimens, but no significant clinical symptoms were observed. Peak consumption of complement occurred at weeks 6 and 12. By weeks 26 and 52, significant complement activation did not occur during infusions.

12.7.2   Phase-3 Study of Aldurazyme

12.7.2.1   Study Objectives and Design

Given the results from the phase-1 study, the ability of rhIDU to reduce storage and improve MPS I disease was demonstrated, but these data were not sufficient to obtain registration in the United States. The approval on a single pivotal trial can be achieved based on FDA guidelines, but the type of endpoints, the nature of the control group, the size of the trial, the multiple site design, and the degree of statistical persuasiveness need to be sufficient to meet expectations. Although phase-1 data were highly significant with $p < 0.001$ for both endpoints, the primary endpoints were considered surrogates and were not validated or proven to be likely to predicting clinical benefit. Given the limited published data on these endpoints during BMT, it was not possible to develop a sufficient body of literature and data to support the relevance of these measures of lysosomal storage to predict clinical outcome. Without a placebo control group, the secondary clinical endpoints could not be considered adequately controlled enough to demonstrate that improvements were not subject to bias during assessments. Based on these issues, a randomized, placebo-controlled, multicenter study was designed using clinical primary endpoints.

The phase-3 study was designed as a randomized, double-blind, placebo-controlled study in 45 MPS I patients treated with weekly infusions of Aldurazyme over a 26-week period [13]. The patient population was restricted to patients over 5 years of age and was predominantly Hurler-Scheie in phenotype. The primary endpoints were the change between baseline and week-26 in the forced vital capacity (FVC), and the 6-min walk test. FVC is a measure of lung capacity, which is severely restricted in MPS I patients such that respiratory insufficiency is a common contributor to death. The 6-min walk test is commonly used in congestive heart failure studies as a measure of endurance. In MPS I, the 6-min walk distance can be severely restricted due to a combination of factors that includes poor respiratory function, cardiac disease, and joint stiffness and pain. In addition to these endpoints, secondary endpoints in the study were liver size, sleep apnea, shoulder flexion, and the Health Assessment Questionnaire (child and adult versions). Other endpoints included urinary GAG excretion, joint range of motion, visual acuity, and quality of life measures.

12.7.2.2 Study Results in the Primary Endpoints

After 26 weeks of the double-blind portion of the study, the difference in the mean change in percent of predicted normal FVC between placebo and drug-treated patients was 5.6 percentage points (median difference 3.0; $p = 0.009$ by Wilcoxon rank sum test). Based on the severity of the 48% of predicted normal FVC in the treated group, the 5.6 percentage point difference reflects an 11% relative change in FVC that is deemed to be clinically significant by the American Thoracic Society. For the 6-min walk test, the mean difference from placebo was 38.1 m (median difference 38.5; $p = 0.066$ by Wilcoxon rank sum test and 0.0039 by an analysis of covariance controlling for certain baseline characteristics). For both FVC and the 6-min walk test, the treated patients in general showed improvements at most interim time points, leading to progressively further separation between the treated and placebo groups as the number of weeks of treatment increased. The effects observed were maintained or improved further at 72 weeks of therapy. When placebo patients crossed over to Aldurazyme, they experienced a similar increase in FVC and walk test distance at 24 and 48 weeks of the extension study, though the FVC had some delay in response.

12.7.2.3. Reductions in Measures of Storage

Liver size reduced 18.9% in treated patients, with a difference from placebo of 20% ($p = 0.001$). Of the 18 patients with abnormal liver size at baseline, 13 (72%) had a reduction in liver to the normal range. Urinary GAG excretion decreased 54% in treated patients whereas placebo patients had a 47% rise ($p < 0.001$). These reductions were maintained after following the patients for 72 weeks. After crossing over to Aldurazyme, the placebo patients experienced a comparable drop in liver size and urinary GAG excretion at 24 weeks.

12.7.2.4 Study Results in Other Endpoints

Sleep apnea was assessed using polysomnograms and the apnea–hypopnea index, a measure of the number of apneic or hypopneic events per h during sleep. When all patients were included, the treated patients had a decrease of about 3.6 events per h ($p = 0.145$). When only patients with clinically significant sleep apnea at baseline were included, the treated patients with sleep apnea ($n = 10$) had a decrease of 6.0 events per h whereas the affected placebo patients ($n = 9$) had an increase of 0.3 events per h. The 11.4 events per h difference (adjusted by ANOVA) between the treated and placebo groups of patients with sleep apnea at baseline was statistically significant ($p = 0.014$). For shoulder flexion, there was no significant difference in the overall group comparison, but for patients with more significant restriction of shoulder flexion at baseline (below the median of 90.5), the treated patients improved 9.6° whereas the placebo patients decreased 4.8°. The Health Assessment Questionnaire did not detect statistically significant differences, but this test is not specific for the problems in MPS I patients and the study was not powered to detect these differences.

12.7.2.5 Safety

There were no significant findings or between-group differences in the variety of standard clinical lab studies. Adverse events occurred at similar frequencies in both control and placebo patients, and the most common adverse events were upper respiratory tract infection, rash, and injection site reaction. The most common adverse reactions requiring intervention were infusion-related reactions, particularly flushing. Clinically significant infusion reactions were observed in some patients that were manageable with premedications and infusion slowing. One patient with severe respiratory insufficiency and airway compromise needed an emergency tracheostomy due to an airway problem during a reaction. This event in one patient did end up in the label for Aldurazyme. Antibodies to rhIDU developed in 20 out of 22 patients (91%), and the mean time to conversion was 52.6 d. By the end of the study, many antibody titers were declining.

12.8 Regulatory Approval

Approval in the United States came after filing a rolling biological license application (BLA) and going through an advisory committee review. The challenges in getting regulatory approval of a drug for a rare disease with no therapeutic or research history are particularly significant. Although the developers of Aldurazyme and the FDA could not have predicted all the steps and issues that would arise, all participants in the process learned a great deal about clinical study design in rare heterogeneous disorders.

12.8.1 Regulatory Strategies and Challenges with Surrogate Endpoints

The original regulatory strategy for the first Aldurazyme trial was to use a single open-label pivotal study with objective measures of lysosomal storage as the primary endpoints. This strategy was based on the precedent provided by the approval of Ceredase in 1991. The strategy ultimately faced many challenges in working through the regulatory process. First was the issue of surrogate primary endpoints [6]. Although there was some published quantitative data on the use of liver size and urinary GAG excretion for the only other accepted therapy for MPS I, BMT, these data were not sufficient to convince the regulatory authorities of the predictive value of the endpoints. Although the biochemical basis of the surrogates was clear and directly relevant to the disease process, these intuitive arguments were not sufficient. The data from the MPS I dog studies were clear regarding the relationship of the surrogate endpoints to the reduction of clinical disease in other tissues, but in the end, animal studies are not given significant weight in these assessments. Even with the combination of the data and information noted above, but without solid and convincing data from human clinical studies that demonstrated correlations between the surrogates and clinical parameters, the surrogates would not be considered likely to predict clinical benefit. In the end, the primary efficacy data on liver size and urine GAG excretion with the strong statistical significance was not accepted as sufficient. The clinical data from the first trial (joint range of motion, sleep apnea, etc.) were considered to be not interpretable because there was no control group and the measures could be affected by the evaluator or operator. A second study was needed. The key added features required were a double-blind, placebo control and a multicenter design to ensure that inadvertent bias did not alter the results. This study was larger and included 45 patients.

12.8.2 Use of Clinical Endpoints in a Novel Disease Target

In the absence of either clinically convincing data relating a surrogate endpoint to clinical outcome or, alternatively, intrinsically meaningful surrogates, it is extremely difficult to design pivotal studies of rare disorders using surrogate endpoints. This is unfortunate, as these are the rare heterogeneous long-standing disorders for which surrogates are most useful and needed, particularly when disease prevention and not reversal is the only achievable endpoint. In some disorders, there are intrinsically meaningful surrogates that can allow their use. For Gaucher's disease, the authorities noted that treated patients showed changes in anemia and thrombocytopenia that were intrinsically meaningful and supported the interpretation of the associated decreases in spleen size. Even though hemoglobin or platelet count endpoints may be laboratory values, the clinical benefit of a higher hemoglobin level or platelet count is established and accepted in other disorders.

In MPS I, this intrinsically meaningful surrogate did not exist. For disorders like MPS I, with its more complex physiology, diverse connective tissues disease, and more chronic progression, the probability of finding an intrinsically meaningful surrogate endpoint is low. Furthermore, the rigor of the regulatory expectations for clinical testing programs may not allow for approval based on single, small, open-label studies for rare disorders as has occurred in the past. This is unfortunate, as many rare disorders could have potential treatments that cannot be developed owing to the cost and risk barrier that long multi-phase clinical development programs entail.

Given this challenge, an appropriate clinical endpoint must be devised when possible. The main choice to make is whether to use a validated clinical endpoint from another disease state or a novel clinical endpoint specific to the disease under consideration. In the former case, the endpoint has been tested in clinical studies and the magnitude of clinical effect has been assessed, but the validation is not for the same disease state and may not measure the same underlying causative disease parameters in the other disease. In the latter case, the novel clinical endpoint might work well directly for the specific disease and be clinically meaningful, but the lack of experience and the ability to interpret the degree of change observed makes the demonstration of a clinically and statistically significant change more uncertain unless specific targets are agreed to beforehand. The Aldurazyme team decided to work with endpoints that had been validated in other studies of other diseases, and hoped to apply them to the MPS I disease assessment. Both FVC and the 6-min walk test have methodology, history, and clinical change benchmarks to assist in the evaluation of the validity of the data as well as the meaning of the changes observed. These issues all proved critical to supporting approval of Aldurazyme in the end. This is not to say that another endpoint designed to fit a disease could not be successful, but it is important to consider the interpretability of the data, and not just that a statistically significant difference can be observed.

12.8.3   Advisory Committee Preparation and Execution

The FDA convened a meeting of the Endocrinologic and Metabolic Advisory Committee on January 15, 2003, to discuss the results of the clinical studies with Aldurazyme. The FDA had received a completed BLA application that included phase-3 data and 6 months of extension data, and these data were reviewed at the committee meeting primarily to assess the clinical meaningfulness of the benefit observed at the primary endpoints. In preparation, the sponsor assembled a briefing document for the panel that included a comprehensive and cogent review of the clinical data and the basis for their interpretation. Most critical to this document was the assessment of the risk–benefit profile for the product and the presentation of the product's profile within the context of the disease being studied. This was particularly important for Aldurazyme given that few physicians have had much more than a just a cursory introduction to the MPS disorders.

The main message of the briefing document from the sponsors was that MPS I was a heterogeneous and complex chronic disease with components of disease that were reversible and others that were not reversible. It is also stated that the treatment effects observed affected multiple systems within the same patients in many cases, and that the totality of the benefit from improved FVC, decreased sleep apnea, increased walk endurance, and improved range of motion must be appreciated as a synthesis of clinical benefits and within the context of a chronic disease without significant therapy.

The FDA produced a briefing document that appropriately intended to question the data and the clinical meaningfulness of the changes observed. The Advisory Committee was asked to vote on whether the change in FVC and the change in the 6-min walk test were clinically meaningful.

In addition to the briefing documents and the presentations, the advisory committee process provided an opportunity for patients on the drug and patient advocacy groups to speak during the public session. The well-prepared and thoughtful presentations by the families of patients about their experience with Aldurazyme for nearly 5 years was compelling testimony as to the value and longevity of the clinical benefit. The families focused on the specific and measurable changes they observed in their children and the importance that these changes had in specific events in their daily lives. Although a public session cannot ever replace an appropriate development plan and good clinical data, a well-prepared and well-expressed public session can be effective in helping the panel appreciate the full story as to how the drug is working from those that know it firsthand. In the case of Aldurazyme, the clinical data and the strong patient support were an important component of the information considered by the panel. The panel voted 12 to 0 that both the FVC and 6-min walk test results were clinically meaningful. Aldurazyme was approved 3 months later.

12.9   Conclusions

The development of a treatment for a rare disorder like MPS I is challenging and rewarding for the drug development team. Aldurazyme is the first ERT for an MPS disorder and represents a major step forward for patients with these rare disorders. The biology and science of enzyme production, uptake, and clinical development is unique in the lysosomal and MPS disorders. The challenges of using surrogate endpoints and the design of studies in heterogeneous populations are most difficult in MPS I precisely because it is so rare. There is also no greater thrill in drug development than the approval of a safe and effective drug that will change the practice of medicine for a rare, untreatable disease like MPS I. The approval of this product represents the combined efforts of scientists, drug development team, regulators, and patients who persistently pursued a solution to a most devastating disease.

Acknowledgements

The author thanks the Ryan Foundation, the iduronidase production laboratory staff managed by Becky Tanamachi, the employees of BioMarin Pharmaceutical Inc. and Genzyme Corporation, and the MPS I patients and families for all of their support during the development of Aldurazyme.

References

1. Neufeld, E.F. and Muenzer, J., The mucopolysaccharidoses, in *The Metabolic and Molecular Bases of Inherited Disease*, Scriver, C., Beaudet, A.L., Valle, D., and Sly, W., Eds., McGraw-Hill, New York, 2001, pp. 3421–3452.
2. Fratantoni, J.C., Hall, C.W., and Neufeld, E.F., Hurler and Hunter syndromes: Mutual correction of the defect in cultured fibroblasts, *Science*, 162, 570–572, 1968.
3. Fratantoni, J.C., Hall, C.W., and Neufeld, E.F., The defect in Hurler and Hunter syndromes. II. Deficiency of specific factors involved in mucopolysaccharide degradation, *Proc. Natl. Acad. Sci., USA*, 64, 360–366, 1969.
4. Bach, G., et al., The defect in Hurler and Scheie Syndromes: Deficiency of α-L-iduronidase, *Proc. Natl. Acad. Sci., USA*, 69, 2048–2051, 1972.
5. Kaplan, A., et al., Phosphohexosyl recognition is a general characteristic of pinocytosis of lysosomal glycosidases by human fibroblasts, *J. Clin. Invest.*, 60, 1088–1093, 1977.
6. Kakkis, E.D., Enzyme replacement therapy for the mucopolysaccharide storage disorders, *Expert. Opin. Investig. Drugs*, 11, 675–685, 2002.
7. Scott, H.S., et al., Human α-L-iduronidase: cDNA isolation and expression, *Proc. Natl. Acad. Sci., USA*, 88, 9695–9699, 1991.
8. Moskowitz, S.M., et al., Cloning and expression of cDNA encoding the human lysosomal enzyme, α-L-iduronidase, *FASEB J.*, 6, A77, 1992.
9. Kakkis, E.D., et al., Overexpression of the human lysosomal enzyme α-L-iduronidase in Chinese hamster ovary cells, *Protein Expr. Purif.*, 5, 225–232, 1994.
10. Shull, R.M., et al., Enzyme replacement in canine model of Hurler syndrome, *Proc. Natl. Acad. Sci., USA*, 91, 12937–12941, 1994.
11. Kakkis, E.D., et al., Long-term and high-dose trials of enzyme replacement therapy in the canine model of mucopolysaccharidosis I, *Biochem. Mol. Med.*, 58, 156–167, 1996.
12. Kakkis, E.D., et al., Enzyme replacement therapy in mucopolysaccharidosis I, *New Engl. J. Med.*, 344, 182–188, 2001.
13 Wraith, J.E., et al., Enzyme replacement therapy for mucopolysaccharidosis I: A randomized, double-blinded, placebo-controlled, multinational study of recombinant human [alpha]-L-iduronidase (laronidase), *J. Pediatr.*, 144, 581–588, 2004.
14. Sando, G.N. and Neufeld, E.F., Recognition and receptor-mediated uptake of a lysosomal enzyme, α-L-iduronidase, by cultured human fibroblasts, *Cell*, 12, 619–627, 1977.

15. Scott, H.S., et al., Structure and sequence of the human α-L-iduronidase gene, *Genomics*, 13, 1311–1313, 1992.
16. Scott, H.S., et al., Multiple polymorphisms within the α-L-iduronidase gene (IDUA): Implications for a role in modification of MPS-I disease phenotype, *Hum. Mol. Genet.*, 2, 1471–1473, 1993.
17. Von Heijne, G., Patterns of amino acids near signal-sequence cleavage sites, *Eur. J. Biochem.*, 133, 17–21, 1983.
18. Durand, P., et al., Active-site motifs of lysosomal acid hydrolases: Invariant features of clan GH-A glycosyl hydrolases deduced from hydrophobic cluster analysis, *Glycobiology*, 7, 277–284, 1997.
19. Zhao, K.W., et al., Carbohydrate structures of recombinant human alpha-L-iduronidase secreted by Chinese hamster ovary cells, *J. Biol. Chem.*, 272, 22758–22765, 1997.
20. Starr, C.M., et al., Fluorophore-assisted carbohydrate electrophoresis in the separation, analysis, and sequencing of carbohydrates, *J. Chromatogr., A*, 720, 295–321, 1996.
21. Hague, C., Masada, R.I., and Starr, C., Structural determination of oligosaccharides from recombinant iduronidase released with peptide N-glycanase F using fluorophore-assisted carbohydrate electrophoresis, *Electrophoresis*, 19, 2612–2620, 1998.
22. Scott, H.S., et al., Molecular genetics of mucopolysaccharidosis type I: Diagnostic, clinical and biological implications, *Hum. Mutat.*, 6, 288–302, 1995.
23. Moskowitz, S.M., Tieu, P.T., and Neufeld, E.F., Mutation in Scheie syndrome (MPS IS): A G→A transition creates new splice site in intron 5 of one IDUA allele, *Hum. Mutat.*, 2, 141–144, 1993.
24. Barton, R.W. and Neufeld, E.F., The Hurler corrective factor: Purification and some properties, *J. Biol. Chem.*, 246, 7773–7779, 1971.
25. Kaplan, A., Achord, D.T., and Sly, W.S., Phosphohexosyl components of a lysosomal enzyme are recognized by pinocytosis receptors on human fibroblasts, *Proc. Natl. Acad. Sci., USA*, 74, 2026–2030, 1977.
26 Stoltzfus, L.J., et al., Cloning and characterization of cDNA encoding canine alpha-L-iduronidase. mRNA deficiency in mucopolysaccharidosis I dog, *J. Biol. Chem.*, 267, 6570–6575, 1992.
27. Hers, H.G., Inborn lysosomal diseases, *Prog. Gastroent.*, 48, 625–633, 1965.
28. Barton, N.W., et al., Replacement therapy for inherited enzyme deficiency — Macrophage-targeted glucocerebrosidase for Gaucher's disease, *New Engl. J. Med.*, 324, 1464–1470, 1991.
29. Kakkavanos, R., Turner, C.T., Hopwood, J.J., Kakkis, E.D., and Brooks, D.A., Immune tolerance after long-term enzyme-replacement therapy among patients who have mucopolysaccharidosis I., *Lancet*, 361, 1608–1613, 2003.

13

Additional Therapeutic Enzymes

Shane O'Connell

CONTENTS

13.1   Introduction

The therapeutic enzymes reviewed in this chapter have either been employed as therapeutic agents in the past or are at a developmental or clinical trial stage as new therapeutics. The anticoagulant ancrod, which is currently at clinical trial stage, is principally
indicated for use in the treatment of ischemic stroke. The results of clinical trials with
ancrod in the treatment of ischemic stroke have been encouraging. Acid α-glucosidase
is currently undergoing clinical trials for the treatment of Pompe disease. It is anticipated that this orphan drug will gain approval in 2005. Superoxide dismutase (SOD) has
been suggested to have many possible beneficial effects in oxidative-associated pathologies.
However, despite its potential, no parenteral SOD-based therapeutic has been centrally
approved for human use. Enzymes have been employed as digestive aids for conditions
such as lactose intolerance and pancreatic exocrine insufficiency to beneficial effect.
However, there are many other enzymes currently marketed as digestive aids for less
clearly defined conditions, which makes determination of their efficacy difficult.
Enzymes such as collagenase, trypsin, and chymotrypsin are frequently constituents of
products marketed as wound-debriding agents and anti-inflammaory agents.
Hyaluronidase has been widely employed as a "spreading factor" for anesthesia and has
a history of safe and effective usage. The thrombolytic agents urokinase, streptokinase,
and staphylokinase, are principally indicated for use in degrading thrombi after ischemic attack and myocardial infarction. Streptokinase and staphylokinase do not possess
catalytic activity of their own, but on forming a complex with plasminogen, they become
catalytically active.

13.1.1   Urokinase

Human urine was first observed to possess the ability to dissolve fibrin clots in 1885.
However, it was not until the 1950s that the agent responsible for this activity was isolated and named urokinase [1]. Urokinase-type plasminogen activator is a specific neutral serine protease. It converts the zymogen plasminogen into plasmin, which
subsequently degrades fibrin clots. Plasminogen activation is involved in a wide variety
of normal and abnormal extracellular physiological processes that require proteolytic
activity [2]. The plasminogen–plasmin enzyme system is highly regulated to be triggered
only where and when plasmin is needed. There are two major plasminogen activators
known. Urokinase is involved in such physiological processes as cell migration and tissue
remodeling, whereas the other major plasminogen activator (tissue plasminogen activator
[tPA]), which is discussed in Chapter 3, is principally involved in thrombolysis [3,4]. The
kidney is the principal site of synthesis and secretion of urokinase *in vivo*, where it is
essential for the prevention of fibrin accumulation leading to blockage of vessels and
tubules. The synthesis of urokinase has been attributed to many renal cell types, two of
which are kidney tubular epithelial cells and glomerular visceral epithelial cells [5]. The
human urokinase plasminogen activator gene is located on chromosome 10, and is 6.4 kb
long. It consists of 11 exons and gives rise to a 2.5 kb long mRNA. Pig and mouse urokinase show strong homologies with the human enzyme; however, mouse urokinase does
not contain an N-glycosylation site while the others do [6]. The production of urokinase
plasminogen activator by various tissues is under hormonal control, and agents that
elevate cellular cAMP levels can increase urokinase plasminogen activator synthesis by
promoting transcription of the gene [7,8].

13.1.1.1 Biochemical Characteristics

There are multiple molecular forms of human urokinase including one-and two-chain high-molecular-mass urokinase, and low-molecular-mass urokinase [3]. Human urokinase plasminogen activator (EC 3.4.21.73) is a glycoprotein and is synthesized as a single-chain prepropolypeptide. It has a molecular mass of 54 kDa, and contains 411 amino acids with 12 disulfide bonds [3,6,9,10]. The calculated molecular mass based on the amino acid sequence is 46 kDa [11]. One-chain high-molecular-mass urokinase is considered a zymogen in that it does not cleave small amide substrates or react with polypeptide plasminogen activator inhibitors [6]. One-chain high-molecular-mass urokinase can be activated by transformation to two-chain high-molecular-mass urokinase by certain proteases such as plasmin, kallikrein, and cathepsin B. These proteases transform the one-chain urokinase to the two-chain form by cleaving the peptide bond between K158 and I159 [12]. The N-terminal 21-kDa A chain (157 amino acids) and the C-terminal 33-kDa B chain (253 amino acids) are held together by a single disulfide bond between C148 and C279 [3]. Two-chain high-molecular-mass urokinase displays catalytic activity. It cleaves small amide substrates and activates plasminogen efficiently [13]. Low-molecular mass-urokinase, which has a molecular mass of 33 kDa, is derived by proteolytic cleavage of one chain high-molecular mass-urokinase between Q143 and L144. The enzyme responsible for the cleavage has been identified as matrix metalloproteinase pump-1 [14]. This form possesses a short interdomain peptide, which is linked to the protease domain by the disulfide bridge between C148 and C279 (Figure 13.1), and is also fully active.

Urokinase is composed of three domains including a Cys-rich N-terminal domain from amino acids I5 to K49, which has a similar sequence to that of human epidermal growth factor. It is by way of this domain that both one- and two-chain high-molecular-mass urokinase bind to a specific receptor on the cell surface known as urokinase plasminogen activator receptor [15]. Sequences from amino acids C50 to K136 are similar to kringle sequence. Kringles are triple-loop structures of about 80 amino acids characteristically constrained by three disulfide bridges. The protease domain at the C terminus of human

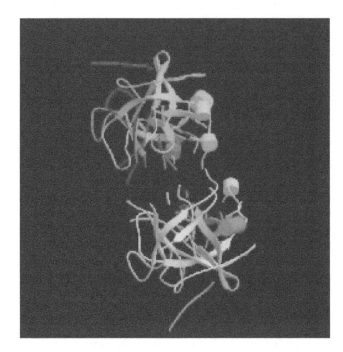

FIGURE 13.1
The three-dimensional structure of low-molecular-mass urokinase plasminogen activator complexed with egrcmk (Glu-Gly-Arg chloromethyl ketone). (From Berman, H., et al., The protein data bank [PDB], *Nucleic Acids Res.*, 28, 235–242, 2000. PDB ID: 1LMW. With permission.)

urokinase contains sequences similar to those in serine proteases [3]. The amino acid residues H46, N97, and S198 forming the active site in human urokinase B chain, correspond to H204, N255, and S356 in single-chain prourokinase, respectively [16]. The principal carbohydrate side chain is attached via N302 in the serine–protease domain of one-chain high-molecular-mass urokinase. Urokinase activates plasminogen to plasmin by cleavage of the R560-V561 peptide bond [17].

13.1.1.2   Sources of Urokinase

Urokinase utilized for medical purposes was principally obtained from human urine in the past. The initial manufacturing steps typically involved concentrating and partially purifying the enzyme by precipitation using sodium benzoate, ammonium sulfate, or ethanol. Chromatography steps employed in further purification of the enzyme include anion-exchange, affinity, and gel-filtration chromatography [18–20]. Current therapeutic urokinase preparations are principally obtained by cell culture methods. One-chain high–molecular-mass urokinase has been produced by recombinant technology in a number of systems, including *Escherichia coli*, mammalian cells, and yeast cells [21]. However, it has been highlighted that urokinase derived from different expression systems do not possess identical fibrinolytic properties. It has been reported that recombinant nonglycosylated one-chain urokinase from *E. coli* had a higher catalytic efficiency against plasminogen than native one-chain urokinase. Similarly, nonglycosylated recombinant one-chain urokinase from mammalian cells had a greater catalytic and fibrinolytic activity than glycosylated recombinant one-chain urokinase from the same cell line [21]. In addition, other studies have found that the carbohydrate component of one-chain urokinase is not important for its fibrinolytic activity in plasma, but provides fibrin specificity [21,22]. Fibrin specificity is an important characteristic of selecting the best form of urokinase (i.e., one-chain, two-chain, or low molecular mass) for utilization as a therapeutic agent to reduce the risk of systemic bleeding. This characteristic also plays a role in identifying the best source of the enzyme for therapeutic applications. One-chain high-molecular-mass urokinase possesses fibrin-specific clot lysis due to its activation to the catalytically active two-chain form primarily at the fibrin clot surface. Neither the high-molecular-mass two-chain form nor the low-molecular-mass form possess this specificity and will therefore activate plasminogen throughout the circulation, whether clot-bound or free [21,23].

Abbokinase (tradename) is one of the principal urokinase-based products on the market and is produced by Abbott Laboratories. Abbokinase is derived from human neonatal kidney cells grown in tissue culture. The urokinase incorporated in this product is the low-molecular-mass form and consists of an A chain of 2 kDa linked by a sulfhydryl bond to a B chain of 30.4 kDa. Abbokinase is supplied as a sterile, lyophilized, white powder containing 250,000 IU urokinase as well as mannitol, albumin, and sodium chloride per vial. The powder is reconstituted in water for injection prior to intravenous infusion [24]. Other urokinase-based products include Actosolv produced by Behringwerke (Marburg, Germany); Ukidan, a two-chain urokinase derived from human male urine, Ukidan produced by Serono Pharma International (Aubonne, Switzerland); and Uronase produced by Mochida (Tokyo, Japan) [19]. Some of these products (particularly those derived from human urine) have been discontinued. New recombinant products include Saruplase (rescupase) produced by Gruenenthal GmbH (Aachen, Germany). This preparation consists of the one-chain urokinase expressed in *E. coli*. Saruplase failed to obtained approval in 1998 due to the increased risk of hemorrhage associated with the preparation [25].

13.1.1.3   Therapeutic Applications

Urokinase is used in a variety of clinical settings in which thrombolytic therapy is required. The clinical applications include treatment of thromboembolic disorders including pulmonary embolism, deep-vein thrombosis, arterial occlusions, and acute myocardial infarction [1]. In addition, it is used for declotting of circulatory access sites in critical care patients and patients with extracorporeal devices (hemodialysis) [26].

Following acute medical events such as pulmonary embolism, urokinase is adminis-tered to the patient by infusion at a high dose for several minutes, with subsequent admin-istration of a lower dose by intravenous injection for up to 12 h [1]. Many studies have been carried out on the efficacy and safety of urokinase in thrombolysis [27]. The effective-ness of urokinase in thrombolytic therapy for arterial occlusion resulting in acute limb ischemia [28] as well as the effective treatment of pulmonary embolism and deep-vein thrombosis has been reported [29,30]. Many of the trials determining the safety and efficacy of urokinase in thrombolytic therapy have compared it to other thrombolytic agents such as streptokinase and tPA. From these trials, no clear advantage of one treatment over the other has been established [27,29,30]. However, the use of urokinase in thrombolytic therapy has risks, with major hemorrhage (intracranial) leading to death chief among them [30]. Applications such as the treatment of chronic saphenous vein graft occlusion have been identified where recombinant one-chain urokinase is more effective and safer than the two-chain low-molecular-mass form in promoting thrombolysis [31]. New recom-binant forms of urokinase possess more fibrin-specific activity as well as longer plasma half-life, which renders them more attractive as potential therapeutic agents.

Urokinase is utilized for the lysis of thrombi in catheters. Lysis of thrombi in the catheter is necessary to prevent bacterial growth, which can flourish on the clot surface, leading to infection and septicemia [32]. In addition, it is utilized as a lytic agent for central venous catheters used in hemodialysis. The restriction in blood flow occurs primarily due to fibrin clot formation in the lumen of the catheter. The lysis of thrombi in this scenario is neces-sary to restore blood flow and allow the continuation of dialysis [33,34].

13.1.2   Streptokinase

The extracellular bacterial protein, streptokinase, is produced by various strains of β-hemolytic streptococci (*Streptococcus haemolyticus*). Billroth first identified streptokinase-producing streptococci in 1874 in exudates of infected wounds. The thrombolytic effect of streptokinase, which was initially called streptococcal fibrinolysin, was first demonstrated in 1933 [1]. In the same year, serological distinctions allowed further differentiation of the β-hemolytic streptococci into groups A to O [35]. Most of the streptokinases are obtained from β-hemolytic streptococci of the groups A, C, and G. The C group is preferred for producing the protein as it lacks erythrogenic toxins. The group C strain *Streptococcus equisimilis* H46A (ATCC 12449) isolated from a human source in 1945 has been widely used for producing streptokinase because it synthesized the most thrombolytically active form. The H46A strain is also the main source of the streptokinase gene (*skc*), which has been studied in detail and expressed in various other microorganisms [35,36].

13.1.2.1   Biochemical Properties

Streptokinase is a single-chain polypeptide and exerts its fibrinolytic action indirectly by activating the circulatory plasminogen to form plasmin, which subsequently lyses the fibrin clot. The translated polypeptide consists of 440 amino acids, including a 26-amino acid N-terminal signal peptide that is cleaved during secretion. The mature 414-amino acid streptokinase displays a molecular mass of 47 kDa [35,37,38]. The protein exhibits its maximum activity at a pH of approximately 7.5 and its pI is 4.7. The protein does not contain conjugated carbohydrates or lipids [35,39]. Streptokinases produced by different groups of streptococci differ considerably in structure [35]. The secondary structure of streptokinase has been quantitatively examined with β-sheet content between 30 and 37%, α-helix content of only 12 to 13%, turns make up 25 to 26%, and "random" structures 15 to 16% [40]. The N-terminal amino acid sequence of streptokinase is NH$_2$-Ile-Ala-Gly-Pro-Glu-Trp-Leu-Leu-Asp-Arg-Pro-Ser, while its entire amino acid sequence suggests that it is closely related to the serine protease family [39,41]. Streptokinase contains three structural domains, α (residues 1 to 150), β (residues 151 to 287), and γ (residues 288 to 414) which all have different associated functional properties. Each domain binds plasminogen, although none can activate plasminogen independently. The domains are separated by coils, and there are small flexible regions at the two ends of the protein [42].

Streptokinase does not possess inherent enzymatic activity [38]. Streptokinase acquires its plasminogen-activating property by complexing with circulatory plasminogen. The resulting high-affinity 1:1 stoichiometric complex (i.e., the streptokinase–plasminogen activator complex) is a high-specificity protease that proteolytically activates other plasminogen molecules to plasmin [35]. Intact plasminogen can be isolated from the streptokinase–plasminogen activator complex. It displays amidolytic activity that cannot activate other plasminogen molecules [43]. This suggests that streptokinase may play three roles in the streptokinase–plasminogen activator complex [44]:

1. Binding to plasminogen to form the complex
2. Generation of the active site in plasminogen
3. Enabling the binding and processing of substrate plasminogen molecules by the streptokinase–plasminogen activator complex

The C-terminal domain of streptokinase is involved in plasminogen substrate recognition and activation [45,46]. Streptokinase binds preferentially to the extended conformation of plasminogen through the lysine-binding site, (residues 256 and 257) to trigger conformational activation of plasminogen [47–49]. A wealth of evidence suggests that residues 1 to 59 of the α domain play a key role in plasminogen activation. Studies have shown that deletion of I1 of streptokinase markedly inhibits its capacity to induce formation of an active site in plasminogen. This supports the hypothesis that establishment of a salt bridge between I1 of streptokinase and N740 of plasminogen is necessary for active-site formation in plasminogen by a nonproteolytic mechanism [38,50]. Streptokinase is known to activate plasminogen both by fibrin-dependent and -independent mechanisms [35]. Residues 1 to 59 are thought to play an important role in determining the capacity of streptokinase to efficiently activate plasminogen in both these scenarios [38]. The streptokinase–plasminogen activator complex interacts and activates circulatory plasminogen through long-range protein–protein interactions to maximize catalytic turnover. The streptokinase of the streptokinase–plasminogen activator complex acts as a protein cofactor of the plasmin active site and facilitates cleavage of the scissile peptide bond in the macromolecular plasminogen substrate [42].

13.1.2.2 Production of Streptokinase

Successful culture of hemolytic streptococci typically requires complex and rich media supplemented with various nutritional factors. A medium used for the production of streptokinase from *S. equisimilis* H46A and *S. haemolyticus* contained peptone, phosphate salts, glucose, biotin, riboflavin, tryptophan, glutamine, and nitrogenous bases (thiamine, adenine, and uracil) [19,35]. A less expensive and complex medium, which consists of yeast autolysate, glucose, and various salts, has also been utilized for the production of high yields of streptokinase. Expression of the *S. equisimilis* H46A streptokinase gene (*ska*) in *E. coli* has resulted in a tenfold increase in production levels [35]. Streptokinase has been purified from the filtrate of a streptococcal fermentation broth using hydrophobic-interaction chromatography on phenyl- or octyl-Sepharose columns. A gradient elution with 21% ammonium sulfate was used to elute the bound streptokinase. Further purification steps included size-exclusion and ion-exchange chromatography. Affinity chromatography using acylated plasminogen has also been employed for purification of streptokinase. Commercial production of streptokinase requires stringent safety protocols, as the protein is potentially immunogenic and the fermenting organism pathogenic. However, the production of the protein by recombinant methods decreases this risk [35].

Commercial preparations of streptokinase include, Streptase, Kabikinase (Pharmacia Upjohn, Stockholm, Sweden), Eskinase (Dabur Pharmaceuticals Ltd., Uttar Pradesh, India), Thrombosolv (VHB Life Sciences, Dadar, Mumbai), Zykinase (Zydus Cadila Healthcare, Ahmedabad, India), Varidase (Wyeth, Madison, New Jersey), and Prokinase (Emcure Pharmaceuticals Ltd., Pune, India). Streptase is produced by Hoechst Marion Roussel (Frankfurt, Germany), and consists of stabilized pure streptokinase derived from the culture filtrate of β-hemolytic streptococci of Lancefield group C [51]. Streptase is in powder form and contains excipients human albumin, sodium-L-hydrogen glutamate monohydrate, and polygeline. The inclusion of human albumin as an excipient prevents flocculation of the streptokinase upon reconstitution and also stabilizes the protein. However, the stabilizing effect of albumin has been shown to be minimal [52]. The powder is reconstituted for intravenous or intra-arterial administration with physiological saline [53].

13.1.2.3 *Therapeutic Applications*

Marketed since 1960, streptokinase is one of the oldest and most cost-effective thrombolytic agents in routine clinical use. It is indicated for use by either the intravenous or intracoronary route in the management of acute myocardial infarction, for the lysis of intracoronary thrombi, and for the improvement of ventricular function. Early administration of streptokinase is correlated with greater clinical benefit, the greatest benefit being evident when streptokinase is administered within the first 4 h of symptom onset. Streptokinase is also employed for the lysis of pulmonary emboli, acute arterial thrombi, and emboli, as well as the lysis of acute and extensive thrombi of the deep veins [51,54]. Along with urokinase, it is also utilized for degrading fibrin clots in arteriovenous catheters, including clots in external arteriovenous shunts of patients on hemodialysis. Varidase (Wyeth) is another commercial preparation containing streptokinase, and is indicated for use in treating wounds and ulcers. This preparation also contains streptodornase, which helps the liquefaction of the components of dead cells and pus. The action of the two enzymes together results in clotted blood, fibrous and infected matter covering a wound to be liquefied, which helps to clean the wound. This process is called desloughing and allows new healthy tissue to grow and the wound to heal more rapidly [55].

Comparative clinical trials of the three major thrombolytic agents available (i.e., tPA, urokinase plasminogen activator, and streptokinase plasminogen activator) show that there are few advantages of using one over the other in certain clinical situations [56,57]. However, on considering the cost of the thrombolytic agents, streptokinase is the least expensive (US$200 per treatment). A major disadvantage of streptokinase is that it elicits an immune response on its introduction into the circulatory systems, which can lead to anaphylactic shock and death. The severity of the immunogenicity is dependent on the level of antibodies against streptokinase in circulation, which restricts multiple administrations of streptokinase [35]. The analysis of three trials reporting the frequency of immune response (ISI-2, ISIS-3, and GUSTO-1) revealed a rate of 4.8% of patients displaying immunogenicity. Allergic symptoms reported ranged from skin reactions and slight temperature elevation to rash and shivering [51]. These symptoms were not deemed severe enough to prevent continuation of streptokinase therapy. Current research on streptokinase has focused on reducing its immunogenicity, prolonging its half-life in plasma, and improving plasminogen activation [35]. Other adverse effects associated with streptokinase are hypotension, arrhythmia, and bleeding. The analysis of published data of five megatrials with almost 70,000 streptokinase patients revealed a frequency of hypotension of 11.3%, arrhythmia 9.4%, and bleeding 6.8%. The rate of intracranial hemorrhage was below 1% for all thrombolytics tested with streptokinase, the lowest rates of all [51].

13.1.3 Staphylokinase

Staphylokinase is a protein secreted by certain *Staphylococcus aureus* strains. Its ability to dissolve fibrin clots has been recognized since the 1940s [58]. In contrast to streptokinase, staphylokinase exhibits fibrin-specific activation of plasminogen. This provides staphylokinase with a theoretical advantage for use in the treatment of thrombosis [59]. Recombinant forms of staphylokinase have been evaluated in recent years for the treatment of myocardial infarction and peripheral arterial occlusion.

13.1.3.1 Biochemical Properties

Translation of the staphylokinase gene yields a protein with 163 amino acids, the first 27 of which represent a signal peptide. The processed mature protein has 136 amino acids, a molecular mass of 16.5 kDa, and is devoid of disulfide bridges. The N-terminal amino acid sequence of the mature protein is Lys-Gly-Asp-Asp-Ala [60]. The three-dimensional structure of staphylokinase has also been elucidated (Figure 13.2). The protein has an elongated conformation with two folded domains of similar size, resulting in the flexible dumbbell-like shape. The protein consists of 9% α-helix and 22 to 39% β-sheet with a central 13-residue α-helix flanked by a two-stranded β-sheet, both of which are located above a five-stranded β-sheet [61–63].

Staphylokinase is a profibrinolytic agent. It is devoid of catalytic activity, but like streptokinase, it forms a 1:1 stoichiometric complex with plasmin and this complex activates

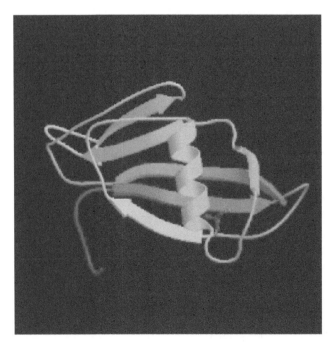

FIGURE 13.2
Three-dimensional structure of Staphylokinase (Sakstar variant). (From Berman, H., et al., The protein data bank [PDB], *Nucleic Acids Res.*, 28, 235–242, 2000. PDB ID: 2SAK. With permission.)

other plasminogen molecules. Staphylokinase and streptokinase display very little homology despite their similar plasminogen activation mechanism [1]. When staphylokinase is added to human plasma containing fibrin clot, it binds to plasminogen, creating the plasminogen–staphylokinase complex. This complex reacts poorly with free plasminogen. However, the staphylokinase–plasminogen complex reacts with traces of plasmin at the clot surface with high affinity, converting it into the plasmin–staphylokinase complex. This complex activates free plasminogen at the clot surface, forming plasmin (process outlined in Figure 13.3). Free plasmin is inhibited from cleaving the plasminogen–staphylokinase complex in plasma by the inhibitor α_2-antiplasmin. The plasmin–staphylokinase complex and plasmin are protected from inhibition by α_2-antiplasmin while they are bound to fibrin. However, once they are liberated from the clot surface or generated in plasma, they are rapidly inhibited. Inhibition by α_2-antiplasmin is mediated by interaction between the plasmin moiety of the plasmin–staphylokinase complex. This interaction results in the plasmin dissociating from staphylokinase and forming an inactive plasmin–α_2-antiplasmin complex [1,64]. Owing to this mechanism, the process of plasminogen activation is confined to the thrombus, preventing excessive plasmin generation and fibrinogen degradation in plasma [62].

R719 of plasminogen plays a pivotal role in the formation of the plasminogen–staphylokinase complex. The amino acid in position 26 appears to be of crucial importance for the activation of plasminogen by staphylokinase. The formation of the highly active plasmin–staphylokinase complex requires the conversion of plasminogen to plasmin and hydrolysis of the K10-K11 peptide bond of staphylokinase by plasmin. The N-terminal amino acids of staphylokinase play a role in conferring plasminogen activation ability on plasmin when bound to staphylokinase. Activation of plasminogen by the preformed plasmin–staphylokinase complex obeys Michaelis–Menten kinetics with a K_m of 7.0 μmol/L [64–67].

Natural strains of *Staphylococcus aureus* produce very low levels of staphylokinase. As a result, many efforts have been made to clone and overexpress the gene [59]. The staphylokinase (*sak*) gene has been cloned from the serotype B bacteriophage *sak*øC, from the serotype F bacteriophage *sak*42D, and from the genomic DNA (*sak*STAR) of a staphylokinase-secreting *Staphylococcus aureus* strain [62]. These three natural staphylokinase gene variants differ at amino acid positions 34, 36, and 43 but have very similar fibrin-dissolving potency [66]. The gene has been cloned into *E. coli*, *Bacillus* sp., and various other recombinant systems. The protein has been produced at high levels (10 to 15% of total cellular protein) intracellularly in *E. coli* TGI cells and has been purified from cytosol fractions by a combination of ion-exchange and hydrophobic-interaction chromatography, with yields of 50 to 70% [1,68]. Natural staphylokinase has been purified by precipitation with ammonium sulfate followed by cation-exchange chromatography on CM-cellulose. Affinity chromatography using a plasmin–Sepharose and a plasminogen–Sepharose ligand has also been successful in obtaining pure staphylokinase [64].

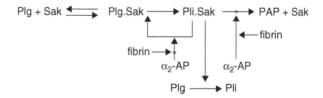

FIGURE 13.3
Mechanism of staphylokinase clot specific generation of plasmin. Plg, plasminogen; Sak, staphylokinase; Pli, plasmin; Pli.Sak, plasmin–staphylokinase complex; α_2-AP, α_2-antiplasmin; PAP, inactive plasmin-α_2-antiplasmin complex. (From Collen, D. and Lijnen, H., *Blood*, 84, 680–686, 1994. With permission)

13.1.3.2   Therapeutic Uses

Staphylokinase is highly fibrin-specific, avoids systemic plasminemia, and is therefore fibrinogen sparing. These properties, along with reduced risk of side effects such as bleeding, and the relatively low product cost, suggest that recombinant staphylokinase has the potential to be widely used in treating thrombosis [69]. Early recombinant forms of staphylokinase were found to be less immunogenic and more active toward platelet-rich arterial blood clots than streptokinase in experimental animal models. However, later trials with human patients revealed that it was as immunogenic as streptokinase [70]. Polyethylene glycol (PEG)-derivitization of staphylokinase increases its circulating half-life in both animals and humans, the extent of which appears to be proportional to the molecular weight of the PEG conjugate. The extended half-life leads to more rapid lysis of the thrombus and better patient outcome. A reduction in immunogenicity has been achieved by site-directed mutagenesis of selected amino acids [71,72].

ThromboGenics, a biopharmaceutical company based in Dublin, Ireland, is developing PEGylated recombinant staphylokinase as a thrombolytic agent. Clinical trials have focused primarily, although not exclusively, on its use as a treatment for acute myocardial infarction. Currently staphylokinase has completed positive phase-IIa clinical trials for the treatment of acute myocardial infarction [73,74]. PEGylated recombinant staphylokinase was administered to patients in a global multicenter trial (CAPTORS II) with an initial dose range varying between 0.025 and 0.20 mg/kg via an intravenous bolus over 1 to 2 min [74]. Results of the trial suggest the agent is at least as effective as tissue-type plasminogen activator in achieving rapid arterial recanalization of acutely occluded coronary arteries in myocardial infarction [69,74].

13.1.4   Ancrod

The thrombin-like serine protease ancrod has been isolated from the venom of the Malayan pit viper *Akistrodon rhodostoma*. Other snake venom proteins with thrombin-like serine protease activity (e.g., defibrase) have also been identified. The principal function of ancrod is its proteolytic effect on the fibrinogen molecule. Ancrod is an enzyme with 234 amino acids and a molecular mass of 35 kDa. It is a glycoprotein containing five potential N-glycosylation sites and about 31% (w/w) neutral carbohydrates. Ancrod has been purified from the crude venom of *Akistrodon rhodostoma* by agmatine–Sepharose affinity chromatography followed by MonoQ anion-exchange chromatography [75]. The 1.54 kb cDNA sequence for ancrod, obtained from the venom glands of *Agkistrodon rhodostoma*, reveals that it is synthesized as a prezymogen of 258 amino acids. This includes a putative secretory peptide of 18 amino acids and a proposed zymogen peptide of 6 amino acid residues [76]. Comparison of the amino acid sequence of ancrod to those of several other thrombin-like serine proteases revealed similarities. The positions of many of the 12 cysteine residues were analogous to trypsin as was the catalytic triad (H43, D88, and S182) [75]. The kinetics of the enzyme has been evaluated using chromogenic substrates, and the optimum pH was 8.0 [77].

The effects of ancrod are mediated by a rapid and effective removal of normal fibrinogen from the bloodstream, without altering other coagulation factors or platelet turnover [75,78,79]. Ancrod cleaves fibrinopeptides A, AP, and AY from the α-chain of fibrinogen, whereas thrombin releases fibrinopeptides A and B. Ancrod does not have any activity on the B fibrinopeptide of the α-chain. The resulting fibrinogen molecule (desAA-fibrin) is incapable of being cross-linked (Figure 13.4), forming easily dispersible clots. Host fibrinolytic/fibrinogenolytic mechanisms are also activated during this process (i.e., tPA and plasmin), which result in the breakdown of fibrin and lowering of the circulating

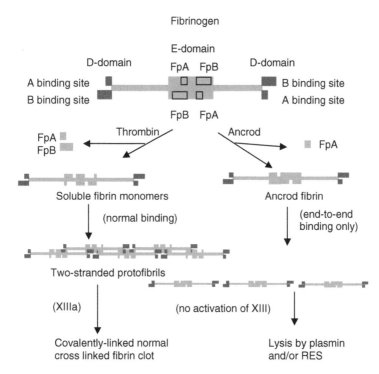

FIGURE 13.4
Ancrod action on fibrinogen. FpA, fibrinopeptide A; FpB, fibrinopeptide B; XIIIa, blood factor XIII; RES, recticuloendothelial system. (Adapted from http://www.strokeonline.net/strok000.htm.)

fibrinogen concentration. By lowering the fibrinogen concentration, the enzyme acts as an anticoagulant and lowers plasma viscosity [75,78,80,81]. In addition, it stimulates the production of prostacyclin by endothelial cells, which inhibits platelet aggregation and formation of thrombi [82,83].

13.1.4.1 Ancrod Development

Repeated administration of natural ancrod to patients suffering from thrombotic diseases results in a stimulation of the immune system, which counteracts the pharmacological activity of the enzyme, limiting its clinical applicability. It has been suggested that the immunogenicity of ancrod may be due to the presence of its nonmammalian-type glycans. However, recombinant production of the enzyme appears to have overcome the problem [84]. Ancrod has been produced by recombinant methods in different expression systems including *E. coli* and mouse fibroblast cells, in glycosylated and nonglycosylated forms. The recombinant protein has been purified from culture media by affinity and ion-exchange chromatography with a purity level greater than 97%. The recombinant protein is considered more effective for therapy than the natural protein owing to its reduced immunogenicity and reduced hemorrhagic complications on its administration [85,86]. Viprinex is a commercial preparation of ancrod, which is licensed to Neurobiologic Technologies Inc. This product has recently completed phase-II clinical trials in the United States and is due to start phase-III trials in 2005. The preparation has been targeted for use in the treatment of acute ischemic stroke within 3 h of symptom onset, for which the only currently approved drug is tPA [87,88].

13.1.4.2 Therapeutic Applications

Ancrod has been used in Europe and Canada since 1968 for various conditions, including heparin-induced thrombocytopenia and deep-vein thrombosis. It was first described for use in stroke patients in 1983. The U.S. Stroke Treatment with Ancrod Trial (STAT) assessed the efficacy and safety of ancrod in the treatment of acute stroke. The study randomized 500 patients to ancrod or placebo treatment initiated within 3 h of symptom onset. Treatment was given as a continuous 72-h infusion, followed by 1-h infusions at 96 h and 120 h. The results of the trial have shown that patients benefit in neurological outcome (placebo 34% vs. ancrod 42%) with only a modest increase in bleeding risk [82,89–92]. The European Stroke Treatment with Ancrod Trial (ESTAT) increased the time of initiating treatment to 6 h after symptom onset, but this trial was terminated as no efficacy was found on interim analysis [93].

13.1.5 Acid α-Glucosidase

Acid α-glucosidase or acid maltase (GAA) (EC 3.2.1.3) is a lysosomal enzyme that hydrolyzes glycogen to glucose by cleavage of 1,4-α-glucosidic linkages [94]. Pompe disease (glycogen storage disease type II) is an autosomal-recessive genetic disorder of glycogen metabolism caused by a deficiency of the lysosomal enzyme acid α-glucosidase. The deficiency of α-glucosidase results in the lysosomal accumulation of glycogen with disruption of cellular function in multiple tissues. The cardiac and skeletal muscles are normally most severely affected. Pompe disease can manifest in different forms, which depend mainly on the age of onset, and include infantile, juvenile, and adult onset. The disease can evolve over a varying period of time with a broad spectrum of clinical severity, which correlates with the extent of enzyme deficiency. The infantile form is characterized by an almost total lack of α-glucosidase activity and has a very poor prognosis, with patients typically dying after 1 year due to cardiac failure [95]. Juvenile and adult onset forms of the disease retain residual enzyme activity [96], therefore clinical symptoms are less severe and they generally exhibit only moderate cardiac involvement. However, the disease progresses with age, leading to deterioration of the respiratory and skeletal muscles. This can result in early mortality, generally from respiratory failure [97]. The combined incidence of all forms of Pompe disease is estimated to be 1:40,000 [98], and many of the genetic mutations associated with its development have been characterized. These mutations vary and can result in altered processing of the enzyme to production of precursor enzyme without catalytic activity [99].

13.1.5.1 Biochemistry

The cDNA for α-glucosidase codes for a protein of 952 amino acids with an apparent molecular mass of 110 kDa. There are seven glycosylation sites, and some of the carbohydrate chains are phosphorylated. In addition to glycosylation and phosphorylation, the maturation of α-glucosidase involves proteolytic processing at both the N- and C-terminal ends [97]. The processing results in the formation of two lysosomal species of 76 and 70 kDa. A 95-kDa protein has also been identified as a processing intermediate. Lysosomal α-glucosidase shares significant sequence similarity with the disaccharidases, sucrase and isomaltase. The amino acid sequence from residues 81 to 130 indicates that the enzyme has a P-type/TFF domain. In addition, the enzyme has three putative disulfide bridges, and the seven N-linked glycosylation sites are at N140, N233, N390, N470, N652, N882 and N925. The structure of the attached glycans have been elucidated [100]. The recombinant enzyme has a K_M of 2.1 mM with the synthetic substrate 4 methylumbelliferyl-α-glucoside. The enzyme has optimal activity between pH 4 and 5 [94]. W516 and D518 residues are critical for catalytic function [94].

The α-glucosidase gene (*GAA*) has been localized to chromosome 17q21-23. The gene spans 20 kb and is composed of 20 exons, including a noncoding exon 1 that is separated by a 2.7-kb intron from exon 2, the site of the initiator codon. It has also been shown that the gene is regulated at the transcriptional level, with the first intron having a prominent role [101]. The enzyme is synthesized and processed via a pathway common to lysosomal enzymes. Like other lysosomal enzymes and secretory proteins, α-glucosidase is synthesized in membrane-bound ribosomes and translocated to the endoplasmic reticulum, where the protein is glycosylated by the transfer of high mannose oligosaccharide chains from a dolichol intermediate to specific asparagine residues. Mannose residues are then phosphorylated, generating the mannose-6-phosphate ligand required for endocytosis and targeting of lysosomal enzymes to their organelle via the cell surface mannose-6-phosphate receptors [102,103].

13.1.5.2 *Production of Acid α-Glucosidase for Therapeutic Use*

Enzyme replacement therapy for Pompe disease directly targets the underlying metabolic defect through the administration of intravenous infusions of recombinant human acid α-glucosidase. The understanding and utilization of cell-surface receptors that can induce endocytosis and deliver lysosomal enzymes to target tissues has now made effective enzyme replacement therapy possible for several lysosomal storage disorders [104]. This therapeutic approach is now commercially available for Gaucher's disease, Fabry's disease, and mucopolysaccharidosis (MPS) type I, and is currently being developed for Pompe disease [98]. The production of recombinant acid α-glucosidase for the treatment of Pompe disease was first attempted by expression of the *GAA* gene in *E. coli*. However, the expressed enzyme was not active, which suggested that glycosylation and posttranslational modification were important for activity. Mammalian expression systems were considered the best option to generate a recombinant human α-glucosidase that would be properly glycosylated, processed, and correctly localized to the lysosome [94]. This was found to be the case, and CHO-cell-produced enzyme was found to be effective in reducing glycogen granules in affected tissues. Therapeutically effective α-glucosidase was also produced as a transgenic enzyme in the milk of rabbits and mice, but this approach has not been commercialized thus far [105,106].

The recombinant acid α-glucosidase-producing CHO cell line was constructed using the cDNA containing the complete coding region for human acid α-glucosidase (*GAA* gene) and cloning it into the mammalian expression plasmid, pMAM, under the control of the SV40 promoter. The recombinant cells were grown in media containing 10% dialyzed fetal bovine serum, proline, glutamine, penicillin—streptomycin, and methotrexate [102]. Ammonium sulfate precipitation and gel filtration with Sephadex G100 were used to purify the enzyme from disrupted CHO cells [102]. Recombinant α-glucosidase has been purified from the milk of transgenic mice using Concanavalin A–Sepharose affinity chromatography and Sephadex G200 chromatography. The purified recombinant enzyme from CHO K1 cells was found to have an N-terminal sequence of Ala-Gln-Ala-His-Pro-Gly-Arg [107]. The only therapeutic agent for Pompe disease currently being evaluated is Myozyme by Genzyme. This product is produced by CHO cells and a marketing application for the EU has been submitted. The sales value of Myozyme have been forecast to reach US$ 65 million by 2007 [108].

13.1.5.3 *Therapeutic Efficacy*

Data from phase I/II clinical trials (recombinant enzyme produced by CHO cells treating infantile onset patients) indicate that cardiac muscle responds well to therapy, while skeletal muscle response is highly variable. Significant glycogen clearance and improvement of skeletal muscle function were observed only in a small number of patients [109]. Preclinical studies in a gene knockout mouse model of the disease also showed that CHO-cell-derived recombinant human α-glucosidase is much more effective in resolving the cardiomyopathy than the skeletal muscle myopathy. However, an additional preclinical study with the Japanese quail (a species of bird that can suffer from Pompe) showed that the CHO recombinant enzyme was also effective in reducing glycogen granules in skeletal muscle [110]. Recombinant enzyme from a transgenic rabbit has also been produced. An open-label study, consisting of four babies with Pompe disease treated with recombinant human α-glucosidase from rabbit milk at starting doses of 15 or 20 mg/kg, and later 40 mg/kg, was carried out. The enzyme was immunologically well tolerated. The transgenic enzyme and the CHO recombinant enzyme were both found to have similar therapeutic effects. Both clear glycogen efficiently from cardiac muscle but are less efficient on skeletal muscle [111]. The clinical trials have focused on the infantile onset form to date, but are to be extended to the adult onset form in future trials. The results of the trials to date have proven the current replacement therapy to be safe and effective.

Manipulation of the recombinant enzyme has been carried out in order to obtain more mannose-6-phospate ligands on the enzyme and therefore more efficient enzyme uptake, particularly into skeletal muscle tissues [112]. This form of the enzyme has had favorable results in the mouse model of the disease [97]. Other therapeutic avenues have also been explored, including gene therapy [113,114]. However, enzyme replacement therapy appears to hold the most promise for the near future.

13.1.6   Superoxide Dismutase

SOD was first identified in 1969. The activity of SOD results in the dismutation of superoxide radicals and their conversion into oxygen and hydrogen peroxide. Elimination of the highly reactive superoxide anion by SOD is essential for the prevention of serious cellular damage. Oxygen is reduced directly to water by respiring aerobic organisms. However, incomplete oxidation results in the formation of highly reactive superoxide, peroxynitrite, hydrogen peroxide, or hydroxyl ions. SOD is responsible for the conversion of superoxide into oxygen and hydrogen peroxide, while catalase is responsible for the subsequent conversion of hydrogen peroxide into water and oxygen, thus eliminating these reactive ions from the cell [18,115]. Superoxide anions are formed by processes other than respiration, including by inflammatory cells, endothelial cells, and during the metabolism of arachidonic acid. Under normal circumstances, formation of superoxide anions is kept under tight control by SOD. However, under conditions such as acute and chronic inflammation, superoxide anions are formed at a faster rate than the capacity of the endogenous SOD enzyme to remove them. This accumulation of superoxide anions results in superoxide-mediated damage [116]. Immunohistochemical and biochemical evidence from tissues affected by acute and chronic inflammation demonstrate the significant role of reactive oxygen species (ROS) such as superoxide. ROS plays a role in the pathophysiology of inflammation as well as shock, ischemia, and reperfusion by initiation of lipid peroxidation, direct inhibition of mitochondrial respiratory chain enzymes, inactivation of glyceraldehyde-3-phosphate dehydrogenase, inhibition of membrane Na^+/K^+ ATPase activity, inactivation of membrane sodium channels, and other oxidative protein modifications [117].

13.1.6.1   Biochemistry

There are three different molecular forms of SOD present in mammalian cells. Two of the isoenzymes are intracellular: the dimeric CuZn-SOD, which is a cytosolic enzyme, and the tetrameric Mn-SOD, which is found in the mitochondrial matrix. The third form is extracellular SOD (EC-SOD), which is found in plasma, lymph, and synovial fluid, but exists primarily in the interstitial space of tissues. The DNA sequences for human CuZn-SOD, Mn-SOD, and EC-SOD have been identified. The genomic organization of CuZn-SOD and Mn-SOD genes consists of five exons and four introns. The CuZn-SOD gene has been mapped to chromosome 21q22, while Mn-SOD has been mapped to chromosome 6q25. The human EC-SOD gene consists of three exons and shares 40 to 60% homology with the CuZn-SOD gene at the exon level, but shows no similarity with Mn-SOD and has been mapped to chromosome 4q21 [118].

CuZn-SOD is a 32 kDa homodimer and contains a zinc and a copper atom at the active site of both subunits. Copper occurs in the oxidized and in the reduced state, both of which are necessary for catalysis. The bovine enzyme has an pI of 4.95 and contains 3.3% α-helix and 36% β-sheet [119]. The three-dimensional structure of the enzyme has also been elucidated [120]. The Mn-SOD enzyme is a homotetramer and has a molecular mass of 96 kDa. Mn-SOD has two associated manganese atoms. The human EC-SOD has been cloned and the recombinant protein has been produced in mammalian cells. The protein has a molecular mass of 135 kDa and is composed of four equal subunits, each containing 222 amino acids with a calculated molecular mass of 24.2 kDa. Each subunit binds one copper and one zinc atom and has a single N-glycosylation site at N89 [121,122]. The protein is synthesized with a signal peptide of 18 amino acids, which is cleaved on secretion. The enzyme also has a strong affinity for heparin, with the C-terminal domain playing a key role in this affinity. Each tetramer of EC-SOD consists of two dimers linked by disulfide bridges between C-terminal cysteine residues of each subunit [122].

Therapeutic SOD has traditionally been derived form bovine liver by enzymatic digestion of an aqueous liver extract. The enzyme was subsequently purified by gel-filtration, ion-exchange chromatography, and ultrafiltration to obtain a product with a purity of greater than 98% [123].

13.1.6.2   Therapeutic Applications

Bovine CuZn-SOD was marketed as an anti-inflammatory drug under the trade name "Orgotein." However, due to adverse immunological side effects, it was withdrawn from the market, and its marketing license was suspended in 1994 [124]. The product has been marketed in Spain by the company OXIS International, where it has been used in humans for the prevention and treatment of radiation-induced tissue inflammation and fibrosis [125,126]. The enzyme was marketed for use in animals in the United States as the active ingredient in Palosein, which is used for the alleviation of musculoskeletal inflammation in dogs and horses. The enzyme is also marketed as a dietary supplement [127], however, there is little evidence to support its therapeutic efficacy in this context. A recombinant CuZn-SOD (Oxsodrol) was registered with the FDA in 1991 by Savient Pharmaceuticals as an orphan drug for the treatment of bronchopulmonary dysplasia in premature infants [128]. The enzyme has undergone phase-II clinical trials for various indications and did show long-term benefits for some, but has not gained approval [125,129–131].

There are numerous pathophysiological conditions associated with the overproduction of superoxide anions and there appears to be a similarity between the tissue injuries that are observed in the various disease states. Disease pathologies arising from this tissue damage include ischemia and reperfusion injuries, radiation injury, hyperoxic lung damage, and atherosclerosis. Loss of SOD activity has also been implicated in the pathogenesis of motor neuron disease [132]. The common etiology of these pathologies provides an opportunity to treat numerous disease states with a single therapeutic for removal of superoxide anions [116]. ROS (e.g., superoxide, peroxynitrite, hydroxyl radical, and hydrogen peroxide) play a significant role in inflammation, enabling SOD to inhibit tissue injury associated with acute and chronic inflammation [117]. SOD injection to patients with osteoarthritis of the knee is one of the most impressive examples of beneficial SOD therapy. The enzyme was considered to have a positive effect in many other conditions as an anti-inflammatory agent and was seeking to gain approval for this use from regulatory authorities in the 1990s [133,134]. Although preclinical and clinical studies were promising, there were drawbacks such as immunogenicity and targeting associated with its use as a therapeutic agent. To overcome or reduce these problems, several approaches have since been attempted. These include entrapment of the enzymes in liposomes and masking of the protein surface by biocompatible natural or synthetic polymers such as PEG. These modifications were principally intended to reduce antigenicity and increase blood residence time [135].

However, these approaches have also had limited success [136]. Low-molecular-mass nonprotein-based SOD mimetics that could overcome some of the limitations of the native enzyme have been designed [137]. One such mimetic is M40403, which is currently in phase I clinical trials. In addition, the use of recombinant EC-SOD as a therapeutic enzyme in many of the conditions associated with free radicals is now being assessed. EC-SOD has a much longer half-life (20 h) than intracellular SOD, and is targeted to endothelial cells by its heparin affinity. The targeting of EC-SOD to the endothelial cells would be very beneficial in the treatment of atherosclerosis and ischemia/reperfusion injury. This beneficial effect has been demonstrated in animal models of these conditions [138]. To date, no SOD-based therapeutic has been approved in the United States.

13.1.7 Hyaluronidase

Hyaluronidases are enzymes that degrade hyaluronan. Hyaluronan is a high-molecular-mass linear polysaccharide, which consists of a repeating disaccharide unit of D-glucuronic acid-β(1-3)-N-acetyl D-glucosamine-β(1-4) [139]. It is widely distributed in the extracellular matrix of higher organisms as well as in the vitreous humor, cartilage, and other tissues. Hyaluronan can also form aggregates with proteoglycans, which contain glycosaminoglycans such as chondroitin and chondroitin sulfate [140,141].

There are three principal groups of enzymes that degrade hyaluronan, all three having different reaction mechanisms [142,143]. The testicular-type hyaluronidase (EC 3.2.1.35) group (also known as hyaluronoglucosaminidase/hyaluronate 4-glycanohydrolase) contains three subdivisions that include testicular hyaluronidase, tissue/lysosomal hyaluronidase, and venom hyaluronidase. This group hydrolyzes the β(1-4) linkages between N-acetyl D-glucosamine and D-glucuronic acid [140]. Transglycosylation activity has also been displayed by this group of enzymes. The leech hyaluronidase group is also known as hyaluronate glycanohydrolase (EC 3.2.1.36) and principally hydrolyzes the β(1-3) linkage between the repeating disaccharide units of hyaluronan. The third group is bacterial hyaluronidase, which is also known as hyaluronate lyase (EC 4.2.2.1 or 4.2.99.1). This group acts like endo-N-acetylhexosaminidases by cleaving the β(1-4) linkages of the hyaluronan polysaccharide [144] (Figure 13.5). This enzyme has been obtained from bacterial sources such as *Aeromonas, Candida*, staphylococci, and streptococci [144].

13.1.7.1 *Testicular-Type Hyaluronidases*

The testicular-type hyaluronidases have thus far been most exploited from a therapeutic standpoint [140]. These enzymes randomly cleave β-N-acetyl-hexosamine-(1-4) glycosidic bonds in glycosaminoglycans such as hyaluronan, chondroitin, and chondroitin sulfates, forming even-numbered oligosaccharides, with mainly tetrasaccharides as the smallest fragments [144]. As previously mentioned, the testicular-type group of enzymes is further subdivided, with hyaluronidases from mammals and humans (testicular and

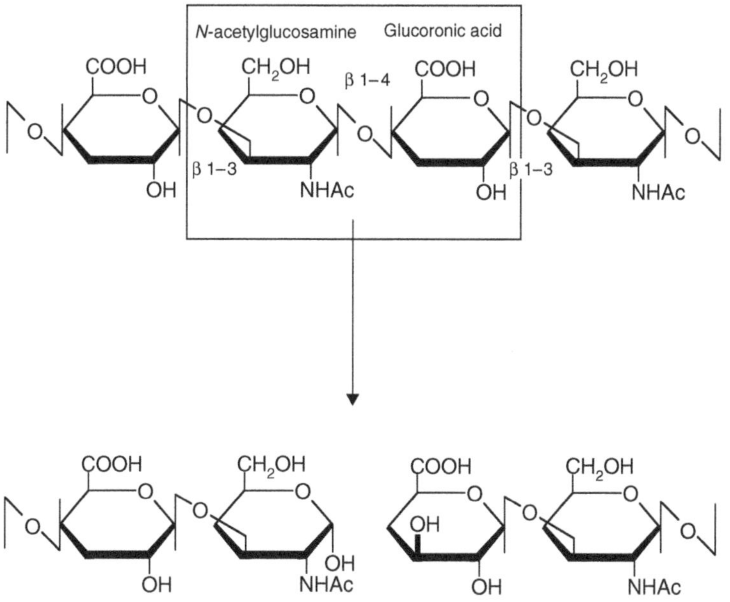

FIGURE 13.5
Hydrolysis of hyaluronan by bacterial hyaluronidase. (Adapted from Hynes, W. and Walton, S., *FEMS Microbiol. Lett.*, 183, 201–207, 2000.)

tissue/lysosomal) constituting two subgroups. In humans, many different molecular forms of the two subgroups of hyaluronidase have been isolated from both organs (testes, spleen, skin, eye, liver, kidney, uterus, and placenta) and body fluids (tears, blood, and sperm) [145]. Six hyaluronidase-like genes have been found in the human genome (*Hyal1*, *Hyal2*, *Hyal3*, *Hyal4*, *Hyalp1*, and *PH-20/Spam*) [146]. The human gene for plasma hyaluronidase (*Hyal1*) has been localized to chromosome 3p21 and has also been cloned. The gene for testicular hyaluronidase (*PH-20*) has been mapped to chromosome 7q31. The plasma enzyme contains 435 amino acids and was found to be 40% homologous to the testicular hyaluronidase (PH-20) [147,148].

Plasma and lysosomal enzymes have acidic pH optima (pH 3.7), whereas the testicular enzyme has a broader pH optimum [143]. The molecular mass of testicular hyaluronidase was determined by gel filtration to be 61 kDa; however, hyaluronidases of lysosomal origin were found to have molecular masses of 81 to 89 kDa [140,142]. All the hyaluronidase gene products are glycosylated. The three-dimensional structure of the bee venom hyaluronidase has been determined and is similar to the testicular and tissue/lysosomal enzyme [141]. Although the various mammalian hyaluronidases are derived from different genes, the enzymes share conserved structural and biological characteristics [149]. Two potential catalytic sites for PH-20 of a macaque have been identified. The region designated peptide 1 includes residues 142 to 172. This region is approximately 86% conserved in human and mouse PH-20. A second region with characteristics of a catalytic site was designated peptide 3, and includes the amino acid sequence 277 to 297. This region of PH-20 is conserved ~70% in the human and mouse enzymes [149].

13.1.7.2 Therapeutic Hyaluronidases

Testicular hyaluronidase is the principal hyaluronidase used as a therapeutic agent. The enzyme has been extracted from both bovine and ovine testicular tissue and semen.

Homogenization followed by centrifugation and precipitation of the supernatant with ammonium sulfate is used to obtain a crude preparation. The enzyme has been further purified to homogeneity by ion-exchange (cation and anion), gel-filtration and affinity (heparin–Sepharose) chromatographies [140].

Bovine testicular hyaluronidase has been used in the cosmetic, pharmaceutical, and medical fields. However, the advent of bovine spongiform encephalitis halted commercial production of bovine hyaluronidase. Wydase from Wyeth was one of the most popular bovine preparations, but production of this product has now ceased. However, a new formulation called Vitrase, by ISTA Pharmaceuticals Inc., has recently gained FDA approval. This enzyme is derived from sheep testicular tissue and is formulated as a sterile lyophilized 6200 USP unit preparation with 5 mg of lactose, 1.92 mg of potassium phosphate dibasic, and 1.22 mg of potassium phosphate monobasic as excipients. The product can be reconstituted with sodium chloride injection, USP [150]. Attempts have been made to clone bovine testicular hyaluronidase in an effective expression system that will yield a correctly glycosylated and functional enzyme [151]. Newer preparations include recombinant human testicular enzyme (rHuPH 20), which has been developed by Halozyme Therapeutics. This enzyme has completed phase-3 trials and is indicated for use in *in vitro* fertilization (to break down the outer hyaluronan layer of the oocyte), and as a spreading factor for anesthesia. These products are being developed to offer safer and purer alternatives to the existing slaughterhouse-derived extracts that carry risks of pathogen contamination, immunogenicity, and toxicity [152].

Hyaluronidase exerts it therapeutic effect by making tissue more permeable to injected fluids, leading to increased speed of drug absorption. Preparations of bovine testicular hyaluronidase have been applied therapeutically in the fields of orthopedics, ophthalmology, and internal medicine for many years with efficacy and safety. A common field of application is its addition to local anesthetic agents, especially ophthalmic anesthesia, to improve the rapidity of onset, dispersion, depth, and duration of the local anesthesia [153,154].

13.1.8   Enzymes as Digestive Aids

An array of products, that contain supplemental digestive enzymes are currently in the market. Some of these preparations exhibit a single enzyme activity aimed at degrading a specific dietary substance, while others exhibit multiple enzymatic activities for the degradation of various dietary components. These supplemental enzymes can be used to complement normal digestion, or to provide an additional digestive capacity. Supplemental digestive enzymes are frequently depolymerases that act on polysaccharides, proteins, and lipids [1,18]. A brief overview of the various enzymes utilized for this purpose is provided here.

A number of enzymes are utilized as digestive aids (Table 13.1), and the majority have been derived from animal (pancreatic extract), microbial (e.g., *Aspergillus oryzae*), and plant (e.g., barley) sources [155]. Amylases are enzymes that catalyze the hydrolysis of α(1-4)-glycosidic linkages of polysaccharides such as starch and glycogen to yield dextrins, oligosaccharides, maltose, and glucose. Amylases are secreted by the pancreas and salivary glands in humans. They are classified according to the manner in which the glycosidic bond is hydrolyzed. α-Amylases hydrolyze endo α(1-4) glycosidic linkages, randomly yielding dextrins, oligosaccharides, and monosaccharides (glucose), which are easier to digest [156]. Amylase is administered as a digestive aid to improve digestion of dietary carbohydrate. Cellulase is not produced by humans and is administered as a digestive supplement to alleviate flatulence and to improve overall digestion, especially

TABLE 13.1

Enzymes Employed as Digestive Aids

Enzyme	Substrate
Amylase	Carbohydrates (e.g., starches)
Cellulase	Cellulose
Invertase	Sucrose
α-Galactosidase	α-Galactosides
Papain, pepsin, bromelains	Protein
Superoxide dismutase	Superoxide
Lactase	Lactose
Pancreatin	Fats, carbohydrate, and protein

in high-fiber diets [1]. Cellulase hydrolyzes the β(1-4) glycosidic bonds of cellulose, an indigestible plant polysaccharaide, releasing glucose. Cellulase can be derived from fungal (*Aspergillus niger*) and bacterial (*Bacillus*) sources [157,158].

Invertase is utilized as a digestive aid in alleviating the symptoms of sucrase–isomaltase deficiency [159]. Invertase alleviates symptoms by hydrolyzing sucrose to glucose and fructose, which are absorbed to portal blood. The enzyme can be derived from *Aspergillus* or *Saccharomyces* species [160]. α-Galactosidase, which is not produce by the body, catalyzes the hydrolysis of the α(1-6) linkages in α-galactoside carbohydrates such as melibiose and raffinose. The enzyme can be derived from selected strains of *Aspergillus niger* [161] and *Saccharomyces cerevisiae* [160]. α-Galactoside carbohydrates are widely found in legumes and cruciferous vegetables including beans, peas, broccoli, and cabbage. These carbohydrates are fermented by bacteria in the colon, with the accompanying production of gas. Supplemental α-galactosidase catabolizes the oligiosaccharides prior to reaching the colon and prevents flatulence and the symptoms associated with it [1].

Papain is a highly active plant protease obtained from the juice of the unripe fruit of the tropical plant *Carica papaya* Linn. It has a broad range of proteolytic activity and is less expensive to produce than microbial enzymes [162]. The proteolytic enzyme pepsin is derived from the zymogen pepsinogen, which is secreted by gastric mucosal cells, and it hydrolyzes dietary protein to shorter polypeptides and peptides. Pepsin used as a digestive aid is typically derived from the gastric mucosa of slaughterhouse animals [18]. Bromelain (EC 3.4.22.32) is a complex natural mixture of proteolytic enzymes derived from pineapple stems. Bromelain is used as a digestive aid to promote healthy digestion by assisting in the hydrolysis of dietary protein [160,163]. SODs play major roles in the protection of cells against ROS. As previously mentioned, CuZn-SOD has been marketed as a nutritional supplement with putative anti-inflammatory activity [127,164].

13.1.8.1 Lactase

Some enzymes are employed as human digestive aids to replace or increase endogenous digestive enzymatic activities. Lactase and pancreatic enzyme replacement therapies are two such examples. The enzyme β-D-galactoside-galactohydrolase (EC 3.2.1.23), commonly known as "β-galactosidase" or "lactase," hydrolyzes lactose, forming glucose and galactose [165]. Lactose, or milk sugar, is a disaccharide found in the milk of most mammals. Lactose is digested *in vivo* in the gastrointestinal tract by lactase-phlorizin hydrolase, a membrane-bound enzyme of the small intestinal epithelial cells. Intestinal lactase insufficiency results in lactose intolerance (maldigestion with negative clinical symptoms). Intestinal β-galactosidase insufficiency can be a result of downregulation in the expression of the β-galactosidase gene, which is a penetrant autosomal gene located on chromosome

2q21, or by injury to the intestinal mucosa [166]. The incidence of β-galactosidase deficiency has been reported to be as large as approximately 75% of the world's population, and is most prevalent among the populations of Asia and the United States [167].

β-Galactosidase-deficient populations have difficulty in consuming milk and other lactose-containing products, as ingestion of lactose can result in abdominal pain, diarrhea, and flatulence. Intestinal β-galactosidase insufficiency is also thought to be a possible etiology for infantile colic. β-Galactosidase has been widely studied, with incidence of its occurrence reported in animal organs, plants, and microorganisms [168]. Microbial β-galactosidases are most extensively utilized for commercial purposes, owing to their high levels of production and desirable physicochemical properties (e.g., pH and temperature optima) [169]. The principal enzymes exploited commercially are obtained from GRAS-listed yeasts and fungi such as *Kluyveromyces lactis* and *Aspergillus oryzae* [170]. The β-galactosidase enzyme derived from *Aspergillus oryzae* is an extracellular protein. The enzyme has a molecular mass of 105 kDa, is a homodimer, and is glycosylated. The enzyme has a pH optimum of 4.5 and also displays transglycosylation activity. It does not require cofactors or metal ions for activity unlike yeast β-galactosidase [171].

Lactose intolerance and infantile colic are two lactose-related conditions whose symptoms can be relieved by dietary hydrolysis of the lactose load via the use of exogenous β-galactosidase enzyme [172–177]. Lactase digestive aids are commonly available as commercial products in pharmacies and health food stores. Some of the most popular products include Lactaid, Dairycare, Lacteeze, and Lifeplan (Table 13.2). The majority of these digestive aids contain *Aspergillus*-derived β-galactosidases. Studies have been carried out *in vivo* to determine the efficacy of lactase digestive aids derived from various sources in alleviating lactose maldigestion and intolerance. Varying results have been obtained with different enzyme administration strategies, but a positive effect was evident for all [177]. In addition, clinical studies assessing the efficacy of lactase-based treatments for colic have reported favorable results in alleviating the condition [172,176].

13.1.8.2 Pancreatin

Pancreatic enzymes are essential for digestion of macromolecules such as protein, fats, and carbohydrates in the small intestine. Malabsorption along with altered upper gastrointestinal secretory and endocrine function are implicated in untreated pancreatic exocrine insufficiency [178]. Pancreatic enzymes are administered to restore nutrient digestion, especially fat absorption (steatorrhea) and proper intestinal function in exocrine pancreatic insufficiency. Sufficient enzymatic activity must be delivered into the duodenal lumen simultaneously with a meal for the digestive enzymes to be effective. Pancreatic enzyme supplementation may be deemed necessary in conditions such as chronic pancreatitis, pancreatic carcinoma, gastric surgery, and cystic fibrosis [179]. Currently, patients with exocrine pancreatic insufficiency are treated with pH-sensitive pancreatin microspheres taken with each meal [180]. Pancreatin is a pancreatic enzyme preparation derived from

TABLE 13.2

Commercial Lactase Digestive Supplements

Tradename	Source of Lactase	Form
Lactaid	*Aspergillus oryzae*	Caplet
Dairycare	*Aspergillus oryzae* and *Lactobacillus acidophilus*	Enteric coated capsule
Lacteeze	*Aspergillus* sp.	Tablet
Lifeplan	*Aspergillus oryzae*	Capsule

porcine pancreas. Pancreatin comprises the pancreatic enzymes trypsin, amylase, nucleases, and lipase. Pancreatin and pancrelipase are similar except that pancrelipase has higher lipase activity than pancreatin. Trypsin hydrolyzes proteins to oligopeptides, amylase hydrolyzes starch to oligosaccharides, and lipase hydrolyzes triglycerides to fatty acids and glycerol [181]. Individual enzyme preparations are also utilized for pancreatic enzyme replacement, with lipase to rectify steatorrhea in cystic fibrosis patients being the most prominent.

Modern preparations of pancreatin are protected within acid-resistant, pH-sensitive microspheres that mix intragastrically with the meal. They are emptied intact into the duodenum within the chyme. Subsequently, increasing pH causes release of the enzyme from the microspheres. These preparations have been shown to be superior to older unprotected pancreatin preparations in controlled studies [180,182,183]. Some of the main pancreatin enzyme preparations available include Creon, Pancrease MT, Cotazyme, and Viokase. The pancreatin preparation Creon is produced by Solvay Pharmaceuticals. Creon capsules are administered orally and contain delayed-release minimicrospheres of pancrelipase, which is of porcine pancreatic origin. Each Creon capsule contains lipase 5,000 USP units, protease 18,750 USP units, and amylase 16,600 USP units. Recent advances in the pancreatic enzyme replacement therapy include using bacterial and recombinant human enzymes to hydrolyze dietary protein, fat, and carbohydrate [184].

13.1.9 Debriding and Anti-Inflammatory Agents

13.1.9.1 Debriding Agents

Debridement is the process of removing necrotic, devitalized tissue and foreign material from a wound to allow prompt healing and minimization of the risk of bacterial infection. Enzymatic debriding-agent formulations have significant value in the treatment of necrotic wounds as an alternative to surgical debridement [185]. The enzyme preparations used as debriding agents are categorized as proteolytics, fibrinolytics, and collagenases. Some of these enzymes include collagenase, papain, sutilains, and fibrinolysin [186]. Given that some of these enzymes do not distinguish between viable and nonviable tissue, their application ideally should be limited to the area of necrosis. Collagenase breaks down collagen, a major and rigid component of wound tissue. Collagen provides the framework to hold necrotic cells to the soft tissue bed. Therefore, when collagen is degraded, necrotic tissue detaches and granulation can occur, providing the surface needed for proper epithelialization. Collagenase is manufactured as a hydrophobic ointment containing the bacterial collagenase Clostridiopeptidase A and other proteases, all derived from cultures of *Clostridium histolyticum* [187,188].

Sutilains are a mixture of serine proteases derived from *Bacillus subtilis*, and are frequently employed in the debriding of wounds, skin ulcers, and burns. These enzymes are nonspecific and are capable of breaking down a variety of necrotic tissue types [189]. Papain, as previously mentioned, is derived form the latex of *Carica papaya* Linn. Papain is a 23-kDa single-polypeptide proteolytic enzyme that is employed as a debriding agent as well as in many other applications [190]. In debriding formulations, it is typically employed with urea. Denaturation by urea renders necrotic tissue and proteins more susceptible to the enzymatic action of papain, leading to more effective debriding of a wound [189]. Bromelain, a plant extract, has been effectively employed in the debriding of wounds [191]. A nonproteolytic component of bromelain may be responsible for this effect. This component, referred to as escharase, has no hydrolytic enzyme activity against normal protein substrates or various glycosaminoglycan substrates, and its level varies from preparation to preparation [192,193]. The proteolytic enzyme fibrinolysin targets fibrin blood clots and fibrinous exudates. Fibrin-degradation products stimulate macrophages to release growth factors into the wound bed. Derived from bovine plasma, fibrinolysin is usually prepared in combination with deoxyribonuclease (DNase) derived from bovine pancreas [188]. As mentioned previously, streptokinase and streptodornase are also used in the debriding of wounds. The proteolytic enzymes trypsin and chymotrypsin can also be employed as debriding agents. Commercial preparations of these enzymes are typically derived from bovine pancreas [189]. Potent debriding enzymes have also been isolated from the digestive system of a small shrimp, Antarctic krill. These krill enzymes constitute a powerful and stable natural system of endopeptidases and exopeptidases that assures a nearly complete breakdown of protein into soluble free amino acids [194].

Three commercially available enzymatic-debriding formulations based on the different types of debriding enzymes include Accuzyme (papain/urea) (Fort Worth, Texas) by Healthpoint Ltd., Collagenase Santyl Ointment by Ross Products Division, Abbolt Laboratories Inc., (Colombus, Ohio). (collagenase from bacterial origin) by Knoll Pharmaceuticals Inc. and Elase Ointment by Fujisawa Pharmaceutical Co. (Tokyo, Japan) [186]. Commercial enzymatic debriding ointments have been evaluated for effective debriding and promotion of healing. For wounds with necrotic eschar induced by heat or chemical insult, papain/urea ointments were most effective in debridement and promotion of healing. Collagenase ointment was less effective, while fibrinolysin/DNase ointment had no effect [195]. In an additional study, collagenase was also found to be more effective than fibrinolysin/DNase [196].

13.1.9.2   Anti-Inflammatory Agents

Bromelain's primary active component is a sulfhydryl proteolytic fraction, but bromelain preparations also contain nonproteolytical enzymes, several protease inhibitors, activators, and organically bound calcium [191]. Bromelain has been demonstrated to have both direct and indirect actions involving other enzyme systems in exerting its anti-inflammatory effect. It has also been shown to remove T-cell CD44 molecules from lymphocytes, thereby affecting T-cell activation and leading to a reduction of inflammation. Bromelain and prednisone have been shown to be comparable in their ability to reduce inflammation in rats [193,197]. Bromelain has been used as an anti-inflammatory and analgesic agent in treating the symptoms of arthritis [198]. Serratiopeptidase is another enzyme preparation used as an anti-inflammatory agent. The enzyme is derived from bacteria belonging to genus *Serratia*. It helps eliminate inflammatory swelling, accelerates liquefaction of pus, and enhances the action of antibiotics [199]. Trypsin and chymotrypsin are thought to induce anti-inflammatory effects by degrading immune-response signaling molecules. Trypsin and chymotrypsin have been used as anti-inflammatory agents in the treatment of bronchial asthma and burns [200].

References

1. Walsh, G., *Biopharmaceuticals: Biochemistry and Biotechnology*, 1st ed., John Wiley & Sons, Chichester, 1998.
2. Dano, K., et al., Plasminogen activators, tissue degradation and cancer, *Adv. Cancer Res.*, 44, 139–266, 1985.
3. Mangel, W., Lins, B., and Ramakrishnan, V., Conformation of one- and two-chain high molecular weight urokinase analyzed by small-angle neutron scattering and vacuum ultraviolet circular dichroism, *J. Biol. Chem.*, 266, 9408–9412, 1991.

4. Mondino, A. and Blasi, F., uPa and uPAR in fibrinolysis, immunity and pathology, *Trends Immunol.*, 25, 450–455, 2004.

5. Beqaj, S., Shah, A., and Ryan, J., Identification of cells responsible for urokinase-type plasminogen activator synthesis and secretion in human diploid kidney cell cultures, *In Vitro Cell. Develop. Biol.*, 40, 102–107, 2004.

6. Blasi, F., Vassalli, J., and Dano, K., Urokinase-type plasminogen activator: Proenzyme, receptor, and inhibitors, *J. Cell Biol.*, 104, 801–804, 1987.

7. Queenan, J., et al., Regulation of urokinase-type plasminogen activator production by cultured human cytotrophoblasts, *J. Biol. Chem.*, 262, 10903–10906, 1987.

8. Marksitzer, R., et al., Role of LFB3 in cell-specific c-AMP induction of the urokinase-type plasminogen activator gene, *J. Biol. Chem.*, 270, 21833–21838, 1995.

9. Fahey, E. and Chaudhuri, J., Molecular characterisation of size exclusion chromatography refolded urokinase-plasminogen activator, *Chem. Eng. Sci.*, 56, 4971–4978, 2001.

10. Nowak, U. and Dobson, C., Unfolding studies of the protease domain of urokinase-type plasminogen activator: The existence of partly folded and stable domains, *Biochemistry*, 33, 2951–2960, 1994.

11. Holmes, W.E., et al., Cloning and expression of the gene for pro-urokinase in Escherichia coli., *Biotechnology*, 3, 923–929, 1985.

12. Sun, Z., et al., Analysis of the forces which stabilise the active conformation of urokinase-type plasminogen activator, *Biochemistry*, 37, 2935–2940, 1998.

13. Petersen, L.C., et al., One-chain urokinase-type plasminogen activator from human sarcoma cells is a proenzyme with little or no intrinsic activity, *J. Biol. Chem.*, 263, 11189–11195, 1988.

14. Marcottes, P., et al., The matrix metalloproteinase pump-1 catalyzes formation of low molecular weight (Pro)urokinase in cultures of normal human kidney cells, *J. Biol. Chem.*, 267, 13803–13806, 1992.

15. Vassalli, J.D., Baccino, D., and Belin, D., A cellular binding site for the Mr 55,000 form of the human plasminogen activator, urokinase, *J. Cell Biol.*, 100, 86–92, 1985.

16. Kasais, T., et al., Primary structure of single-chain pro-urokinase, *J. Biol. Chem.*, 260, 12382–12389, 1985.

17. Lijnen, R., et al., Activation of Plasminogen by Pro-urokinase, *J. Biol. Chem.*, 261, 1253–1258, 1986.

18. Walsh, G., *Proteins: Biochemistry and Biotechnology*, 2nd ed., John Wiley & Sons, Chichester, 2002.

19. Sittig, M., *Pharmaceutical Manufacturing Encyclopedia*, 2nd ed., Vol. 2, Noyes Publications, NJ, 1568–1569, 1988.

20. Takahashi, R., et al., Affinity chromatography for the purification of two urokinases from human urine, *J. Chromatogr., B*, 742, 71–78, 2000.

21. Wang, P., et al., Catalytic and fibrinolytic properties of recombinant urokinase plasminogen activator from E. coli, mammalian, and yeast cells, *Thromb. Res.*, 100, 461–467, 2000.

22. Li, X., et al., Biochemical properties of recombinant mutants of nonglycosylated single chain urokinase type plasminogen activator, *Biochim. Biophys. Acta*, 1159, 37–43, 1992.

23. Herfindal, E. and Gourley, D., (Eds.), *Textbook of Therapeutics: Drug and Disease Management*, 6th ed., Williams and Wilkins, Baltimore, 847–849, 1996.

24. Anonymous, *Abbokinase*, Abbott Laboratories, Abbott Park, Illinois, 2002.

25. http://www.emea.eu.int/pdfs/general/direct/listprod/3032703en.pdf

26. Kohles, et al., Stability of reconstituted urokinase solutions, *Curr. Ther. Res. Clin. Exp.*, 61, 1–6, 2000.

27. Wardlaw, J., et al., *Thrombolysis for acute ischaemic stroke* (*Cochrane Review*) in *The Cochrane Library*. John Wiley & Sons: Chichester, UK, 1–57, 2003.

28. Suggs, W., et al., When is urokinase treatment an effective sole or adjunctive treatment for acute limb ischemia secondary to native artery occlusion, *Am. J. Surg.*, 178, 103–106, 1999.

29. Katchan, B., Thrombolytic therapy for pulmonary embolism, *Can. J. Surg.*, 43, 411–416, 2000.

30. Deitcher, S. and Jaff, M., Pharmacologic and clinical characteristics of thrombolytic agents, *Rev. Cardiovasc. Med.*, 3, 25–33, 2002.

31. Teirstein, P.S., et al., Low- versus high-dose recombinant urokinase for the treatment of chronic saphenous vein graft occlusion, *Am. J. Cardiol.*, 83, 1623–1628, 1999.

32. Solomon, B., et al., Lack of efficacy of twice weekly urokinase in the prevention of complications associated with Hickmann catheters, *Eur. J. Cancer*, 37, 2379–2384, 2001.

33. Mc Farland, H., et al., Lytic therapy in central venous catheters for hemodialysis, *Nephrol. Nurs. J.*, 29, 355–362, 2002.

34. Hyman, G., et al., The efficacy and safety of reteplase for thrombolysis of hemodialysis catheters at a community and academic regional medical center, *Nephron*, 96, 39–42, 2004.

35. Banerjee, A., Chisti, Y., and Banerjee, U., Streptokinase — A clinically useful thrombolytic agent, *Biotechnol. Adv.*, 22, 287–307, 2004.

36. Malke, H., et al., Expression and regulation of the streptokinase gene, *Methods*, 21, 111–124, 2000.

37. Malke, H. and Ferretti, J., Streptokinase: Cloning, expression and excretion by *Escherichia coli*, *Proc. Natl. Acad. Sci., USA*, 81, 3557–3561, 1984.

38. Mundada, L., et al., Structure–function analysis of the streptokinase amino terminus (residues 1–59), *Biochemistry*, 278, 24421–24427, 2003.

39. Brockway, W. and Castellino, F., A characterization of native streptokinase and altered streptokinase isolated from a human plasminogen activator complex, *Biochemistry*, 13, 2063–2070, 1974.

40. Fabian, H., et al., Secondary structure of streptokinase in aqueous solution: A fourier transform infrared spectroscopic study, *Biochemistry*, 31, 6533–6538, 1992.

41. Jackson, K. and Tang, J., Complete amino acid sequence of streptokinase and its homology with serine proteases, *Biochemistry*, 21, 6620–6625, 1982.

42. Sundram, V., et al., Domain truncation studies reveal that the streptokinase-plasmin activator complex utilizes long range protein-protein interactions with macromolecular substrate to maximize catalytic turnover, *J. Biol. Chem.*, 278, 30569–30577, 2003.

43. Reed, G., et al., Identification of a plasminogen binding region in streptokinase that is necessary for the creation of a functional streptokinase-plasminogen activator complex, *Biochemistry*, 34, 10266–10271, 1995.

44. Buck, F. and Boggiano, E., Interaction of streptokinase and human plasminogen, *J. Biol. Chem.*, 246, 2091–2096, 1971.

45. Kim, D., et al., Specificity role of streptokinase C-terminal domain in plasminogen activation, *Biochem. Biophys. Res. Commun.*, 290, 585–588, 2002.

46. Zhai, P., et al., Functional roles of streptokinase C-terminal flexible peptide in active site formation and substrate recognition in plasminogen activation, *Biochemistry*, 42, 114–120, 2003.

47. Lin, L., et al., Mutation of lysines in a plasminogen binding region of streptokinase identifies residues important for generating a functional activator complex, *Biochemistry*, 35, 16879–16885, 1996.

48. Boxrud, P. and Bock, P., Streptokinase binds preferentially to the extended conformation of plasminogen through lysine binding site and catalytic domain interactions, *Biochemistry*, 39, 13974–13981, 2000.

49. Loy, J., et al., Domain interactions between streptokinase and human plasminogen, *Biochemistry*, 40, 14686–14695, 2001.

50. Wang, S., Reed, G., and Hedstrom, L., Zymogen activation in the streptokinase-plasminogen complex ILe1 is required for the formation of a functional active site, *Eur. J. Biochem.*, 267, 3994–4001, 2000.

51. http://www.streptase.com

52. Lopez, M., et al., Stabilization of a freeze-dried recombinant streptokinase formulation without serum albumin, *J. Clin. Pharm. Ther.*, 29, 367–373, 2004.

53. Trissel, L., *Handbook on Injectable Drugs*, 12th ed., American Soceity of Health Pharmacists Inc., Bethesda, 1257–1258, 2003.

54. Rogers, L. and Lutcher, C., Streptokinase therapy for deep vein thrombosis: A comprehensive review of the English literature, *Am. J. Med.*, 88, 389–395, 1990.

55. http://www.netdoctor.co.uk/medicines/100002717.html

56. Tebbe, U., et al., Randomised, double-blind study compairing saruplase with streptokinase therapy in acute myocardial infarction: The COMPASS equivalence trial, *J. Am. Coll. Cardiol.*, 31, 487–493, 1998.

57. Mielke, O., Wardlaw, J., and Liu, M., Thrombolysis (different doses, routes of administration and agents) for acute ischaemic stroke, *Cochrane Database Syst. Rev.*, 1, 1–37, 2004.

58. Lack, C., Staphylokinase: An activator of plasma protease, *Nature*, 161, 559–560, 1948.

59. Lee, S., et al., Enhancement of secretion and extracellular stability of staphylokinase in *Bacillus subtilis* by *wprA* gene disruption, *Appl. Environ. Microbiol.*, 66, 476–480, 2000.

60. Collen, D., et al., Isolation and characterisation of natural and recombinant staphylokinase, *Fibrinolysis*, 6, 203–213, 1992.

61. Ohlenschlager, O., et al., Nuclear magnetic resonance solution structure of the plasminogen-activator protein staphylokinase, *Biochemistry*, 37, 10635, 1998.

62. Collen, D. and Lijnen, H., Recent developments in thrombolytic therapy, *Fibrinol. Proteol.*, 14, 66–72, 2000.

63. Rabijns, A., De Bondt, H., and De Ranter, C., Three-dimensional structure of staphylokinase, a plasminogen activator with therapeutic potential, *Nat. Struct. Biol.*, 4, 357–360, 1997.

64. Collen, D. and Lijnen, H., Staphylokinase, a fibrin-specific plasminogen activator with therapeutic potential? *Blood*, 84, 680–686, 1994.

65. Jespers, L., et al., Arginine 719 in human plasminogen mediates formation of the staphylokinase: Plasmin activator complex, *Biochemistry*, 37, 6380–6386, 1998.

66. Schlott, B., et al., NH_2-terminal structural motifs in staphylokinase required for plasminogen activation, *J. Biol. Chem.*, 273, 22346–22350, 1998.

67. Rajamohan, G. and Dikshit, K., Role of the N-terminal region of staphylokinase (SAK): Evidence for the participation of the N-terminal region of SAK in the enzyme-substrate complex formation, *FEBS Lett.*, 474, 151–158, 2000.

68. Schlott, B., et al., High yield production and purification of recombinant staphylokinase for thrombolytic therapy, *Biotechnology (N.Y.)*, 12, 185–189, 1994.

69. Armstrong, P., et al., Collaborative angiographic patency trial of recombinant staphylokinase (CAPTORS II), *Am. Heart J.*, 146, 484–488, 2003.

70. Collen, D. and Van de Werf, F., Coronary thrombolysis with recombinant staphylokinase in patients with evolving myocardial infarction, *Circulation*, 87, 1850–1853, 1993.

71. Toombs, C., New directions in thrombolytic therapy, *Curr. Opin. Pharmacol.*, 1, 164–168, 2001.

72. Vanwetswinkel, S., et al., Pharmacokinetic and thrombolytic properties of cysteine-linked polyethylene glycol derivatives of staphylokinase, *Blood*, 95, 936–942, 2000.

73. http://www.thrombogenics.com/flash.html

74. Moreadith, R. and Collen, D., Clinical development of PEGylated recombinant staphylokinase (PEG-Sak) for bolus thrombolytic treatment of patients with acute myocardial infarction, *Adv. Drug Deliv. Rev.*, 55, 1337–1345, 2003.

75. Burkhart, W., et al., Amino acid sequence determination of Ancrod, the thrombin-like α-fibrinogenase from the venom of *Akistrodon rhodostoma*, *FEBS Lett.*, 297, 297–301, 1992.

76. Au, L., et al., Molecular cloning and sequence analysis of the cDNA for ancrod, a thrombin-like enzyme from the venom of Calloselasma rhodostoma, *Biochem. J.*, 294, 387–390, 1993.

77. Ascenzi, P., Bertollini, A., and Bolognesi, M., Catalytic properties of ancrod, the thrombin-like proteinase from the malayan pit viper (*Akistrodon rhodostoma*) venom., *Biochim. Biophys. Acta*, 829, 415–423, 1985.

78. http://www.strokeonline.net/strok000.htm

79. Kelton, J., et al., The interaction of ancrod with human platelets, *Platelets*, 10, 24–29, 1999.

80. Pizzo, S., et al., Mechanism of ancrod anticoagulation a direct proteolytic effect on fibrin, *J. Clin. Invest.*, 51, 2841–2850, 1972.

81. Dempfle, C., et al., Analysis of fibrin formation and proteolysis during intravenous administration of ancrod, *Blood*, 96, 2793–2802, 2000.

82. Albers, G., et al., Antithrombotic and thrombolytic therapy for ischemic stroke., *Chest*, 119, 300S–320S, 2001.

83. Krishnamurti, C., et al., Pharmacology and mechanism of action of ancrod: Potential for inducing thrombosis, *Blood*, 79, 2492–2501, 1992.

84. Geyer, H., et al., Glycosylation of recombinant ancrod from *Akistrodon rhodostoma* after expression in mouse epithelial cells, *Eur. J. Biochem.*, 237, 113–127, 1996.

85. Behrens, S. and Hennerici, M., Ancrod BASF, *Curr. Opin. Anti-Inflam. Immunomod. Investi. Drugs*, 2, 249–256, 2000.
86. Bach, A., Strube, K., and Koerwer, W., Ancrod Proteins, Their Preparation and Use, U.S. Patent application 690957, 6,015,685, BASF Aktiengesellschaft, 2000.
87. http://www.ntii.com/company/index.shtml
88. Madhavan, R., Jacobs, B., and Levine, S., Stroke trials: What have we learned? *Neurol. Res.*, 24 (Suppl. 1), S27–S32, 2002.
89. Sherman, D., Ancrod, *Curr. Med. Res. Opin.*, 18, s48–s52, 2002.
90. Samsa, G., et al., Cost-effectiveness of ancrod treatment of acute ischaemic stroke: Results from the Stroke Treatment with Ancrod Trial (STAT), *J. Eval. Clin. Pract.*, 8, 61–70, 2002.
91. Liu, M., et al., Fibrinogen depleting agents for acute ischaemic stroke, *Cochrane Database Syst. Rev.*, 3, 1–30, 2003.
92. Atkinson, P., Ancrod in the treatment of acute ischemic stroke, *Cerebrovasc. Dis.*, 8, 23–28, 1997.
93. Dempfle, C., et al., Plasminogen activation without changes in tPA and PAI-1 in response to subcutaneous administration of ancrod, *Thromb. Res.*, 104, 433–438, 2001.
94. Hermans, M., et al., Human lysosomal α-Glucosidase: Characterisation of the catalytic site, *J. Biol. Chem.*, 266, 25–28, 1991.
95. Hirschhorn, R., Pompe disease, in *The Metabolic and Molecular Basis of Inherited Disease*, Scriver, C., et al., Eds., McGraw-Hill, New York, 2001, 3389–3420.
96. Mehler, M. and DiMauro, S., Residual acid maltase activity in late-onset acid maltase deficiency, *Neurology*, 27, 178–184, 1977.
97. Zhu, Z., et al., Conjugation of mannose 6-phosphate-containing oligosaccharides to acid α-glucosidase improves the clearance of glycogen in Pompe mice, *J. Biol. Chem.*, 279, 50336–50341, 2004.
98. Kishnani, K. and Howell, R., Pompe disease in infants and children, *J. Pediatr.*, 144, S35–S43, 2004.
99. Huie, M., et al., Mutation at the catalytic site (M519V) in glycogen storage disease type II (Pompe disease), *Hum. Mutat.*, 4, 291–293, 1994.
100. Mutsaers, J., et al., Determination of the structure of the carbohydrate chains of acid alpha-glucosidase from human placenta, *Biochim. Biophys. Acta*, 911, 244–251, 1987.
101. Yan, B., et al., Transcriptional regulation of the human acid α-glucosidase gene, *J. Biol. Chem.*, 276, 1789–1793, 2001.
102. Martiniuk, F., et al., Correction of glycogen storage disease type II by enzyme replacement with a recombinant human acid maltase produced by over-expression in a CHO-DHFRneg cell line, *Biochem. Biophys. Res. Commun.*, 276, 917–923, 2000.
103. Wisselaar, H., et al., Structural and functional changes of lysosomal acid α-glucosidase during intracellular transport and maturation, *J. Biol. Chem.*, 286, 2223–2231, 1993.
104. Chen, Y. and Amalfitano, A., Towards a molecular therapy for glycogen storage disease type II (Pompe disease), *Mol. Med. Today*, 6, 245–251, 2000.
105. Reuser, A., et al., Enzyme therapy for Pompe disease: From science to industrial enterprise, *Eur. J. Pediatr.*, 161, S106–S111, 2002.
106. Bijvoet, A., et al., Recombinant human acid α-glucosidase: High level production in mouse milk, biochemical characteristics, correction of enzyme deficiency in GSDII KO mice, *Hum. Mol. Genet.*, 7, 1815–1824, 1998.
107. Fuller, M., et al., Isolation and characterisation of a recombinant, precursor form of lysosomal acid α-glucosidase, *Eur. J. Biochem.*, 234, 900–903, 1995.
108. Werber, Y., Lysosomal storage diseases market, *Nat. Rev. Drug Discov.*, 3, 9, 2004.
109. Raben, N., et al., Replacing acid α-glucosidase in Pompe disease: Recombinant and transgenic enzymes are equipotent, but neither completely clears glycogen from type II muscle fibers, *Mol. Ther.*, 11, 1, 48–56, 2004.
110. Kikuchi, T., et al., Clinical and metabolic correction of pompe disease by enzyme therapy in acid maltase-deficient quail, *J. Clin. Invest.*, 101, 827–833, 1998.
111. Van den Hout, H., et al., Recombinant human α-glucosidase from rabbit milk in Pompe patients, *Lancet North Am. Ed.*, 356, 397–833, 2000.
112. Canfield, M., Methods of Treating Lysosomal Storage Diseases, 6,537,785, Genzyme Glycobiology Research Institute Inc., U.S. Patent application 636077, 2003.

113. Nicolino, M., et al., Adenovirus-mediated transfer of the acid α-glucosidase gene into fibroblasts, myoblasts and myotubes from patients with glycogen storage disease type II leads to high level expression of enzyme and corrects glycogen accumulation, *Hum. Mol. Genet.*, 7, 1695–1702, 1998.

114. Byrne, B., et al., Intercellular transfer of the virally derived precursor form of acid α-glucosidase corrects the enzyme deficiency in inherited cardioskeletal myopathy Pompe disease, *Hum. Gene Ther.*, 12, 527–538, 2001.

115. Mc Cord, J. and Fridovich, I., Superoxide dismutases: A history, in *Superoxide and Superoxide Dismutases*, Michelson, A., McCord, J., and Fridovich, I., Eds., Academic Press, London, 1–8, 1977.

116. Salvemini, D., Riley, D., and Cuzzocrea, S., SOD mimetics are coming of age, *Nat. Rev. Drug Discov.*, 1, 367–374, 2002.

117. Cuzzocrea, S., Thiemermann, C., and Salvemini, D., Potential therapeutic effect of antioxidant therapy in shock and inflammation, *Curr. Med. Chem.*, 11, 1147–1162, 2004.

118. Zelko, I., Mariani, T., and Folz, R., Superoxide dismutase multigene family: A comparison of the CuZn-SOD (SOD1), Mn-SOD (SOD2), AND EC-SOD (SOD3) gene structures, evolution, and expression, *Free Radic. Biol. Med.*, 33, 337–349, 2002.

119. Banci, L., et al., The solution structure of reduced dimeric copper zinc superoxide dismutase: The structural effects of dimerization, *Eur. J. Biochem.*, 269, 1905–1915, 2002.

120. Berman, H., et al., The protein data bank, *Nucleic Acids Res.*, 28, 235–242, 2000.

121. Hansson, L., et al., Expression and characterization of biologically active human extracellular superoxide dismutase in milk of transgenic mice, *J. Biol. Chem.*, 269, 5358–5363, 1994.

122. Fattman, C., Schaefer, L., and Qury, T., Extracellular superoxide dismutase in biology and medicine, *Free Radic. Biol. Med.*, 35, 236–256, 2003.

123. Rodriguez-Lopez, M., et al., Multicenter clinical trial of epidural orgotein versus placebo in patients with chronic intractable spinal pain, *The Pain Clinic*, 15, 7–15, 2003.

124. http://www.un.org/esa/coordination/ecosoc/Consolidated.List.of.Products.final.pdf

125. Campana, F., et al., Topical superoxide dismutase reduces post-irradiation breast cancer fibrosis, *J. Cell. Mol. Med.*, 8, 109–116, 2004.

126. http://www.oxis.com/therapeutics/sod.shtml

127. http://www.mqrx.com/?id=52&sku=2144

128. http://www.fda.gov/

129. Jobe, A., An unanticipated benefit of the treatment of preterm infants with CuZn superoxide dismutase, *Pediatrics*, 111, 680, 2003.

130. Iselin, N., Bio-Technology General Corp. announces encouraging SOD phase II study results in premature infants, *Business Wire*, July, 12, 1999.

131. Suresh, G., Davis, J., and Soll, R., Superoxide dismutase for preventing chronic lung disease in mechanically ventilated preterm infants, *Cochrane Database Syst. Rev.*, 1, 1–18, 2001.

132. Charles, T. and Swash, M., Amyotrophic lateral sclerosis: Current understanding, *J. Neurosci. Nurs.*, 33, 245–253, 2001.

133. Emerit, J., et al., Phase II trial of copper zinc superoxide dismutase (CuZnSOD) in treatment of Crohn's disease, *Free Radic. Biol. Med.*, 7, 145–149, 1989.

134. Copsey, D. and Delnatte, S., *Genetically Engineered Human Therapeutic Drugs*, Stockton Press, New York, 1990.

135. Veronese, F., et al., Polyethylene glycol-superoxide dismutase, a conjugate in search of exploitation, *Adv. Drug Deliv. Rev.*, 54, 587–606, 2002.

136. Butterworth, J., et al., A randomized, blinded trial of the antioxidant pegorgotein: No reduction in neuropsychological deficits, inotropic drug support, or myocardial ischemia after coronary artery bypass surgery, *J. Cardiothorac. Vasc. Anesth.*, 113, 690–695, 1999.

137. Muscoli, C., et al., On the selectivity of superoxide dismutase mimetics and its importance in pharmacological studies, *Br. J. Pharmacol.*, 140, 445–460, 2003.

138. Fukai, T., et al., Extracellular superoxide dismutase and cardiovascular disease, *Cardiovasc. Res.*, 55, 239–249, 2002.

139. Laurent, T. and Fraser, J., Hyaluronan, *FASEB J.*, 6, 2397, 1992.

140. Demeester, J. and Vercruysse, K., Hyaluronidase, in *Pharmaceutical Enzymes*, Lauwers, A., and Scharpe, S., Eds., Marcel Dekker, New York, 155–186, 1997.

141. Housley, Z., et al., Crystal structure of hyaluronidase, a major allergen of bee venom, *Structure*, 8, 1025–1035, 2000.

142. Menzel, E. and Farr, C., Hyaluronidase and its substrate hyaluronan: Biochemistry, biological activities and therapeutic uses, *Cancer Lett.*, 131, 3–11, 1998.

143. Kreil, G., Hyaluronidases — A group of neglected enzymes, *Protein Sci.*, 4, 1666–1669, 1995.

144. Hynes, W. and Walton, S., Hyaluronidases of Gram-positive bacteria, *FEMS Microbiol. Lett.*, 183, 201–207, 2000.

145. Fiszer-Szafarz, B., Litynska, A., and Zou, L., Human hyaluronidases: Electrophoretic multiple forms in somatic tissues and body fluids Evidence for conserved hyaluronidase potential N-glycosylation sites in different mammalian species, *J. Biochem. Biophys. Methods*, 45, 103–116, 2000.

146. Csoka, A., Frost, G., and Stern, R., The six hyaluronidase-like genes in the human and mouse genomes, *Matrix Biol.*, 20, 499–508, 2001.

147. Csoka, T., et al., The hyaluronidase gene HYAL1 maps to chromosome 3p21.2-p21.3 in human and 9F1-F2 in mouse, a conserved candidate tumor suppressor locus, *Genomics*, 48, 63–70, 1998.

148. Frost, G., et al., Purification, cloning, and expression of human plasma hyaluronidase1, *Biochem. Biophys. Res. Commun.*, 236, 10–15, 1997.

149. Cherr, G., Yudin, A., and Overstreet, J., The dual functions of GPI-anchored PH-20: Hyaluronidase and intracellular signaling, *Matrix Biol.*, 20, 515–525, 2001.

150. http://www.istavision.com/index.asp

151. Chowpongpang, S., Shin, S., and Kim, E., Cloning and characterization of the bovine testicular PH-20 hyaluronidase core domain, *Biotechnol. Lett.*, 26, 1247–1252, 2004.

152. http://www.halozyme.com

153. Oettl, M., et al., Comparative characterization of bovine testicular hyaluronidase and a hyaluronate lyase from *Streptococcus agalactiae* in pharmaceutical preparations, *Eur. J. Pharm. Sci.*, 18, 267–277, 2003.

154. http://www.ashp.org/shortage/hyaluronidase.cfm

155. Rachman, B., Unique features and application of non-animal derived enzymes, *Clin. Nutr. Insights*, 5, 1–4, 1997.

156. Hoover, R. and Zhou, Y., *In vitro* and *in vivo* hydrolysis of legume starches by alpha-amylase and resistant starch formation in legumes-a review, *Carbohyd. Polym.*, 54, 401–417, 2003.

157. Bhat, M., Cellulases and related enzymes in biotechnology, *Biotechnol. Adv.*, 18, 355–383, 2000.

158. Mawadza, C., et al., Purification and characterization of cellulases produced by two Bacillus strains, *J. Biotechnol.*, 83, 177–187, 2000.

159. Anonymous, New molecular entities: Sucraid, *Formulary*, 33, 505, 1998.

160. Cheetham, P., The applications of enzymes in industry, in *Handbook of Enzyme Biotechnology*, Wiseman, A., Ed., Ellis Horwood Limited, Chichester, 1987, p. 335.

161. Ademark, P., et al., Multiple α-galactosidases from *Aspergillus niger*: Purification, characterization and substrate specificities, *Enzyme Microb. Technol.*, 29, 441–448, 2001.

162. Khaparde, S. and Singhal, R., Chemically modified papain for applications in detergent formulations, *Bioresour. Technol.*, 78, 1–4, 2001.

163. Hale, L., Proteolytic activity and immunogenicity of oral bromelain within the gastrointestinal tract of mice, *Int. Immunopharmacol.*, 4, 255–264, 2004.

164. http://www.pdrhealth.com

165. Nagy, Z., et al., β-galactosidase of *Penicillium chrysogenum*: Production, purification and characterisation of the enzyme, *Protein Expres. Purif.*, 21, 24–29, 2001.

166. Suarez, F., Savaiano, D., and Levitt, M., A comparison of symptoms after consumption of milk or lactose hydrolyised milk by people with self reported severe lactose intolerance, *New Engl. J. Med.*, 333, 1–4, 1995.

167. Gaska, J., Treatment of lactose intolerance, *Am. Drug.*, 202, 36–43, 1990.

168. Wallenfalls, K. and Weil, R., β–galactosidase, in *The Enzymes*, Boyer, P., Ed., Academic Press, New York, 1972, 617–662.

169. Greenberg, N. and Mahoney, R., Immobilisation of lactase (β–galactosidase) for use in dairy processing: A review, *Process Biochem.*, 16, 2–8, 1981.

170. Geskas, V. and Lopez-Levia, M., Hydrolysis of lactose: A literature review, *Process Biochem.*, February, 20, 2–12, 1985.

171. Nakayama, T. and Amachi, T., β–Galactosidase, enzymology, in *Encyclopedia of Bioprocess Technology, Fermentation, Biocatalysis and Bioseparation*, Flinckinger, M. and Drew, S., Eds., John Wiley & Sons, New York, 1999, 1291–1305.

172. Kanabar, D., Randhawa, M., and Clayton, P., Improvement of symptoms in infant colic following reduction of lactose load with lactase, *J. Hum. Nutr. Diet*, 14, 359–363, 2001.

173. Gao, K., et al., Effect of lactase preparations in asymphomatic individuals with lactase deficiency — Gastric digestion of lactose and breath hydrogen analysis, *Nagoya J. Med. Sci.*, 65, 21–28, 2002.

174. Lin, M., et al., Comparative effects of exogenous lactase (β-galactosidase) preparations on *in vivo* lactose digestion, *Dig. Dis. Sci.*, 38, 2022–2027, 1993.

175. Solomons, N., Guerrero, A., and Torun, B., Effective *in vivo* hydrolysis of milk lactose by beta-galactosidases in the presence of solid food, *Am. J. Clin. Nutr.*, 41, 222–227, 1985.

176. Lucassen, P., et al., Effectivness of treatments for infantile colic: Systematic review, *Br. Med. J.*, 316, 1563–1569, 1998.

177. Barillas, C. and Solomons, N., Effective reduction of lactose maldigestion in preschool children by direct addition of β-galactosidases to milk at meal time, *Pediatrics*, 79, 766–772, 1987.

178. DiMagno, E., Clain, J., and Layer, P., Chronic pancreatitis, in *Pancreas: Biology, Pathobiology, and Diseases*, Go, V., Ed., Raven Press, New York, 1993, 665–706.

179. Sarner, M., Treatment of pancreatic exocrine deficiency, *World J. Surg.*, 27, 1192–1195, 2003.

180. Layer, P., Keller, J., and Lankisch, P., Pancreatic enzyme replacement therapy, *Curr. Gastroenterol. Rep.*, 3, 101–108, 2001.

181. Scharpe, S., Uyttenbroeck, W., and Samyn, N., Pancreatic enzyme replacement, in *Pharmaceuticals Enzymes*, Lauwers, A. and Scharpe, S., Eds., Marcel Dekker, New York, 1997, 187–222.

182. Willson, N., Ghosal, T., and Pickering, M., Reducing pancreatic enzyme dose does not compromise growth in cystic fibrosis, *J. Hum. Nutr. Diet*, 11, 487–492, 1998.

183. Bruno, M., et al., Placebo controlled trial of enteric coated pancreatin microsphere treatment in patients with unresectable cancer of the pancreatic head region, *Gut*, 42, 92–96, 1998.

184. Keller, J. and Layer, P., Pancreatic enzyme supplementation therapy, *Curr. Treat. Options Gastroenterol.*, 6, 369–374, 2003.

185. Sieggreen, M. and Maklebust, J., Debridement: Choices and challenges, *Adv. Wound Care*, 10, 32–37, 1997.

186. Hobson, D., et al., Development and use of a quantitative method to evaluate the action of enzymatic wound debriding agents *in vitro*, *Wounds*, 10, 105–110, 1998.

187. Zacur, H. and Kirsner, R., Debridement: Rationale and therapeutic options, *Wounds*, 14, 2S–6S, 2002.

188. Singhal, A., Reis, E., and Kerstein, M., Options for nonsurgical debridement of necrotic wounds, *Adv. Wound Care*, 14, 96, 2001.

189. Wright, J. and Shi, L., Accuzyme papain-urea debriding ointment: A historical review, *Wounds*, 15, 2S–12S, 2003.

190. Lauwers, A. and Dekeyser, The cysteine proteinases from the latex of *Carica papaya* L., in *Pharmaceutical Enzymes*, Lauwers, A. and Scharpe, S., Eds., Marcel Dekker, New York, 1997, 107–129.

191. Vanhoof, G. and Cooreman, W., Bromelain, in *Pharmaceutical Enzymes*, Lauwers, A. and Scharpe, S., Eds., Marcel Dekker, New York, 1997, 131–153.

192. Anonymous, Bromelain monograph, *Altern. Med. Rev.*, 3, 302–305, 1998.

193. Kelly, G., Bromelain: A literature review and discussion of its therapeutic applications, *Altern. Med. Rev.*, 1, 243–257, 1996.

194. Mekkes, J., et al., Efficient debridement of necrotic wounds using proteolytic enzymes derived from Antarctic krill: A double-blind, placebo-controlled study in a standardized animal wound model, *Wound Repair Regen.*, 6, 50–57, 1998.

195. Hebda, P., Flynn, K., and Dohar, J., Evaluation of the efficacy of enzymatic debriding agents for removal of necrotic tissue and promotion of healing in porcine skin wounds, *Wounds*, 10, 83–96, 1998.

196. Mekkes, J., Zeegelaar, J., and Westerhof, W., Quantitative and objective evaluation of wound debriding properties of collagenase and fibrinolysin/desoxyribonuclease in a necrotic ulcer animal model, *Arch. Dermatol. Res.*, 290, 152–157, 1998.

197. Vellini, M., et al., Possible involvement of eicosanoids in the pharmacological action of brome-lain, *Arzneimittelforschung*, 36, 110–112, 1986.
198. Walker, A., et al., Bromelain reduces mild acute knee pain and improves well-being in a dose-dependent fashion in an open study of otherwise healthy adults, *Phytomedicine*, 9, 681–686, 2002.
199. Moriya, N., Nakata, M., and Nakamura, M., Intestinal absorption of serrapeptase (TSP) in rats, *Biotechnol. Appl. Biochem.*, 20, 101–108, 1994.
200. RaviKumar, T., et al., Effect of trypsin–chymotrypsin (Chymoral Forte D.S.) preparation on the modulation of cytokine levels in burn patients, *Burns*, 27, 709–716, 2001.

Index